Oral Microbiology
Fourth edition

Philip Marsh BSc PhD
Centre for Applied Microbiology & Research, Porton Down, Salisbury and University of Leeds

and

Michael V. Martin BDS BA PhD FRCPath
Department of Clinical Dental Sciences, University of Liverpool

wright

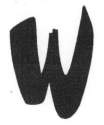

OXFORD AUCKLAND BOSTON JOHANNESBURG MELBOURNE NEW DELHI

Wright
An imprint of Butterworth–Heinemann
Linacre House, Jordan Hill, Oxford OX2 8DP
225 Wildwood Avenue, Woburn, MA 01801-2041
A division of Reed Educational and Professional Publishing Ltd

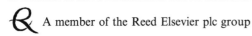 A member of the Reed Elsevier plc group

First edition 1980
Second edition 1984
Reprinted 1985, 1988, 1989
Third edition 1992
Reprinted 1994, 1996
©P.D. Marsh and M. V. Martin 1980, 1984, 1992

Fourth edition 1999
©Reed Educational and Professional Publishing Ltd 1999

British Library Cataloguing in Publication Data
A catalogue record for this book is available from the British Library

Library of Congress Cataloguing in Publication Data
A catalogue record for this book is available from the Library of Congress

ISBN 0 7236 1051 7

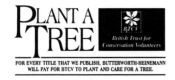

FOR EVERY TITLE THAT WE PUBLISH, BUTTERWORTH-HEINEMANN
WILL PAY FOR BTCV TO PLANT AND CARE FOR A TREE.

Typeset by Bath Typesetting
Printed and bound in Great Britain by MPG Books Ltd, Bodmin, Cornwall

To Jane, Katherine, Thomas, Jonathan and Mary

Contents

Preface

The aim of this book is to describe the complex relationship between the resident oral micro-flora and the host, both in health and disease. The Fourth Edition has been completely rewritten and enlarged, while retaining its philosophy of explaining this relationship by the application of ecological principles. This approach is of benefit to the reader by providing a clear understanding of the under-lying issues (rather than having to remember an ever-increasing number of facts) that determine whether the microflora will have a pathogenic or a commensal relationship at a site. This information can then be applied to a range of problems by health professionals and researchers alike.

In this latest edition, greater emphasis has been placed on the properties of dental plaque as a biofilm, and on the role of oral micro-organisms in disease, as well as on descriptions of current thinking on their control. The inter-relationship between the commensal microflora and opportunistic infection is considered in detail, as is the role of true pathogens. The book incorporates the latest ideas on the relationship between oral health and general health, and reflects the impact that molecular biology has had on the ability to identify oral micro-organisms that are currently difficult to grow, and to determine their virulence determi-nants. This edition also considers the current global concerns on the use and misuse of antimicrobial agents, and guidelines are pro-vided for their use in oral infections. The impact of the growing number of medically compromised patients with oral problems on treatment design is also discussed.

The book provides a comprehensive coverage of the field of oral microbiology which will be essential to those with specific interests in dentistry as well as those with a more general interest in host–microbe interactions and in microbial ecology. The book will be suitable for undergraduate and postgraduate students, re-search workers, and a wide range of clinical dental professionals.

We would like to thank our colleagues who have helped us by providing information, especially David Beighton, Diane Biddle, George Bowden, Dave Bradshaw, Mike Curtis, Deirdre Devine, Andrew Featherstone, Ian Hamilton, Jeremy Hardie, Nick Jacques, Mogens Kilian, Mark Maiden, Eileen Thiel, William Wade, Rob Whiley and Mike Wilson. Particular thanks also go to our families, who have supported us during the preparation of this edition.

P. D. Marsh, Salisbury
M. V. Martin, Liverpool

Glossary

Several scientific disciplines are involved in the study of oral microbiology. Inevitably, specialist terminology will have been used in this book that is unfamiliar to students of different subjects. This glossary has been provided to help overcome these problems. Specialist terms are given a simple explanation in relation to their usage in this book. Such explanations should not be regarded as strict definitions.

Angina:	choking or suffocation
Antisialogogue:	substance which prevents salivation
Apicectomy:	an operation in which the apex of a tooth is removed
Approximal:	surface between adjacent teeth (*see* Figure 2.2)
Atrophy:	shrinkage in size of an organ or tissue by reduction in size of its cells
Autoclave:	an instrument that uses steam under pressure to sterilize instruments
Autochthonous population:	a characteristic member of the microbial community of a habitat
Autogenic succession:	bacterial succession influenced by microbial factors, e.g. the metabolism of pioneer species lowers the redox potential during plaque development; this allows obligate anaerobes to colonize
Bacteraemia:	micro-organisms present in the bloodstream
Bacterial succession:	pattern of development of a microbial community (*see* Figure 4.1)
Bacteriophage:	a virus that can infect bacteria
Candidosis:	infection with *Candida* spp.
Cariogenic:	dental caries-inducing (e.g. bacterium, diet etc.)
Cellulitis:	inflammation of the tissues
Circumvallate papillae:	structures on the back of the tongue which are involved in taste
Climax community:	stable complex microbial community that develops by, and is the final product of, the process of bacterial succession (*see* Figure 4.1)
Co-aggregation:	the attachment of a cell to a pre-attached organism by specific molecular interactions
Colonization resistance:	the ability of the resident microflora to prevent colonization by exogenous species
Commensalism:	an inter-bacterial interaction beneficial to one population but with a neutral effect on the other
Competition:	rivalry among bacteria for growth-limiting nutrients
Conjugation:	the transfer of genetic material from one bacterium to another through sex pilli
Cryptitope:	a receptor on a host molecule for a microbial adhesin that is exposed only under certain conditions, e.g. when adsorbed to a surface or after enzyme cleavage
Cyst:	a fluid-filled pathological cavity lined by epithelium
Demineralization:	dissolution of enamel or cementum by acid
Dental caries:	localized dissolution of the enamel or root surface by acid derived from the microbial degradation of dietary carbohydrates
Dental plaque:	tenacious deposit on the tooth surface comprising bacteria, their extracellular products and polymers of salivary origin
Endoprosthesis:	an artificial device put inside a joint to replace a diseased part of the joint

Empirical therapy:	therapy (usually antibiotics) prescribed without the benefit of laboratory tests
Ganglion:	a collection of nerve cells forming a semi-independent nerve centre
Genotype:	a set of alleles inherited by an individual or organism
Gingival crevice:	protected habitat formed where the teeth rise out of the gum (*see* Figures 2.1 and 2.2)
Gingival crevicular fluid:	serum-like exudate bathing and flushing the gingival crevice. It has a considerable influence on the ecology of this region by introducing (1) nutrients for the microbial community and (2) components of the immune system and other host defences
Gnotobiotic animal:	germ-free animal deliberately infected with a known bacterial population or microflora
Hepatitis:	inflammation of the liver
Hyperplasia:	increase in the size of an organ by increase in the number of cells
Immunocompromised:	the state of being susceptible to infection by virtue of impairment or malfunction of the immune system
Infective endocarditis:	infection of the lining of the heart (endocardium)
Metastasis:	spread through bloodstream or lymphatic system to another organ or tissue
Microbial homeostasis:	the natural stability of the resident microflora of a site
Microbial taxonomy:	study of the classification of micro-organisms according to their resemblances and differences
Minimum infective dose:	the minimum number of micro-organisms required to cause an infection
Mitral valve:	valve between the left ventricle and atrium
Mucocutaneous:	*affects both* skin and mucous membranes
Necrosis:	death of tissues or cells
Neoplasia:	literally new growth of cells but usually applied to benign or malignant cancers
Niche:	the function or role of an organism in a habitat. Species with identical niches will, therefore, be in competition
Occlusal:	surface on the top of the tooth (*see* Figure 2.2)
Opportunistic pathogen:	an organism normally enjoying a commensal relationship with the host but which has the potential to cause disease under extraordinary circumstances, such as when the resistance of the host is reduced or when the organism is found in a new habitat
Osseointegrated:	the intregration of bone with artificial material
Osteomyelitis:	inflammation of bone caused usually by infection
Paraesthesia:	disordered sensation such as tingling or pins and needles
Pericoronitis:	infection around the crown of an erupting tooth
Periodontal disease:	general term for several diseases in which the supporting tissues of the teeth are attached
Periodontal pocket:	formed by the migration of the junctional epithelium at the base of the gingival crevice down the root of the tooth (*see* Figures 2.1 and 7.1). The migration and subsequent tissue destruction is caused by a host inflammatory response to the microbial challenge and by the production of virulence factors (*see* Table 7.9) by periodontopathogens
Periodontopathogen:	an organism implicated in the aetiology of periodontal diseases
Phenotype:	the properties shown by a body or cell which are due to expression of its genotype
Pheromones:	substances produced to attract other cells or bodies
Polymerase chain reaction (PCR):	a method of producing multiple copies of DNA using polymerase enzymes; this amplification process can be use to detect a microbe when present in low cell numbers

Prion:	a protein associated with transmissible spongiform encephalopathies
Prodromal phase:	the time period between infection and the appearance of the symptoms
Proto-cooperation:	an interbacterial interaction beneficial to all populations involved
Protonmotive force (pmf):	a vectorial gradient of cations, principally protons, across a membrane that generates potential energy. This energy can be harnessed to ATP synthesis, motility and transport of solutes
Pus:	a collection of micro-organisms, fluid and cellular debris
Redox potential:	Eh, the oxidation–reduction potential of a site; anaerobic bacteria prefer an environment with a low Eh
Resident microflora:	the microbial community associated with a particular habitat; this microflora usually lives in harmony with the host and has several beneficial functions to the host, e.g. colonization resistance
Restriction fragment length polymorphism (RFLP):	a technique for the enzymic digestion of DNA which is then resolved electrophoretically and can give a unique pattern of fragments. It is a form of genetic 'fingerprinting'
Retrovirus:	a virus that transcribes its RNA into DNA and back again; this is accomplished by the presence of a reverse transcriptase
Reverse transcriptase:	an enzyme found in HIV which can turn RNA into a complementary strand of DNA and *vice versa*
Ribotyping:	a molecular method to determine the similarity of (bacterial) strains
16S ribosomal RNA:	16S rRNA contains conserved and variable base sequences that can be used to determine the genetic relatedness of bacteria; a benefit of this approach is that bacteria do not need to be culturable, and can be present as part of a mixed culture
Sequestrum:	a necrotic piece of bone
Sialadenitis:	infection of the salivary glands
Sialogogue:	substance that encourages saliva production
Sialoliths:	stones in the salivary gland
Sinus:	a tissue tract or space lined with epithelium from which pus or fluids drain
Sjögren's syndrome:	a syndrome that involves dry mouth and eyes
Sub-gingival:	below the gingival (gum) margin e.g. as in a sample taken from the gingival crevice or periodontal pocket (*see* Figures 2.1 and 2.2)
Thrombus:	a blood clot
Transformation:	the insertion of DNA directly from one cell to another
Transmissible spongiform encephalopathies (TSE):	diseases of the central nervous tissue that result in vacuolation or spongiform changes in neural tissue
Vegetations:	blood clots on the heart lining or endocardium
Xerostomia:	dryness of the mouth, usually due to impairment of salivary gland function

1

Introduction

It has been estimated that the human body is made up of over 10^{14} cells of which only around 10% are mammalian. The remainder are the micro-organisms that comprise the resident microflora of the host. This resident microflora does not have merely a passive relationship with its host, but contributes directly and indirectly to the normal development of the physiology, nutrition and defence systems of the organism. In general, these microfloras live in harmony with humans and animals and, indeed, all parties benefit from the association. It has been proposed recently that this harmonious relationship is a result of complex molecular signalling between members of the resident microflora and host cells.

The microbial colonization of all environmentally exposed surfaces of the body (both external and internal) begins at birth. Such surfaces are exposed to a wide range of micro-organisms derived from the environment and from other persons. Each surface, however, because of its physical and biological properties, is suitable for colonization by only a proportion of these microbes. This results in the acquisition, selection and natural development of diverse but characteristic microfloras at particular sites. For example, following extensive studies comparing the microflora of dental plaque (in health and disease) and the gastro-intestinal tract, only 29 out of over 500 taxa found in the mouth were recovered from faecal samples, despite the continual passage of these bacteria into the gut.

The oral microflora in health and disease

The mouth is similar to other sites in the body in having a natural microflora with a characteristic composition and existing, for the most part, in a harmonious relationship with the host. Perhaps more commonly than elsewhere in the body, this relationship can be altered, and disease can occur in the mouth. This is usually associated with:

(a) major disturbances to the habitat which perturb the stability of the microflora. These disturbances can be from exogenous sources (e.g. following antibiotic treatment or the frequent intake of fermentable carbohydrates) or they can be a result of endogenous changes (e.g. alterations in the integrity of the host defences);

or

(b) the unexpected presence of bacteria at sites not normally accessible to them (e.g. following tooth extraction or other trauma, and when oral bacteria enter tissues or the bloodstream and are disseminated around the body).

Micro-organisms with the potential to cause disease in this way are termed '**opportunistic pathogens**', and many from the oral cavity have the capacity to behave in this manner. Indeed, most individuals suffer at some time in their life from localized episodes of disease in the mouth caused by imbalances in the composition of their resident oral microflora. The commonest clinical manifestations of such imbalances include dental caries and periodontal diseases, both of which are highly prevalent in industrialized societies, and are on the increase in developing countries. Dental caries is the dissolution of enamel (demineralization) by acid, produced primarily from the metabolism of dietary carbohydrates by the bacteria attached to the tooth surface in dental plaque. Dental plaque is also associated with the aetiology of periodontal diseases. Periodontal diseases are a group of disorders in which the supporting tissues of the teeth are attacked; this can eventually lead to the loss of the tooth.

Although rarely life-threatening, dental caries and periodontal diseases have a major clinical significance because of their high prevalence within the general population and the huge costs to health services associated with their treatment. Individuals are retaining their dentition for longer periods due to scientific and clinical advances, and also due to a greater dental awareness among the public, which means that potentially susceptible sites and surfaces are at risk of disease for a much longer period (perhaps for a lifetime).

Statistics on the prevalence of dental disease can be found on the Home Page of the World Health Organization (WHO) Oral Care Unit: *http://www.who.ch/programmes/ncd/orh_www.-htm.* For example, in the United Kingdom in 1993, 46% of 5-year-old children examined had caries in their primary dentition (mean decayed, missing and filled teeth, dmft = 2.0), while this figure rose to 61% in the permanent dentition of 14-year-olds (mean DMFT = 2.2). The mean DMFT in 35–44-year-old individuals in developed countries can range from 19.0 (UK, 1990), 13.6 (USA, 1991), to 20.8 (Australia, 1990). Although the incidence of dental caries has fallen over the past two decades in young children in Western countries, the prevalence still remains unacceptably high in the general population, and the decline seems to have halted in countries that have now reached a low incidence of caries, i.e. caries is not disappearing, and is on the increase in developing countries. The retention of teeth into later life means that surfaces are vulnerable to disease for longer. Periodontal diseases are more common in older age (*see* Chapter 7), and their prevalence can be gauged from the following UK data. Although only 3% of 15–19-year-olds had pockets up to 5 mm deep, over 60% of those aged 35 years and older had pockets of that depth. Caries of the root surface is also an increasing problem in the elderly, and follows on from recession of the gums in old age and exposure of vulnerable cementum to microbial colonization (*see* Chapter 6).

Another way of assessing the impact of dental diseases is by calculating the cost of their treatment. They represent the most costly diseases that the majority of individuals will have to contend with in their lifetime. In 1995, in the USA, the cost of dental treatment was estimated at approximately 46 billion dollars

while the cost to the National Health Service (NHS) of the United Kingdom in 1995–96 was £1292 million. The number of specific treatment items provided by the NHS in 1995–96 is also shown in Table 1.1; in addition to the direct costs of treatment can be added the expense of the accumulated time lost from employment. Not surprisingly, therefore, the main thrust of research in oral microbiology is directed towards understanding the processes involved in the two major groups of dental diseases: caries and periodontal diseases.

Table 1.1 Number of treatments carried out by the National Health Service of England & Wales (1995–96)

Procedure	Number
Amalgam fillings	19 348 052
Crowns	4 940 938
Bridges	782 787
Dentures	1 936 918
Root canals	1 297 553
Extractions	2 736 231
Total cost of treatment	£1 292 million

Dental caries and periodontal diseases result from a complex interaction of environmental triggers (such as diet), the resident microflora and the host (Figure 1.1). In order to determine the mechanisms behind these diseases it is necessary to understand the factors that influence the ecology of the oral cavity. In this book, the relationships among oral micro-organisms, and between these oral micro-organisms and the host, will be examined. The general composition of the oral microflora is reasonably well characterized, but less is understood of the influence of the mouth as a habitat for micro-organisms, and how the properties of this environment influence the composition and metabolism of the resident microflora in health and disease.

Ecological terminology

Much of the terminology used in this book to describe events in microbial ecology will be as defined by Alexander (1971). The site where micro-organisms grow is the **habitat**. The micro-organisms growing in a particular habitat constitute a **microbial community** made up of populations of individual species or less well-

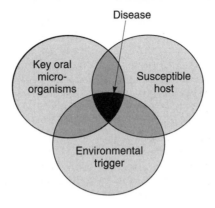

Environmental triggers include:
• poor diet
• poor oral hygiene

Confounding factors include:
• fluoride
• length of time of exposure

Figure 1.1 The inter-relationships that lead to dental disease

defined groups (taxa). The microbial community in a specific habitat together with the abiotic surroundings with which these organisms are associated is known as the **ecosystem**. The most misused ecological term of all, the **niche**, describes the function of an organism in a particular habitat. Thus, the niche is not the physical position of an organism but is its role within the community. This role is dictated by the biological properties of each microbial population. Species with identical functions in a particular habitat will compete for the same niche, while the coexistence of many species in a habitat is due to each population having a different role (niche) and thus avoiding competition.

A number of terms have been used to describe the characteristic mixtures of micro-organisms associated with a site. These include the **normal**, **indigenous** or **commensal** microflora, but some difficulties in nomenclature can arise if some of the organisms are associated with disease on occasions. Alexander (1971) proposed that species found characteristically in a particular habitat should be termed **autochthonous** micro-organisms. These multiply and persist at a site and contribute to the metabolism of a microbial community (with no distinction made regarding disease potential), and can be contrasted with **allochthonous** organisms which originate from elsewhere and are generally unable to colonize successfully unless the ecosystem is severely perturbed.

Similarly, the term **'resident microflora'** is used to describe any organisms that are regularly isolated from a site; again, no distinction concerning disease potential is made. Micro-organisms that have the potential to cause disease are termed **pathogens**. As stated earlier, those that cause disease only under exceptional circumstances are described as **opportunistic pathogens**, and can be distinguished from **true pathogens** which are consistently associated with a particular disease.

The properties of the mouth that influence its function as a microbial habitat together with the major groups of micro-organisms that reside there will be described in the next two chapters. The acquisition and development of the oral microflora, especially dental plaque, will be covered in Chapters 4 and 5, while the remainder of the book will consider the role of the oral microflora in disease.

The oral microflora and general health

The significance of dental diseases is generally considered only in the context of oral health, but evidence is accumulating suggesting that these conditions may impact on the general health of an individual. Periodontal diseases may represent a risk factor for cardiovascular disease, or to pre-term low-birthweight babies (either as a direct consequence of pre-term labour or to premature rupture of membranes) (*see* Chapter 7). Periodontal pockets harbour large numbers of Gram-negative bacteria that produce virulence factors such as lipopolysaccharide (LPS), cytotoxic metabolites and immunoreactive molecules. The host mounts an inflammatory response to the microbial 'insult', and prostaglandins and pro-inflammatory cytokines are produced. These bacterial and host factors enter the bloodstream due to the high vascularity of the periodontium and may affect distant sites in the body.

The mouth can also affect general health by acting as a reservoir for opportunistic pathogens. Oral hygiene is poor among patients in intensive care, and their dental plaque contains large numbers of potential respiratory pathogens. Aspiration of these pathogens into the lower respiratory tract can increase the likelihood of serious lung infection, especially in immunocompromised or elderly people. *Helicobacter pylori* has also been detected in dental plaque on occasions, and this organism is strongly associated with chronic gastritis and peptic ulcers, and is a risk factor for gastric cancer. *H. pylori* is not a normal bacterial inhabitant of the mouth, and its presence is probably associated with gastro-oesophagal reflux. Its intermittent persistence in the mouth may aid its transmission from person-to-person. This pathogen may be retained in dental plaque by selective adherence to already attached bacteria, namely *Fusobacterium* spp., by a process called co-aggregation (*see* Chapter 5).

Summary

The mouth has a resident microflora with a characteristic composition that exists, for the most part, in harmony with the host. This microflora is of benefit to the host and contributes to the normal development of the physiology and host defences of animals and humans. Components of this microflora can act as opportunistic pathogens when the habitat is disturbed or when micro-organisms are found at sites not normally accessible to them. Dental diseases, caused by imbalances in the resident microflora, are highly prevalent and extremely costly to treat. Dental diseases may act as risk factors for more serious medical conditions; the mouth can also act as a reservoir for exogenous pathogens such as H. pylori.

Bibliography

Alexander, M. (1971) *Microbial Ecology*, John Wiley, New York.

Andersen, R.N., Ganeshkumar, N. and Kolenbrander, P.E. (1998) *Helicobacter pylori* adheres selectively to *Fusobacterium* spp. *Oral Microbiol. Immunol.,* **13**, 51–54.

Henderson, B. and Wilson, M. (1998) Commensal communism and the oral cavity. *J. Dent. Res.,* **77**, 1674–1683.

Madinier, I.M., Fosse, T.M. and Monteil, R.A. (1997) Oral carriage of *Helicobacter pylori*: A review. *J. Periodontol.,* **68**, 2–6.

Marthaler, T.M., O'Mullane, D.M. and Vrbic, V. (1996) The prevalence of dental caries in Europe 1990–1995. *Caries Res.,* **30**, 237–255.

Offenbacher, S., Katz, V., Fertik, G. *et al.* (1996) Periodontal infection as a possible risk factor for preterm low birth weight. *J. Periodontol.,* **67**, 1103–1113.

Seymour, R.A. and Steele, J.G. (1998) Is there a link between periodontal disease and coronary heart disease? *Br. Dent. J.,* **184**, 33–38.

2

The mouth as a microbial habitat

The mouth as a habitat for microbial growth

Not all of the micro-organisms that enter the mouth are able to colonize. The properties of the mouth make it ecologically distinct from all other surfaces of the body, and dictate the types of microbe able to persist. Moreover, distinct habitats exist even within the mouth, each of which will support the growth of a character-istic microbial community because of their biological features. Habitats that provide ob-viously different ecological conditions include mucosal surfaces (such as the lips, cheek, palate and tongue) and teeth (Table 2.1). The proper-ties of some of these habitats will change during the life of an individual; for example, only mucosal surfaces are available for colonization during the first few months of life, and then tooth eruption provides hard (non-shedding) surfaces and introduces gingival crevicular fluid as an additional source of nutrients (Figures 2.1 and 2.2). Ecological conditions within the mouth will also vary during the change from the primary to the permanent dentition, and following the extraction of teeth, the insertion of prostheses such as dentures, and any dental treatment, including scaling, polishing and fillings. Transient fluctuations in the stability of the oral ecosystem may be induced by the frequency and type of food ingested, variations in saliva flow and periods of antibiotic therapy.

Four features that make the oral cavity distinct from other areas of the body are: teeth, specialized mucosal surfaces, saliva and gingi-val crevicular fluid (GCF).

Teeth

The mouth is the only normally accessible site in the body that has hard non-shedding surfaces

Table 2.1 Distinct microbial habitats within the mouth

Habitat	Comment
Lips, cheek, palate	Biomass restricted by desquamma-tion; different surfaces have specialized host cell types
Tongue	Highly papillated surface; acts as a reservoir for anaerobes
Teeth	Non-shedding surface enabling large masses of microbes to accumulate (e.g. biofilms such as dental plaque). Teeth have distinct surfaces for microbial colonization; each surface (e.g. fissures, smooth surfaces, approximal, gingival crevice) will support a distinct microflora because of their intrinsic biological properties

for microbial colonization. These unique tissues allow the accumulation of large masses of micro-organisms (predominantly bacteria) and their extracellular products, termed dental plaque. Plaque is an example of a biofilm, and, while it is found naturally in health, it is also associated with dental caries and period-ontal disease. In disease, there is a shift in the composition of the plaque microflora away from the species that predominate in health. The properties of dental plaque will be de-scribed in detail in Chapter 5, and its relation-ship to disease in Chapters 6 and 7.

Each tooth is composed of four tissues: **pulp**, **dentine**, **cementum** and **enamel** (Figure 2.1). The pulp receives nerve cells and blood supplies from the tissues of the jaw via the roots. Thus the pulp is able to nourish the dentine and act as a sensory organ by detecting pain. Dentine makes up the bulk of the tooth and functions by supporting the enamel and protecting the pulp. Dentine is composed of bundles of

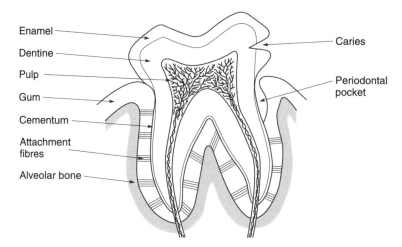

Figure 2.1 Tooth structure in health and disease

collagen filaments surrounded by mineral crystals. Enamel is the most highly calcified tissue in the body and is normally the only part of the tooth exposed to the environment. Cementum is a specialized calcified connective tissue that covers and protects the roots of the tooth. Embedded in the cementum are the fibres of the periodontal ligament which anchor each tooth to the periodontal bone of the jaw. With ageing, recession of the gingival tissues can occur exposing cementum to microbial colonization and attack. Root surface caries can be a consequence, and is an increasing problem in the burgeoning elderly population (*see* Chapter 6).

Teeth do not appear in the mouth until after the first few months of life. The primary dentition is usually complete by the age of 3 years, and around 6 years the permanent teeth begin to erupt. This process is complete by about 12 years of age. Local ecological conditions will vary during these periods of change, which will in turn influence the resident microbial community at a site. The ecological complexity of the mouth is increased still further by the range of habitats associated with the tooth surface. Teeth do not provide a uniform habitat but possess several distinct surfaces (Table 2.1, Figure 2.2), each of which is optimal for colonization and growth by different populations of micro-organisms. This is due to the physical nature of the particular surface and the resulting biological properties of the area. The areas between adjacent teeth (approximal) and in the gingival crevice afford protection from adverse conditions in the mouth.

Both sites are also anaerobic and, in addition, the gingival crevice region is bathed in the nutritionally rich GCF, particularly during inflammation, and so these areas support a more diverse community. Smooth surfaces are more exposed to the environment and can be colonized by only a limited number of bacterial species adapted to such extreme conditions. The properties of a smooth surface will differ according to whether it faces the cheek (buccal surface) or the inside (lingual surface) of the mouth. Pits and fissures of the biting (occlusal) surfaces of the teeth also offer protection from the environment. Such protected areas are associated with the largest microbial communities and, in general, the most disease.

The relationship between the environment and the microbial community is not unidirectional. Although the properties of the environment dictate which micro-organisms can occupy a given site, the metabolism of the microbial community can modify the physical and chemical properties of their surroundings. Thus, the environmental conditions on the tooth will vary in health and disease (Figure 2.1). As caries progresses, the advancing front of the lesion penetrates the dentine. The nutritional sources will change and local conditions may become acidic and more anaerobic due to the accumulation of products of bacterial metabolism. Similarly, in periodontal disease, the gingival crevice develops into a periodontal pocket and the production of GCF is increased. These new environments will select the microbial community most suitably adapted to the prevailing conditions.

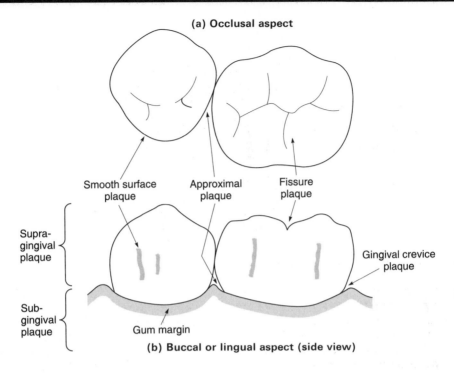

(a) Occlusal aspect

Smooth surface plaque

Approximal plaque

Fissure plaque

Supra-gingival plaque

Gingival crevice plaque

Sub-gingival plaque

Gum margin

(b) Buccal or lingual aspect (side view)

Figure 2.2 Diagram illustrating the different surfaces of a tooth, and the terminology used to describe plaque sampling sites

Mucosal surfaces

Although the mouth is similar to other ecosystems in the digestive tract in having mucosal surfaces for microbial colonization, the oral cavity does have specialized surfaces which contribute to the diversity of the microflora at certain sites. The papillary structure of the dorsum of the tongue provides refuge for many micro-organisms which would otherwise be removed by mastication and the flow of saliva. Such sites on the tongue can also have a low redox potential, which enables obligately anaerobic bacteria to grow. Indeed, the tongue may act as a reservoir for some of the Gram-negative anaerobes that are implicated in the aetiology of periodontal diseases (*see* Chapter 7). The mouth also contains keratinized (e.g. the palate) as well as non-keratinized, stratified squamous epithelium which may affect the intra-oral distribution of micro-organisms.

Saliva

The mouth is kept moist and lubricated by saliva which flows over all the internal surfaces of the oral cavity. Saliva enters the oral cavity via ducts from the major paired parotid, submandibular and sublingual glands as well as from the minor glands of the oral mucosa (labial, lingual, buccal and palatal glands) where it is produced. There are differences in the chemical composition of the secretions from each gland, but the complex mixture is termed 'whole saliva'. Saliva contains several ions including sodium, potassium, calcium, chloride, bicarbonate and phosphate (Table 2.2); their concentrations vary in resting and stimulated saliva. Some of these ions contribute to the buffering property of saliva which can reduce the cariogenic effect of acids produced from the bacterial metabolism of dietary carbohydrates. Bicarbonate is the major buffering system in saliva but phosphates, peptides and proteins are also involved. The mean pH of saliva is between pH 6.75 and 7.25, although the pH and buffering capacity will vary with the flow rate. Within a mouth, the flow rate and the concentration of components such as proteins and calcium and phosphate ions have circadian rhythms, with the slowest flow of saliva occurring during sleep.

Table 2.2 The mean concentration (mg/100 ml) of selected constitutents of whole saliva and gingival crevicular fluid (GCF) from humans

Constituent	Whole Saliva		GCF
	Resting	Stimulated	
Protein	220	280	7×10^3
IgA	19		110*
IgG	1		350*
IgM	<1		25*
C_3	tr	tr	40
Amylase	38		—
Lysozyme	22	11	+
Albumin	tr	tr	+
Sodium	15	60	204
Potassium	80	80	70
Calcium	6	6	20
Magnesium	<1	<1	1
Phosphate	17	12	4
Bicarbonate	31	200	—

tr = trace amounts.
*Determined in GCF samples from patients with periodontitis.

The major organic constituents of saliva are proteins and glycoproteins, such as mucin.

These proteins and glycoproteins influence the oral microflora by:

(a) adsorbing to the tooth surface to form a conditioning film (the acquired pellicle) to which micro-organisms can attach (*see* Chapters 4 and 5);
(b) acting as primary sources of nutrients (carbohydrates and proteins) for the resident microflora;
(c) aggregating micro-organisms and thereby facilitating their clearance from the mouth by swallowing; and
(d) inhibiting the growth of some exogenous micro-organisms.

Other nitrogenous compounds provided by saliva include urea and numerous free amino acids. Not all of the amino acids essential for the growth of oral bacteria are present, and these are derived from the enzymic breakdown of salivary proteins and peptides by the action of various microbial proteases and peptidases. The concentration of free carbohydrates is low in saliva, and most have to be derived from the

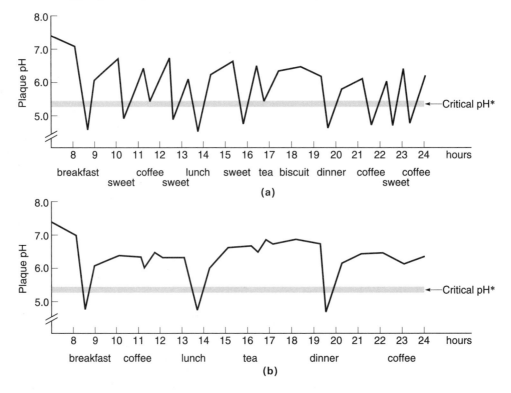

Figure 2.3 Schematic representation of the changes in plaque pH in an individual who (a) has frequent intakes of fermentable carbohydrate during the day, or (b) limits their carbohydrate intake to main meals only
* The critical pH is the pH below which demineralization of enamel is favoured.

Table 2.3 Specific and non-specific host defence factors of the mouth

Defence factors	Main function
Non-specific	
Saliva flow	Physical removal of micro-organisms
Mucin/agglutinins	Physical removal of micro-organisms
Lysozyme-protease-anion	Cell lysis
Lactoferrin	Iron sequestration
Apo-lactoferrin	Cell killing
Sialoperoxidase system	Hypothiocyanite production (neutral pH)
	Hypocyanous acid production (low pH)
Histidine-rich peptides	Antibacterial and anti-fungal activity
Specific	
Intra-epithelial lymphocytes & Langerhans cells	Cellular barrier to penetrating bacteria and/or antigens
sIgA	Prevents microbial adhesion and metabolism
IgG, IgA, IgM	Prevent microbial adhesion; opsonins; complement activators
Complement	Activates neutrophils
Neutrophils/macrophages	Phagocytosis

metabolism of glycoproteins by the production of glycosidases. The metabolism of amino acids, peptides, proteins and urea can lead to the net production of base, which contributes to the rise in pH following acid production after the dietary intake of fermentable carbohydrates (Figure 2.3). In particular, a salivary tetrapeptide with the sequence gly-gly-lys-arg (termed sialin) can be converted to ammonia and putrescine by oral bacteria and can cause a pH-rise effect in the presence of low sugar concentrations.

Several anti-bacterial factors are present in saliva (Table 2.3) which are important in controlling bacterial and fungal colonization of the mouth, and include lysozyme, lactoferrin and the sialoperoxidase system. Antibodies have been detected, with secretory IgA (sIgA) being the predominant class of immunoglobulin; IgG and IgM are also present but in lower concentrations. Peptides with anti-microbial activity, e.g. histidine-rich peptides (histatins), are also present in saliva. The properties of these factors will be described later in this chapter.

Gingival crevicular fluid (GCF)

Serum components can reach the mouth by the flow of a serum-like fluid through the junctional epithelium of the gingivae (Table 2.3). The flow of GCF is relatively slow at healthy sites (*ca* 0.3 μl/tooth/hour), but increases during inflammation. GCF can influence the site by acting as a novel source of nutrients, while its flow will remove non-adherent microbial cells. Many bacteria from sub-gingival plaque are proteolytic and interact synergistically to break down the host proteins and glycoproteins to provide peptides, amino acids and carbohydrates for growth. Essential co-factors, including haemin for black-pigmented anaerobes, can also be obtained from the degradation of haeme-containing molecules such as transferrin, haemopexin, haemoglobin and haptoglobin.

GCF also contains components of the host defences (Tables 2.2 and 2.3) which play an important role in regulating the microflora of the gingival crevice in health and disease. In contrast to saliva, IgG is the predominant immunoglobulin; IgM and IgA are also present, as is complement. GCF contains leucocytes, of which 95% are neutrophils, the remainder being lymphocytes and monocytes. The neutrophils in GCF are viable and can phagocytose bacteria within the crevice. Enzymes such as collagenase, elastase, trypsin etc., derived both from phagocytic host cells and from bacteria, can be detected in GCF. These enzymes can degrade host tissues and thereby contribute to the destructive processes associated with periodontal diseases (Chapter 7). Several of these enzymes are under evaluation as candidates for use as diagnostic markers of active periodontal breakdown, e.g. for applications such as chairside kits.

Factors affecting the growth of micro-organisms in the oral cavity

Temperature

The human mouth is kept at a relatively constant temperature (35–36 °C), which provides conditions suitable for the growth and metabolism of a wide range of micro-organisms. Temperature can also affect key parameters associated with the habitat, such as pH, ion activity, aggregation of macro-molecules and gas solubility.

Periodontal pockets with active disease have a higher temperature (up to 39 °C) compared with healthy sites (mean value 36.8 °C). Such changes in temperature affect gene expression in periodontal pathogens, such as *Porphyromonas gingivalis*. A large rise in temperature down-regulates expression of fimbriae (which mediate attachment of the bacterium to host cells) and the major proteases of this micro-organism, and up-regulates synthesis of superoxide dismutase, which neutralizes toxic oxygen metabolites. Temperature has been shown to vary between different sub-gingival sites, even within the same individual, and may influence the proportions of certain bacterial species, such as the putative periodontal pathogens *P. gingivalis*, *'Bacteroides forsythus'* and *Campylobacter rectus*.

Redox potential/anaerobiosis

Despite the easy access to the mouth of air with an oxygen concentration of approximately 20%, it is perhaps surprising that the oral microflora comprises few, if any, truly aerobic (oxygen-requiring) species. The majority of organisms are either facultatively anaerobic (i.e. can grow in the presence or absence of oxygen) or obligately anaerobic (i.e. require reduced conditions, and oxygen can be toxic to these organisms). In addition, there are some capnophilic (CO_2-requiring) and micro-aerophilic species (requiring low concentrations of oxygen for growth). Anaerobiosis is frequently described in rigid terms: micro-organisms are separated into aerobes and anaerobes on their ability to grow in the presence or absence of oxygen. However, sharp distinctions cannot be made between these groups, and a wide spectrum of oxygen tolerances occurs.

Oxygen concentration is considered the main factor limiting the growth of obligately anaerobic bacteria. It is the commonest and most readily reduced electron acceptor in the majority of microbial habitats, and its presence results in the oxidation of the environment. Anaerobic species require reduced conditions for their normal metabolism; therefore, it is the degree of oxidation-reduction (redox potential, Eh) at a site that governs their survival. In general, the distribution of anaerobes in the mouth will be related to the redox potential at a particular site, although some survive at overtly aerobic habitats by existing in close partnership with oxygen-consuming species. Obligate anaerobes also possess specific molecular defence mechanisms that enable them to cope with low levels of oxygen.

The oxygen tension of the anterior surface of the tongue was found to be 16.4%, the posterior surface 12.4% and the buccal folds of the upper and lower jaw only 0.3–0.4%. Micro-electrodes have measured the redox potential at specific sites in the oral cavity. The redox potential falls during plaque development on a clean enamel surface from an initial Eh of over +200 mV (highly oxidized) to −141 mV (highly reduced) after 7 days. The development of plaque in this way is associated with a specific succession of micro-organisms (*see* Chapters 4 and 5). Early colonizers will utilize O_2 and produce CO_2; later colonizers may produce H_2 and other reducing agents such as sulphur-containing compounds and volatile fermentation products. Thus, as the Eh is gradually lowered, sites become suitable for the survival and growth of a changing pattern of organisms, and particularly anaerobes. Differences have been found between the Eh of the gingival crevice in health and disease. Periodontal pockets are more reduced (mean value −48 mV) than healthy gingival crevices in the same individuals (mean value +73 mV). Approximal areas (between teeth) will also have a low Eh although values for the redox potential at these sites have not been reported. Gradients of O_2 concentration and Eh will exist in the oral cavity, particularly in a thick biofilm such as plaque. Thus, plaque will be suitable for the growth of bacteria with a range of oxygen tolerances. The redox potential at various depths will be influenced by the metabolism of the organisms present and the ability of gases to diffuse in and out of plaque. Similarly, the redox potential will also affect bacterial metabolism, e.g. the activity of intracellular glycolytic enzymes and the pattern of fermentation products of *Streptococcus mutans* varies under strictly anaerobic conditions. Thus, modifications to the habitat that disturb such gradients may influence the composition and metabolism of the microbial community.

pH

Many micro-organisms require a pH around neutrality for growth, and are sensitive to extremes of acid or alkali. The pH of most surfaces of the mouth is regulated by saliva (mean pH, unstimulated whole saliva = 6.75–7.25) so that, in general, optimum pH values for microbial growth are provided at sites bathed by this fluid.

Bacterial population shifts within the plaque microflora can occur following fluctuations in environmental pH. After sugar consumption, the pH in plaque can fall rapidly to below pH 5.0 by the production of acids (predominantly lactic acid) by bacterial metabolism (Figure 2.3); the pH then recovers slowly to base-line values. Depending on the frequency of sugar intake, the bacteria in plaque will be exposed to varying challenges of low pH. Many of the predominant plaque bacteria from healthy sites can tolerate only brief conditions of low pH, and are inhibited or killed by more frequent or prolonged exposures to acidic conditions. These latter conditions are likely to occur in subjects who commonly consume sugar-containing snacks or drinks between meals (Figure 2.3*b*). This can result in the enhanced growth of, or colonization by, acid-tolerant (aciduric) species, especially mutans streptococci and *Lactobacillus* species, which are normally absent or only minor components in dental plaque at healthy sites. Such a change in the bacterial composition of plaque predisposes a surface to dental caries. The acid tolerance of these bacteria is achieved by the possession of particular metabolic strategies and the induction of a specific set of stress response proteins (*see* Chapter 4).

In contrast, the pH of the gingival crevice becomes alkaline during the host inflammatory response in periodontal disease, e.g. following deamination of amino acids and ammonia production. The mean pH may rise to between pH 7.2 and 7.4 during disease, with a few patients having pockets with a mean pH of around 7.8. This degree of change may perturb the balance of the resident microflora of the gingival crevice by favouring the growth and metabolism of periodontal pathogens, such as *Porphyromonas gingivalis*, that have pH optima for growth above pH 7.5.

Nutrients

Populations within a microbial community are dependent solely on the habitat for the nutrients essential for their growth. Therefore, the association of an organism with a particular habitat is direct evidence that all of the necessary growth-requiring nutrients are present. The mouth can support a microbial community of great diversity and satisfy the requirements of many nutritionally demanding bacterial populations (*see* Chapters 3 and 4).

Endogenous nutrients

The persistence and diversity of the resident oral microflora is due primarily to the metabolism of the endogenous nutrients provided by the host, rather than by exogenous factors in the diet. The main source of endogenous nutrients is saliva, which contains amino acids, peptides, proteins and glycoproteins (which also act as a source of sugars and aminosugars), vitamins and gases. In addition, the gingival crevice is supplied with GCF which, in addition to delivering components of the host defences, contains potential sources of novel nutrients, such as albumin and other host proteins and glycoproteins, including haeme-containing molecules. The difference in source of endogenous nutrients is one of the reasons for the variation in the microflora of the gingival crevice compared with other oral sites, particularly on teeth.

Evidence for the importance of endogenous nutrients has also come from the observation that a diverse microbial community persists in the mouth of humans and animals fed by intubation (stomach tube). Also, the oral microflora of animals with dietary habits ranging from insectivores and herbivores to carnivores is broadly similar at the genus level. Likewise, it was found that the growth rate of bacteria colonizing teeth of experimental animals was relatively unaffected by the addition of fermentable carbohydrate to their drinking water. Plaque bacteria produce glycosidases (which release carbohydrates from the oligosaccharide side chains of salivary mucins) and proteases, and interact synergistically to break down these endogenous nutrients as no single species has the full enzyme complement to totally metabolize these nutrients.

Exogenous (dietary) nutrients

Superimposed upon these endogenous nutrients is the complex array of foodstuffs ingested periodically in the diet. Fermentable carbohydrates are the main class of compounds that influence markedly the ecology of the mouth. Such carbohydrates can be broken down to acids while, additionally, sucrose can be converted by bacterial enzymes (glucosyltransferases, GTF, and fructosyltransferases, FTF) into two classes of polymer (glucans and fructans) which can be used to consolidate attachment or act as extracellular nutrient storage compounds, respectively. The frequent consumption of dietary carbohydrates is associated with a shift in the proportions of the microflora of dental plaque. The levels of mutans streptococci and lactobacilli increase, while those of acid-sensitive species (e.g. *Streptococcus sanguis, S. gordonii*) decrease. The metabolism of plaque changes so that the predominant fermentation product becomes lactate. Such alterations in the microflora and its metabolism predispose a site to dental caries. Laboratory studies suggest that it is the repeated low pH generated from sugar metabolism rather than the availability of excess carbohydrate *per se* that is responsible for these perturbations to the microflora.

Dairy products (milk, cheese) have some influence on the ecology of the mouth. The ingestion of milk or milk products can protect the teeth of animals against caries. This may be due to the buffering capacity of milk proteins or due to decarboxylation of amino acids after proteolysis since several bacterial species can metabolize casein. Milk proteins (casein) and casein derivatives can also adsorb on to the tooth surface, in exchange for albumin in the enamel pellicle, and reduce the adhesion of mutans streptococci by modifying the structure of this conditioning film; they can also sequester calcium phosphate and enhance remineralization. Similarly, kappa-casein can inhibit GTF adsorption into the pellicle and reduce enzyme activity, thereby suppressing glucan formation. Cheese has been shown to increase salivary flow rates in animals and to rapidly elevate plaque pH changes in humans following a sucrose rinse.

Sugar substitutes are sweet-tasting compounds that cannot be metabolized to acid by oral bacteria. They have been added to some confectionery; xylitol, for example, is inhibitory to the growth of *S. mutans*, and lower levels of this species are found in plaque and saliva of those that frequently consume products containing this alternative sweetener.

Adherence and agglutination

Chewing and the natural flow of saliva (mean rate = 19 ml/h; range = 0.5–111.0 ml/h) will detach micro-organisms not firmly attached to an oral surface. Although saliva contains between 10^8 and 10^9 viable micro-organisms per ml, these organisms are all derived from the teeth and mucosa, with plaque and the tongue being the main contributors. Salivary components can aggregate certain bacteria which facilitates their removal from the mouth by swallowing. Bacteria are unable to maintain themselves in saliva by cell division because they are lost at an even faster rate by swallowing.

The molecules responsible for agglutination have been characterized. Mucins are high molecular weight glycoproteins containing > 40% carbohydrate. Their protein backbone has oligosaccharide side chains of different length and composition; some of these side chains are branched and sialic acid and fucose are common terminal sugars. Two chemically distinct mucins have been identified in human saliva, and are termed mucin glycoproteins 1 and 2 (MG1 and MG2, respectively); MG1 has a molecular weight $> 10^3$ kDa while MG2 is only 130–150 kDa. These mucins not only agglutinate oral bacteria, but can also interact with exogenous pathogens such as *Staphylococcus aureus* and *Pseudomonas aeruginosa*, as well as viruses (e.g. influenza virus). Mucin binding to bacteria appears to involve blood group reactive components (e.g. N-acetylgalactose) and sialic acid. Removal of sialic acid by neuraminidase reduces the ability of mucins to agglutinate *S. sanguis*, although not *S. mutans*. Mucins such as MG2 may require an interaction with other salivary components, e.g. sIgA, in order to retain their agglutinating activity. Other agglutinins include a fucose-rich glycoprotein, β-2 microglobulin and lysozyme.

Desquamation ensures that the bacterial load on most mucosal surfaces is light, and indeed,

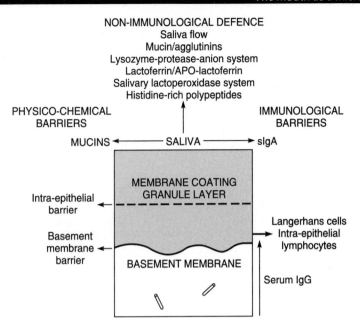

Figure 2.4 The host defences associated with oral mucosal surfaces

only a relatively few species are able to adhere (*see* Chapter 4). In contrast, relatively thick biofilms (dental plaque) are able to accumulate on teeth, particularly at stagnant or retentive sites like fissures, approximal regions and the gingival crevice (*see* Figure 2.2). Dental plaque formation involves an ordered colonization (microbial succession, *see* Chapter 4) by a range of bacteria. The early colonizers interact with, and adhere to, saliva-coated enamel, while later colonizers bind to already attached species (co-aggregation). Many specific mechanisms of cell-to-host surface and cell-to-cell adherence have been determined for oral bacteria and will be described in Chapter 4.

Antimicrobial agents and inhibitors

In addition to the components of the host defences present in saliva and GCF, the resident oral microflora is regularly challenged with modest concentrations of antimicrobial and anti-plaque agents. Anti-plaque agents are distinguished from antimicrobials on the basis of their mode of action. Anti-plaque agents remove already attached cells, or prevent adhesion of new cells to the tooth surface, unlike antimicrobials which are designed to kill (bactericidal) or inhibit the growth (bacteriostatic) of the bacteria. Both types of agent can be delivered from toothpastes (dentifrices) and mouthwashes, and are described in Chapters 6 and 7.

Antibiotics given systemically or orally for problems at other sites in the body will enter the mouth via saliva or GCF and affect the stability of the oral microflora. Within a few hours of taking prophylactic high doses of penicillins, the salivary microflora can be suppressed permitting the emergence of antibiotic-resistant bacteria. These bacteria can persist at significant levels for several weeks before returning to their low base-line values. The antibiotic should be changed if several courses of treatment are necessary and the interval between courses is less than one month. Resistant bacteria have been observed following the use of penicillins and erythromycin. These aspects will be considered in more detail in Chapter 13.

Host defences

The health of the mouth is dependent on the integrity of the mucosa (and enamel) which acts as a physical barrier to prevent penetration by micro-organisms or antigens (Figure 2.4). The host has a number of additional defence mechanisms which play an important role in maintaining the integrity of these oral surfaces; these are listed in Table 2.3 and their sphere of

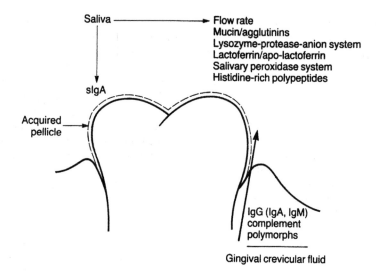

Figure 2.5 Host defences associated with the tooth surfaces

influence is shown diagrammatically in Figures 2.4 and 2.5. These defences are divided into non-specific (or **innate**) and specific (or **immune**) factors. The former, unlike antibodies, do not require prior exposure to an organism or antigen for activity and so provide a continuous, broad spectrum of protection. An alternative terminology is for the non-specific and specific factors to be termed **innate immunity** and **adaptive immunity**, respectively.

Non-specific factors
The physical removal by swallowing of microorganisms either by aggregation or by the flow of saliva (or GCF) is an important defence mechanism. Lysozyme, a 14 kDa basic protein found in several bodily secretions including saliva, can bind to and aggregate oral bacteria, but it also has the potential to hydrolyse peptidoglycan which confers rigidity to bacterial cell walls. At acid pH, the lytic action of lysozyme is enhanced by monovalent anions (bicarbonate, fluoride, chloride, or thiocyanate) and proteases found in saliva. Members of the resident oral microflora are relatively insensitive to the action of lysozyme, so that its role may be targeted more at inhibiting the growth of exogenous bacteria.

Other non-specific factors in oral secretions include lactoferrin (mol. wt = 75 kDa), a high affinity, iron-binding glycoprotein. Since microbial pathogens grow in the host under iron-restricted conditions, the protective role of this molecule was presumed to be due primarily to iron sequestration. However, iron-free lactoferrin (apo-lactoferrin) can also be bactericidal to a range of Gram-positive and Gram-negative bacteria. In addition, the salivary peroxidase enzyme system (sialoperoxidase) can generate hypothiocyanite at neutral pH or hypothiocyanous acid at low pH in the presence of H_2O_2, and both can inhibit glycolysis by plaque bacteria. H_2O_2 is generated during metabolism by several resident bacterial species, including *S. sanguis* and *S. mitis*.

Antimicrobial peptides have been identified in saliva, including histatins and cystatins. Histatins are a family of histidine-rich basic peptides found in human parotid and submandibular/sublingual gland saliva that help regulate the levels of yeasts in the mouth. There are at least seven major histatins in human saliva, each of which may have a different role. For example, histatin 5 is more active than histatins 3 and 1 in terms of killing germinated yeast cells, while histatin 3 is a more potent inhibitor of yeast germination. Cystatins comprise a diverse group of thiol protease inhibitors, and at least seven are present in human saliva. They differ slightly in molecular weight (14–15 kDa), charge and degree of phosphorylation. They are able to form complexes with mucins, which may enable cystatins to be targeted to different oral surfaces where they may play a role in modulating de-/re-mineralization processes on enamel; they may also suppress the growth and protease activity of periodontal pathogens. Certain types of human defensin may be produced by oral mucosal cells; defensins are antibacterial peptides that have been shown to be important in the defence of mucosal surfaces at other sites.

Specific factors

Components of the specific host defences (intra-epithelial lymphocytes and Langerhans cells, IgG and IgA) are found within the mucosa (*see* Figure 2.4), where they act as a barrier to penetrating antigens. The predominant immunoglobulin in the healthy mouth is sIgA; it is composed of IgA heavy and light chains (300 kDa), secretory component (70 kDa), and the J chain (15 kDa). The J chain connects the two IgA molecules into a dimer, while the secretory component stabilizes the molecule and reduces its susceptibility to attack by acids or general proteases. sIgA can agglutinate oral bacteria, modulate enzyme activity and inhibit the adherence of bacteria to oral surfaces. sIgA is usually considered to be a first line of defence by virtue of its local dispersal of environmental antigens. Compared with other classes of immunoglobulin, sIgA is only weakly complement-activating and opsonizing and, therefore, is less likely to cause damage to tissues by any indirect effect of an inflammatory response. Other components, e.g. IgG, IgM, IgA and complement, can be found in saliva but are almost entirely derived from GCF (*see* Table 2.2). GCF also contains phagocytic cells, which are predominantly neutrophils, with some lymphocytes and monocytes.

Specific antibody production can be stimulated by bacterial antigens associated with plaque at the gingival margin or on the oral mucosa. Salivary and circulating antibodies have been detected with activity against a range of oral bacteria, even in health. The pattern of the host response in GCF, saliva, or serum is being explored as a method of improved diagnosis of disease or as a means of recognizing at-risk individuals.

The antimicrobial factors described above do not necessarily operate in isolation. Combinations of specific and non-specific host defence factors can function synergistically so that, for example, lysozyme and sIgA can react with salivary agglutinins (mucins) and so be pre-sented directly to immobilized cells. Other synergistic combinations include mucins or sIgA and salivary peroxidase.

Despite this rich array of antimicrobial factors, the mouth naturally harbours a diverse collection of micro-organisms. Indeed, this resident microflora confers several beneficial functions on the host. A full description of the indigenous oral microflora, together with a consideration of how it might persist in spite of the host defences, and the benefits it provides will be considered in subsequent chapters.

Host genetics

Studies of periodontal disease have suggested that gender and race can influence disease susceptibility, and possibly also affect the microflora. In an adult periodontitis group, *P. gingivalis* and *Peptostreptococcus anaerobius* were associated more with black subjects whereas *Fusobacterium nucleatum* was found more commonly in white individuals. The reasons for this are unknown, but may reflect some variation in the local immune response. In other studies, some strains of *Actinobacillus actinomycetemcomitans* (a pathogen in juvenile periodontitis; *see* Chapter 7) were found to over-produce a particular virulence factor (a leukotoxin), all of which were isolated from people who could be traced to North West Africa.

The sub-gingival microflora of twins has also been compared. The microflora of twin children living together was more similar than that of unrelated children of the same age. Further analysis showed that the microflora of identical twins was more similar than that of fraternal twins, suggesting some genetic control.

Concluding remarks

Despite the potential for regular environmental perturbations involving some of the factors described above, once established at a site, the oral microflora remains relatively stable in composition and proportions over time. This stability is termed **microbial homeostasis** and the mechanisms that support this homeostasis are discussed in Chapter 5.

Summary

The mouth is not a uniform habitat for microbial growth and colonization. Several distinct surfaces provide different habitats due to their physical nature and biological properties. These include a variety of mucosal surfaces as well as teeth; the latter are unique for microbial colonization being hard and non-shedding. The surfaces of the mouth are lubricated by saliva, while the gingival crevice is bathed with GCF. Both fluids help remove weakly attached micro-organisms, and deliver specific and non-specific components of the host defences that help regulate bacterial and fungal colonization. Saliva and GCF are also the primary sources of nutrients for oral micro-organisms. Consortia of different bacterial species with complementary patterns of glycosidase and protease activities are required to break down host glycoproteins. Dietary components have much less of an influence on the microflora of the mouth, although fermentable carbohydrates can lead to increases in acidogenic and aciduric organisms that are potentially cariogenic, due to the low pH generated from their metabolism. Other factors that influence the growth of micro-organisms in the mouth include the Eh and pH of a site, the ability of cells to adhere to oral surfaces, and the presence of antimicrobial agents (from both endogenous and exogenous sources).

Bibliography

Arnold, R.R., Russell, J.E., Devine, S.M. *et al.* (1985) Antimicrobial activity of the secretory innate defence factors lactoferrin, lactoperoxidase and lysozyme. In *Cariology Today* (B. Guggenheim, ed.), Karger, Basel, pp. 75–88.

Cimasoni, G. (1983) *The Crevicular Fluid Updated* (H.M. Myers, ed.), Karger, Basel.

Edgar, W.M. and O'Mullane, D.M. (eds) (1996) *Saliva and Dental Health,* 2nd edn, British Dental Journal, London.

Igarashi, K., Lee, I.K. and Schachtele, C.F. (1989) Comparison of *in vivo* human dental plaque pH changes within artificial fissures and at interproximal sites. *Caries Res.,* **23**, 417–422.

Jenkins, G.N. (1978) *The Physiology and Biochemistry of the Mouth,* 4th edn, Blackwell, Oxford.

Mandel, I.D. and Ellison, S.A. (1985) The biological significance of the non-immunological defence factors. In *The Lactoperoxidase System: Chemistry and Biological Significance* (K.M. Pruitt and J. Tenovuo, eds), Marcel Dekker, New York, pp. 1–14.

Lehner, T. (1993) *Immunology of Oral Diseases,* 3rd edn, Blackwell, Oxford.

Scannapieco, F.A. (1994) Saliva–bacterium interactions in oral microbial ecology. *Crit. Revs Oral Biol. Med.,* **5**, 203–248.

Schenkein, H.A., Burmeister, J.A., Koertge, T.E. *et al.* (1993) The influence of race and gender on periodontal microflora. *J. Periodontol.,* **64**, 292–296.

3

The resident oral microflora

The resident oral microflora is diverse and consists of a wide range of species of viruses, mycoplasma, bacteria, yeasts and even, on occasions, protozoa. This diversity is due to the fact that the mouth is composed of a number of varied habitats supplied with a range of different nutrients. In addition, in dental plaque gradients develop in parameters of ecological significance, such as oxygen tension and pH, providing conditions suitable for the growth and coexistence of micro-organisms with a wide spectrum of requirements. Plaque also functions as a true microbial community and synergistic metabolic interactions occur, enabling some fastidious bacteria to survive and grow under conditions they would be unable to tolerate if in pure culture. The mouth can be contrasted with ecosystems in which the intensity of one or more parameters approaches the extreme; such sites have a lower species diversity.

Before the microbial community at individual sites in the mouth will be considered (Chapters 4 and 5), the types and properties of the organisms found commonly in health and disease will be described. First, however, it may be instructive to discuss the principles of microbial classification and identification, and describe briefly some of the methods used.

Classification is the arrangement of organisms into groups (taxa) on the basis of their similarities and differences. In contrast, **identification** is the process of determining that a new isolate belongs to a particular taxon; the aim of classification is to define these taxa at the **genus** or **species** level. Traditionally, a hierarchical system has existed for the naming of bacteria so that groups of closely related organisms form a

species, and related species are placed in a genus etc. (Table 3.1); species are designated by Latin or latinized binomials (e.g. *Streptococcus mutans*; the genus is '*Streptococcus*' and the species is '*mutans*', Table 3.1). If an isolate does not belong to an existing taxon, then a new species can be proposed. The naming of bacteria to reflect this classification (**nomenclature**) is regulated by an international committee. Once an organism has been placed in a species, it may be possible to sub-type individual strains; this can be valuable in epidemiological studies investigating transmission of strains between individuals (*see* Figure 3.1). The classification, nomenclature and identification of micro-organisms is referred to as **taxonomy,** although, sometimes, the terms classification and taxonomy are used interchangeably.

Table 3.1 Hierarchical ranks in microbial classification

Taxonomic rank	Example
Kingdom	Procaryotae
Division	Firmicutes
Sub-division	low G + C content of DNA
Order	—
Family	Streptococcaceae
Genus	*Streptococcus*
Species	*Streptococcus mutans*
Serotype*	*Streptococcus mutans* serotype *c*
Strain*	*Streptococcus mutans* NCTC 10449

*These ranks are not formally recognized in taxonomy, but are of great practical importance.

Principles of microbial classification

As stated above, the purpose of classification

schemes is to develop a logical arrangement of organisms based on their similarities and relatedness. This requires the determination and comparison of as many characteristics as possible, though in identification schemes, only a few key discriminatory tests may be needed to distinguish between organisms. Early classification schemes relied heavily on morphological and simple physiological criteria, e.g. the shape of the cell, and the pattern of fermentation of simple sugars. In effect, these approaches analysed only a fraction of the genetic material of the cell **(genome)**. In contrast, contemporary classification schemes are based more on chemical analyses of cells **(chemotaxonomy)** and on measuring the genetic relatedness among strains. Chemotaxonomy compares the molecular composition of major components of whole cells (e.g. membrane lipids, peptidoglycan structure, whole cell protein profiles, fermentation products), and hence a greater number of gene products. Likewise, the antigenic profile of cell surfaces can be compared using serological techniques **(serology)**, using specific antibodies (polyclonal or monoclonal).

As the properties of an organism are dictated by what is coded in its genome, the ultimate comparison is to determine the similarity in **DNA base composition**. Initially, the mole percentage of guanine (G) plus cytosine (C) in the total DNA is determined. Organisms with markedly different $G+C$ contents are unrelated, while organisms that have similar $G+C$ values are closely related, although similarity in gross DNA composition is not unequivocal proof of close relatedness because the base pairs could be organized in a different sequence. In such a situation, genotypic similarity can be confirmed by determining the degree of homology between the DNA from two strains, i.e. the abilities of heat-denatured, single strands of DNA from different strains to re-anneal with each other, or to a reference strain, during slow cooling **(DNA–DNA hybridization).** High levels of homology reflect an overall similarity in the nucleotide sequences from the DNA of the two strains, and hence confirms their close taxonomic relationship. The genetic relatedness of micro-organisms can also be determined by comparing **16S ribosomal RNA** (16S rRNA) sequences. This approach has clarified the classification of many heterogeneous groups. These gene sequences have also been exploited in the design of species-specific probes or primers for identification purposes. For example, discriminatory regions of DNA can be amplified by the polymerase chain reaction (PCR) using primers that flank the region of interest. Only a proportion of bacteria from a site can be cultured in the laboratory. The extraction, amplification (by PCR techniques using universal primers) and sequencing of 16S rRNA genes from micro-organisms present in clinical samples (e.g. sub-gingival plaque, pus from abscesses), and comparison against known sequences in databases, can lead to the recognition of new genera or species without the need for culture. The advent of molecular approaches to classification has allowed bacteria to be grouped for the first time according to their 'natural' relationships, thereby showing their evolutionary relationships as **phylogenetic trees**.

A consequence of classification is the generation of internationally approved species. A species represents a collection of strains that share many features in common, and which differ considerably from other strains. Once a species has been recognized, then a **type strain** is nominated that has properties representative of the species. Type strains are held in national collections, such as the American Type Culture Collection (ATCC), and the National Collection of Type Cultures (NCTC), which is located in the United Kingdom. A species may be divided into sub-species if minor but consistent phenotypic variations can be recognized. Likewise, groups of strains within a species can sometimes be distinguished by a special characteristic, and are termed biovars or **biotypes**, while strains with a distinctive antigenic composition are described as serovars or **serotypes,** and can be recognized using appropriate antibodies.

Principles of microbial identification

Once organisms have been correctly classified using rigorous techniques, then more simple identification schemes can be devised in which limited numbers of key discriminatory properties are compared (Figure 3.1). These might include physiological tests, e.g. sugar fermentation patterns, enzyme synthesis, or the pattern of acidic fermentation products following glucose metabolism. The type of tests will vary

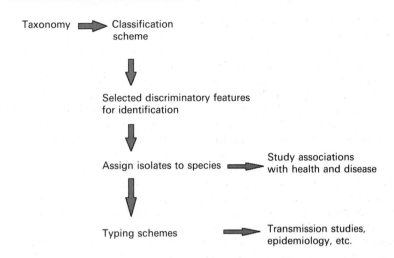

Figure 3.1 Diagrammatic representation to distinguish classification, identification and typing of bacterial strains

with the particular groups (taxa) of micro-organisms being examined. Furthermore, monoclonal antibodies and nucleic acid probes have been developed for the rapid identification of a limited number of species, but primarily those associated with disease. Such antibodies and probes can be labelled with a signalling group to aid in detection, e.g. with fluorescein, a radiolabel, or horseradish peroxidase. These techniques have the advantage that organisms can be detected directly in plaque or clinical samples without the need for lengthy culturing, although a potential drawback is that they can detect dead as well as viable cells. In general, the first stage in identification of bacteria is the reaction of an organism with the Gram stain, and the determination of cellular morphology. Bacteria are described as being, for example, Gram-positive cocci or Gram-negative rods, etc. Some distinguishing parameters used in microbial identification are listed in Table 3.2.

Some of the molecular approaches described earlier can be adapted for sub-typing strains within a species. Whole genomic DNA can be digested by different restriction enzymes (endonucleases), which cut the nucleic acid in specific places; these digests are then electrophoresed on an agarose gel to generate a chromosomal fingerprint. Different strains generate different patterns (**restriction fragment length polymorphisms, RFLPs**), although strains that appear to give similar patterns need to be compared after digestion with more than one enzyme. This approach, however, can yield

Table 3.2 Some characteristics used in microbial classification and identification schemes

Characteristic	Examples
Cellular morphology	Shape; Gram stain reaction; flagella; spores; size
Colonial appearance	Pigment; haemolysis; shape
Carbohydrate fermentation	Acid or gas production
Amino acid hydrolysis	Ammonia production
Pattern of fermentation products	Butyrate; lactate; acetate
Pre-formed enzymes	Glycosidases (e.g. α-glucosidase)
Antigen	Monoclonal/polyclonal antibodies to cell surface proteins
Lipids	Menaquinones, long-chain fatty acids
DNA	Base composition (G+C ratio); sequence homology; oligonucleotide probes
Enzyme profile	Presence, or electrophoretic mobility of malate dehydrogenase
Peptidoglycan	Amino acid composition, e.g. lysine

complex patterns; simpler profiles can be obtained by blotting the restriction fragments onto nitrocellulose or nylon membranes, and hybridizing them with a suitably labelled probe (**ribotyping**). This can yield different patterns within a species, and has allowed insights to be made into the transmission of strains among family members (Figure 3.1), and in the persistence of specific ribotypes at a site (*see* Chapter 4).

Difficulties arising from recent advances in microbial classification

Although recent advances have led to improvements in the classification of oral bacteria, this has also created problems when interpreting early data when a previous nomenclature was in use. The classification of many groups of oral bacteria has been revolutionized in a relatively short time period, with many new genera and species described. An organism discussed in an early study may now justify reclassification and hence renaming. As it is not always clear how such an organism would be classified in modern schemes, new and old terminologies may co-exist in the scientific literature. For example, *Streptococcus sanguis* has been described for many decades, but as of 1989, its description became more limited, and organisms previously included within this species were found to be sufficiently different as to warrant the formation of a distinct species, e.g. *S. gordonii*. Some strains reported in earlier studies as *S. sanguis* may not have the same properties as strains more recently identified as *S. sanguis sensu stricto*.

Microbial taxonomy is a dynamic area with existing species being reclassified due to the application of more stringent tests, together with the recognition of genuinely newly discovered species. The emphasis paid to the classification and identification of the oral microflora is necessary because without valid sub-division and accurate identification of isolates, the specific association of species with particular diseases (**microbial aetiology**) cannot be recognized. Likewise, it has to be accepted that further changes in microbial classification schemes will occur in the future. The properties of the main groups of micro-organism found in the mouth will now be discussed.

Gram-positive cocci

Streptococcus

Streptococci have been isolated from all sites in the mouth and comprise a large proportion of the resident oral microflora. Traditionally, oral streptococci have been differentiated by simple biochemical and physiological tests. More recent studies comparing DNA homology, whole cell protein profiles and the detection of glycosidase activity has clarified the taxonomic relationship between many species. Oral streptococci have been divided into four main species groups (Table 3.3).

Table 3.3 Current recognized species of oral streptococci

Group	Species
mutans-group	*S. mutans*, serotypes *c, e, f*
	S. sobrinus, serotype *d, g*
	S. cricetus, serotype *a*
	S. rattus, serotype *b*
	S. ferus
	S. macacae
	S. downei, serotype *h*
salivarius-group	*S. salivarius*
	S. vestibularis
anginosus-group	*S. constellatus*
	S. intermedius
	S. anginosus
mitis-group	*S. sanguis*
	S. gordonii
	S. parasanguis
	S. oralis
	S. mitis
	S. crista

S. mutans-*group (mutans streptococci)*

There is great interest in this group because of their role in the aetiology of dental caries. *S. mutans* was originally isolated from carious human teeth by Clarke (1924) and, shortly afterwards, was recovered from a case of infective endocarditis (growth of bacteria on damaged heart valves). Little attention was paid to this species until the 1960s when it was demonstrated that caries could be experimentally induced and transmitted in animals artificially infected with strains resembling *S. mutans*. Its name derives from the fact that cells can lose their coccal morphology and often appear as short rods or as cocco-bacilli (Figure 3.2). Eight serotypes were recognized (*a–h*), based on the serological specificity of carbohydrate antigens located in the cell wall. Subsequent work showed that sufficient differences

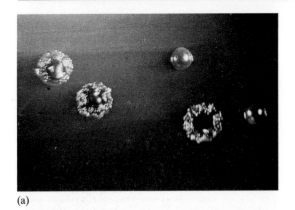

(a)

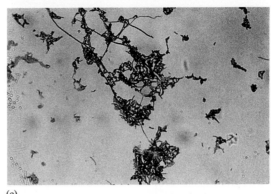

(c)

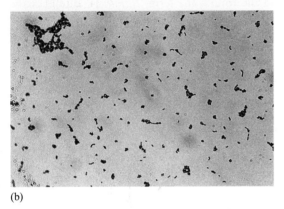

(b)

Figure 3.2 (a) The colony morphology of *S. mutans* growing on sucrose-containing agar, and the cell morphology of selected oral micro-organisms when viewed by light microscopy; (b) *S. mutans*, and (c) *A. naeslundii*.

existed between clusters of these serotypes to warrant their sub-division into seven distinct species (Table 3.3); these are described collectively as mutans streptococci.

The specific epithet, *S. mutans*, is now limited to human isolates previously belonging to serotypes *c, e* and *f*. This is the most commonly isolated species of mutans streptococci from dental plaque, and epidemiological studies have implicated *S. mutans* as the primary pathogen in the aetiology of enamel caries in children and young adults, root surface caries in the elderly and nursing (or bottle) caries in infants (*see* Chapter 6). The next most commonly isolated species of the mutans streptococci group is *S. sobrinus* (serotypes *d* and *g*), which has also been associated with human dental caries. However, there is less known about the role of *S. sobrinus* in disease than *S. mutans* because some studies do not attempt to distinguish between these species, while some commonly used selective media for the isolation of mutans streptococci from dental plaque contain bacitracin which can be inhibitory to the growth of both *S. sobrinus* and *S. cricetus* (serotype *a*). *S.*

cricetus is recovered only rarely from humans. Some subjects harbour more than one species of mutans streptococci in their mouth. These range from *S. mutans/S. sobrinus* combinations which are found together in 3% (UK children) to 49% (Saudi Arabian adults) of individuals, to combinations of *S. mutans* and *S. rattus*, and *S. mutans* and *S. cricetus*, which were found together in 1% of elderly individuals in the USA.

The antigenic structure of mutans streptococci has been studied in detail for use in caries vaccine development (*see* Chapter 6) or in serological typing schemes. Mutans streptococci possess cell wall carbohydrate antigens, lipoteichoic acid, lipoproteins and cell wall or cell wall-associated proteins (*see* Chapter 4). Antigen I/II (also termed antigen B or P1) has generated considerable interest because of its inclusion in a possible sub-unit vaccine. This antigen may be involved in the initial adherence of *S. mutans* to the tooth surface by interacting with components of the salivary pellicle (*see* Chapters 4 and 5).

Mutans streptococci make extracellular soluble and insoluble extracellular polysaccharides (glucans and fructans) from sucrose (*see* Figure 3.2) that are associated with plaque formation and cariogenicity (*see* Chapters 4 and 6). They can also synthesize intracellular polysaccharides which act as carbohydrate reserves, and can be converted to acid during periods when dietary carbohydrates are unavailable. Mutans streptococci produce acid at an extremely rapid rate from pulses of fermentable carbohydrate, and this contributes to their pathogenic potential in caries. However, of equal significance is their ability to grow and survive under the acidic conditions they so generate, by the expression of a specific molecular stress response (*see* Chapter 4).

S. salivarius-*group*

This group comprises *S. salivarius*, the closely related *S. thermophilus* (which is not found in the mouth), and recently described *S. vestibularis*. *S. salivarius* preferentially colonizes mucosal surfaces, especially the tongue. Strains produce an extracellular fructan (polymer of fructose with a levan structure; Chapter 4), and this gives rise to characteristically large mucoid colonies when grown on sucrose-containing agar. *S. salivarius* also produces extracellular soluble and insoluble glucans from sucrose. *S. salivarius* is not considered a significant opportunistic pathogen.

S. vestibularis is isolated mainly from the vestibular mucosa of the human mouth. These strains do not synthesize extracellular polysaccharides from sucrose, but do produce a urease (which can generate ammonia and hence raise the local pH) and hydrogen peroxide (which can contribute to the salivary peroxidase system, and inhibit competing bacteria).

S. anginosus-*group*

This group is readily isolated from dental plaque and mucosal surfaces, but members are also an important cause of purulent disease in humans. They are commonly found in abscesses of internal organs, especially of the brain and liver, and have also been recovered from cases of appendicitis, peritonitis and endocarditis. The classification and nomenclature of this group has been resolved recently. Early work in Europe had grouped various haemolytic and non-haemolytic streptococci, including those with Lancefield group F and G antigens, as *S. milleri*. In the USA, an alternative classification had been proposed and two groups were

formed, designated *S. MG-intermedius* and *S. anginosus-constellatus*. It was subsequently proposed that strains should be divided on the basis of lactose fermentation into *S. constellatus* (non-lactose fermenters), *S. intermedius* (lactose fermenters), with *S. anginosus* to include a collection of β-haemolytic strains possessing various Lancefield grouping antigens. These divisions were confirmed by chemotaxonomic and genetic studies, although their precise descriptions were emended. The general term, 'anginosus-group', has been applied when the identity of individual species is uncertain and, in the future, the term '*S. milleri*' should cease to be used. These streptococci are potential opportunistic pathogens; *S. intermedius* is isolated mainly from liver and brain abscesses, while *S. anginosus* and *S. constellatus* are derived from a wider range of sources. Pathogenic strains of *S. intermedius* produce a protein toxin, termed intermedilysin. No strains from this group make extracellular polysaccharides from sucrose.

S. mitis-*group*

The recent application of chemotaxonomic and genetic techniques (especially DNA–DNA hybridization studies, and the determination of 16S rRNA sequences) has resolved many of the previous anomalies in the classification of this group. Strains originally designated *S. sanguis* I have been sub-divided into *S. sanguis* and *S. gordonii*; both produce extracellular soluble and insoluble glucans (*see* Chapter 4) from sucrose. *S. sanguis* produces a protease that can cleave sIgA, while *S. gordonii* can bind α-amylase enabling these strains to break down starch. Amylase-binding may also mask bacterial antigens and allow the organism to avoid recognition by the host defences.

Strains originally described as *S. sanguis* II were termed '*S. mitior*' by most European workers. Some strains produced glucans from sucrose; those that did not were designated by some as *S. mitis*. Unfortunately, the widely used name '*S. mitior*' is not officially recognized and has been replaced by the internationally valid name *S. oralis*. Strains of *S. oralis* produce neuraminidase and an IgA protease but cannot bind α-amylase. Extracellular glucan production from sucrose is a variable characteristic. Members of the *S. mitis*-group are opportunistic pathogens, e.g. in infective endocarditis.

S. parasanguis can be isolated from clinical

specimens (throat, blood, urine). Strains can hydrolyse arginine but not urea, and can bind salivary α-amylase, but cannot produce extracellular polysaccharides from sucrose. The name 'S. crista' has been proposed for strains that resemble *S. sanguis* but which are characterized by tufts of fibrils on their cell surface (*see* Chapter 4). *S. pneumoniae* is isolated from the nasopharynx, and can acquire and transfer antibiotic resistance genes among other members of the *S. mitis*-group.

Other streptococci

Lancefield group A streptococci (*S. pyogenes*) are not usually isolated from the mouth of healthy individuals, although they can often be cultured from the saliva of people suffering from streptococcal sore throats, and may be associated with a particularly acute form of gingivitis (*see* Chapter 7).

Strains that were originally described as being nutritionally variant streptococci (NVS; *S. adjacens* and *S. defectivus*) have been isolated from the mouth when appropriate isolation media were used. Following analysis of 16S rRNA sequences of these bacteria, they have been placed in a new genus, *Abiotrophia*, as *A. adiacens* and *A. defectiva*, respectively.

Anaerobic Gram-positive cocci are commonly recovered from teeth, especially from carious dentine, infected pulp chambers and root canals (Chapter 6), advanced forms of periodontal disease (Chapter 7), and from dental abscesses (Chapters 8 and 9). They are also found in deep-seated abscesses elsewhere in the body, and are usually isolated in mixed culture, i.e. from a polymicrobial infection. Most strains are placed in the genus *Peptostreptococcus*, and representative species include *P. micros*, *P. magnus* and *P. anaerobius*. *Peptostreptococcus micros* is strongly proteolytic, while *P. anaerobius* can produce a β-lactamase. The genus *Peptostreptococcus* is heterogeneous and will undergo radical revision at some time. For this reason, these organisms are sometimes referred to only as Gram-positive anaerobic cocci (GPAC).

Enterococcus

Little information is available on the presence of enterococci in the healthy mouth. They have been recovered in low numbers from several oral sites when appropriate selective media were used; the most frequently isolated species is *Enterococcus* (formerly *Streptococcus*) *faecalis*. Enterococci can be isolated from the mouth of immuno- and medically-compromised patients. Some strains can induce dental caries in gnotobiotic rats while others have been isolated from infected root canals and from periodontal pockets.

Staphylococcus, *Micrococcus* and *Stomatococcus*

Staphylococci and micrococci are not commonly isolated in large numbers from the oral cavity, although the former have been reported in plaque samples from subjects with dentures, as well as in immunocompromised patients and individuals suffering from a variety of oral infections (*see* Chapter 8). Although these bacteria are not usually considered to be members of the resident oral microflora, they may be present transiently, and they have been isolated from some sites with root surface caries (*see* Chapter 6) and from some periodontal pockets that fail to respond to conventional therapy (*see* Chapter 7). Interestingly, this is in sharp contrast to other surfaces of the human body in close proximity to the mouth, such as the skin surface and the mucous membranes of the nose, where they are among the predominant components of the microflora. This finding emphasizes the major differences that must exist in the ecology of these particular habitats. Skin and nasal flora must be passed consistently into the mouth and yet these organisms are normally unable to colonize or compete against the resident oral microflora.

Stomatococcus (formerly *Micrococcus*) *mucilagenosus* is a catalase-positive, Gram-positive coccus that is isolated almost exclusively from the tongue. It produces an extracellular slime which may play a significant role in the association of this species with that site.

Gram-positive rods and filaments

Gram-positive rods and filaments are commonly isolated from dental plaque. Chemotaxonomic methods (e.g. cell wall composition, profile of acidic fermentation products) and serological approaches have always played a fundamental role in the identification and classification of these bacteria.

Actinomyces

Actinomyces species form a major portion of the microflora of dental plaque, particularly at approximal sites and the gingival crevice (*see* Chapter 5). They have been associated with root surface caries and are known to increase in numbers during gingivitis (*see* Chapters 6 and 7, respectively).

Cells of *Actinomyces* species appear as short rods, but are often pleomorphic in shape (Figure 3.2); some cells show a true branching morphology, while those of *A. israelii* can be filamentous. Some species (particularly *A. naeslundii*) are heavily fimbriated, while others have relatively smooth surfaces. All *Actinomyces* spp. ferment glucose to a characteristic pattern of metabolic end products, namely, succinic, acetic and lactic acids, and this profile is exploited in identification schemes. Six species have been definitely recovered from the oral cavity of humans (Table 3.4); distinct species have also been recovered from animals. Some newly described species have been identified in a variety of clinical specimens (e.g. *A. bernardiae*, *A. radingae*, *A. neuii*, *A. europaeus*, *A. graevenitzii* and *A. turicensis)*, but their source and habitat is as yet unknown.

Table 3.4 Classification of human *Actinomyces* species

Present nomenclature	Previous designation
Actinomyces georgiae	Untypable subgingival *Actinomyces* sp.
Actinomyces gerencseriae	*A. israelii* serotype II
A. israelii	*A. israelii* serotype I
A. odontolyticus	*A. odontolyticus*
A. naeslundii genospecies 1	*A. naeslundii* serotype I
A. naeslundii genospecies 2	*A. naeslundii* serotypes II & III
	A. viscosus serotype II
A. meyeri	*A. meyeri*
A. bernardiae	
A. radingae	
A. neuii	
A. europaeus	
A. graevenitzii	
A. turicensis	

The species currently described as *A. naeslundii* is now made up of strains previously classified as *A. viscosus* and *A. naeslundii*; these species were previously distinguished primarily on the basis that *A. viscosus* strains were catalase-positive. Earlier phenotypic and serological studies had demonstrated considerable heterogeneity within the *A. naeslundii/A. viscosus* group. Following the application of genetic techniques, such as DNA–DNA hybridization, it was proposed that there should be a single species (*A. naeslundii*), but with two genospecies (*A. naeslundii* genospecies 1 and genospecies 2) (Table 3.4). This is because two species could be recognized at the genetic level, but no phenotypic markers could be found to distinguish between them. At present, serology is the only means of distinguishing between these two genospecies, using antisera recognizing cell wall antigens.

Some strains of *A. naeslundii* produce an extracellular slime and a fructan from sucrose; some strains also produce a urease that may modulate pH in plaque. Two types of fimbriae can be found on the surface of cells of *A. naeslundii*. Each type serves a specific function, and is implicated either in cell-to-cell contact (co-aggregation) or in cell-to-surface interactions (Chapters 4 and 5).

A. naeslundii has been implicated in root surface caries and gingivitis, although its role in the former is still under debate (*see* Chapter 6). Strains can also be recovered from cervico-vaginal secretions of women, irrespective of the presence of intra-uterine contraceptive devices.

Actinomyces israelii can act as an opportunistic pathogen causing a chronic inflammatory condition called actinomycosis (*see* Chapter 9). The disease is usually associated with the cervicofacial region, but it can disseminate to cause deep seated infections in other sites in the body such as the abdomen. Strains of *A. israelii* characteristically form 'granules' and such granules may contribute to their ability to disseminate around the body by affording cells physical protection from the environment, from the host defences and from antibiotic treatment. *A. israelii* has also been found in cervical smears of women using intra-uterine devices.

Following comparisons of 16S rRNA sequences, strains originally classified as *A. israelii* serotype II have been designated as a separate species, *A. gerencseriae*, which is a common but minor component of the microflora of the healthy gingival crevice, although it has also been isolated from abscesses. *A. israelii* and *A. gerencseriae* are both obligately anaerobic but can be differentiated on the basis of whole cell protein profiles, serological reactions, and the inability of the latter to ferment L-arabinose.

A. georgiae is a facultatively anaerobic organism that is found occasionally in the healthy gingival crevice. Other species include *A. odontolyticus*, of which about 50% of strains form colonies with a characteristic red-brown pigment. This species has been correlated with the very earliest stages of enamel demineralization, and with the progression of small caries lesions (*see* Chapter 6). *A. meyeri* has been reported occasionally and in low numbers from the gingival crevice in health and disease, and from brain abscesses.

Eubacterium

This is a poorly defined genus which contains a variety of obligately anaerobic, filamentous bacteria that are often Gram-variable. Traditionally, this genus has been a 'dumping-ground' for strains not belonging to other genera of anaerobic, non-spore-forming bacilli. They can be difficult to cultivate and many laboratories have not isolated them from plaque while others have found numerous 'taxa' (>25) in various forms of periodontal disease. When recovered and identified, asaccharolytic *Eubacterium* species can comprise over 50% of the anaerobic microflora of periodontal pockets.

The classification and identification of these strains is severely hampered by the general lack of reactivity of isolates. Consequently, whole cell protein profiles, patterns of fermentation products and the presence of preformed enzymes have been used in an attempt to differentiate between species. Furthermore, culture-independent, molecular analyses, for example, comparing 16S rRNA sequences, are being used to identify as yet unculturable *Eubacterium* species from dento-alveolar abscesses. Among the current asaccharolytic species are *E. brachy*, *E. timidum*, *E. nodatum* and *E. saphenum*, and these are strongly implicated in advanced forms of periodontal disease; saccharolytic strains such as *E. saburreum* and *E. yurii* can also be found in subgingival plaque in both health and disease. New species such as *E. tardum*, *E. infirmum* and *E. minutum* have been proposed. Asaccharolytic strains do not produce proteases but possess acid phosphatase, esterase and aminopeptidase

activities. *E. yurii* is involved in some of the 'corn-cob' and 'test-tube brush' arrangements with coccal bacteria seen in dental plaque (*see* Chapter 5). This genus requires further study, especially as these organisms can be frequently isolated from infections of the head, neck and lung, and from carious dentine and necrotic dental pulp.

Recent 16S rRNA sequencing of oral asaccharolytic *Eubacterium* species have shown that the genus *Peptostreptococcus* is their closest relative, while some other, as yet un-named taxa, appear to be related to members of the genus, *Clostridium*. *E. alactolyticum* has now been reclassified as *Pseudoramibacter alactolyticus*. It is likely that there will be further taxonomic changes in this area.

Lactobacillus

Lactobacilli are commonly isolated from the oral cavity although they usually comprise less than 1% of the total cultivable microflora. However, their proportions and prevalence increase in advanced caries lesions both of the enamel and of the root surface. A number of homo- and hetero-fermentative species have been identified, producing either lactate or lactate and acetate, respectively, from glucose. The most common species are *L. casei*, *L. fermentum* and *L. acidophilus*, with *L. salivarius*, *L. plantarum*, '*L. brevis*', *L. cellobiosus* and *L. buchneri* also reported. Comparisons of the properties of *L. brevis*-like strains from the mouth and from cheese showed that the oral strains were distinct, and these have now been placed in a new species, *L. oris*. Recently, some *Lactobacillus* species have been shown to be heterogeneous. For example, *L. acidophilus* has been sub-divided into *L. acidophilus sensu stricto*, *L. crispatus* and *L. gasseri*, while within the *L. casei*-group, several distinct species have been recognized, including *L. rhamnosus* and *L. paracasei*. Whether all of these species are found in the mouth has yet to be determined, although preliminary studies suggest that the majority of oral isolates are *L. rhamnosus* and *L. paracasei* subspecies *paracasei*. Genetic studies of some of these strains, together with analysis of whole cell protein profiles, have led to the proposal that *L. casei* subsp. *casei* and *L. rhamnosus* should be reclassified as *L. zeae*, and that the name *L. paracasei* be rejected. These revisions have not been widely adopted yet.

L. uli has been isolated from periodontal pockets.

Despite these advances in classification, little is known of the preferred habitat of these species in the normal mouth, and most studies still merely refer to them as 'lactobacilli' or *Lactobacillus* spp. They are highly acidogenic organisms, and are associated more with carious dentine and the advancing front of carious lesions than with the initiation of the disease. Simple tests with selective media have been designed for estimating the numbers of lactobacilli in patients' saliva to give an indication of the cariogenic potential of a mouth. Although these tests are often unreliable, they are useful for monitoring the dietary behaviour of a patient because levels of lactobacilli correlate well with the intake of dietary carbohydrate.

Propionibacterium

Several species of propionibacteria have been reported from the mouth, including *P. acnes* in dental plaque. These bacteria are obligately anaerobic and this genus now includes *P. propionicus,* which was formerly classified as *Arachnia propionica. P. propionicus* is morphologically indistinguishable from *A. israelii* but the two species can be differentiated by the production of propionic acid from glucose by the former. Strains of *P. propionicus* have been isolated from cases of actinomycosis and lacrimal canaliculitis (infection of the tear duct), and so are opportunist pathogens; they have also been isolated from samples overlying root surface caries.

Other genera

Corynebacterium (formerly *Bacterionema*) *matruchotii* has an unusual cellular morphology having a long filament growing out of a short, fat rod-like cell, thus earning its description of 'whip-handle' cell. This species is found only in the mouth and appears to be the only true coryneform in the oral cavity. *Rothia dentocariosa* is found in dental plaque, and is also isolated occasionally from cases of infective endocarditis. *Bifidobacterium dentium* is also regularly isolated from dental plaque. Two new species of bifidobacteria have been recognized recently (*B. inopinatum* and *B. denticolens*), but their role in the mouth is yet to be determined. Occasionally, strains of mycobacteria, *Coryne-*

bacterium xerosis and some *Bacillus* and *Clostridium* species are detected, but these probably represent transient visitors from other habitats.

Gram-negative cocci

Neisseria and *Moraxella*

Neisseria are isolated in low numbers from most sites in the oral cavity, and are among the earliest colonizers of a clean tooth surface. *Neisseria* spp. are generally saccharolytic and can grow well aerobically, although their growth is stimulated by carbon dioxide and retarded under anaerobic conditions. The taxonomy of this group remains confused. The most common species is *N. subflava* which is saccharolytic and polysaccharide producing. *N. sicca* is closely related and also produces polysaccharides and is saccharolytic. *N. mucosa* is found in the nasopharynx, and some strains possess a capsule. Other neisseriae are asaccharolytic and non-polysaccharide forming. *Neisseria* may consume oxygen during the very early stages of plaque formation, and produce atmospheric conditions more suitable for the growth of facultative and obligately anaerobic species. Some strains of *Neisseria* metabolize lactic acid, and the significance of this property is discussed in the next section on *Veillonella*; *Neisseria* are rarely associated with disease.

In general, aerobic isolates that are asaccharolytic, non-polysaccharide formers, and whose colonies lack pigment, fall within the genus *Moraxella* (formerly *Branhamella*). *M. catarrhalis* is a commensal of the upper respiratory tract but is also a well-established opportunistic pathogen; many strains produce a β-lactamase which can complicate antibiotic treatment.

Veillonella

Veillonellae are strictly anaerobic Gram-negative cocci; three species are recognized: *V. parvula, V. dispar* and *V. atypica.* Veillonellae have been isolated from most surfaces of the oral cavity, although they occur in highest numbers in dental plaque. Veillonellae lack glucokinase and fructokinase and are unable to metabolize carbohydrates. They utilize several intermediary metabolites, in particular lactate, as energy sources and consequently may play an important role in the ecology of dental plaque and in the aetiology of dental caries. Lactic acid is the strongest acid produced in quantity by oral bacteria and, therefore, is implicated in the dissolution of enamel. *Veillonella* might reduce this harmful effect by metabolizing lactic acid and converting it to weaker acids (predominantly propionic acid).

Gram-negative rods

Facultatively anaerobic and capnophilic genera

The majority of facultatively anaerobic Gram-negative rods in the mouth belong to the genus *Haemophilus*. These organisms were not detected in early studies until, as with the enterococci, use was made of appropriate isolation media that contained the essential growth factors required by members of this genus, i.e. haemin (X-factor) and nicotinamide adenine dinucleotide (V-factor). Haemophili are commonly present in saliva, on epithelial surfaces and in dental plaque, and include: *H. parainfluenzae* biotypes I, II and III (V-factor requiring), *H. segnis* (V), *H. paraphrophilus* (V), *H. aphrophilus* (X) and *H. haemolyticus* (X and V factors). In addition, *H. parahaemolyticus* is isolated from soft tissue infections of the oral cavity, but is probably not a regular member of the oral microflora. Strains have been isolated from jaw infections and cases of infective endocarditis but, in general, the pathogenic potential of these organisms is low. *H. influenzae* (X- and V-factor requiring) is not usually isolated from the mouth, although it is found in the pharyngeal region.

Other facultatively anaerobic Gram-negative rods include *Eikenella corrodens*. Colonies of this species characteristically pit the surface of agar plates. *E. corrodens* has been isolated from a range of oral infections, including infective endocarditis and abscesses, and has been implicated in periodontal disease. *Capnocytophaga* (formerly classified as *Bacteroides ochraceus*) are CO_2-dependent Gram-negative rods, with a gliding motility, and are found in subgingival plaque, and increase in proportions in gingivitis. Species include *C. gingivalis*, *C. ochracea*, *C. sputigena*, *C. granulosa* and *C. haemolytica*, but no simple tests can differentiate them. *Capnocytophaga* are opportunistic pathogens and have been isolated from a number of infections in immunocompromised patients; strains produce an IgA1 protease.

Actinobacillus actinomycetemcomitans (Figure 3.3) has been implicated in the aetiology of particularly aggressive forms of periodontal disease in adolescents (localized juvenile periodontitis). It has been described as being microaerophilic, capnophilic or facultatively anaerobic, although it appears to grow best in an aerobic atmosphere enriched with 5–10% CO_2. It possesses cell surface layers that contain molecules that stimulate bone resorption, as well as a range of serotype-determining polysaccharides (*a–e*). Freshly isolated strains possess fimbriae, although these are lost on subculture. *A. actinomycetemcomitans* produces a range of virulence factors, including a powerful leukotoxin, collagenase, immunosuppressive factors and proteases capable of cleaving IgG; in addition, strains can be invasive. *A. actinomycetemcomitans* is also an opportunistic pathogen, being isolated from cases of infective endocarditis, brain and subcutaneous abscesses, osteomyelitis and periodontal disease (*see* Chapter 7). A highly virulent clone of *A. actinomycetemcomitans* has been recognized, whose distribution is restricted to only certain adolescents with juvenile periodontitis, all of whom have an African origin.

The gliding bacterium *Simonsiella* has been isolated from epithelial surfaces of the oral cavity of man and a variety of animals. These organisms have a unique cellular morphology, being composed of unusually large, multicellular filaments in groups, or multiples of eight cells.

Obligately anaerobic Gram-negative rods

Obligately anaerobic Gram-negative rods comprise a large proportion of the microflora of dental plaque. The classification of many of these organisms has proved difficult. For example, some strains grow so poorly that clear results in fermentation tests are not obtained, and the concentration of metabolites is too low to be analysed satisfactorily. As a consequence, difficulties can arise in discriminating between a strain that is growing poorly in a range of tests and one that is truly asaccharolytic. The development and application of new tests such as lipid analyses and enzyme mobilities has been necessary for the speciation of isolates that appeared non-

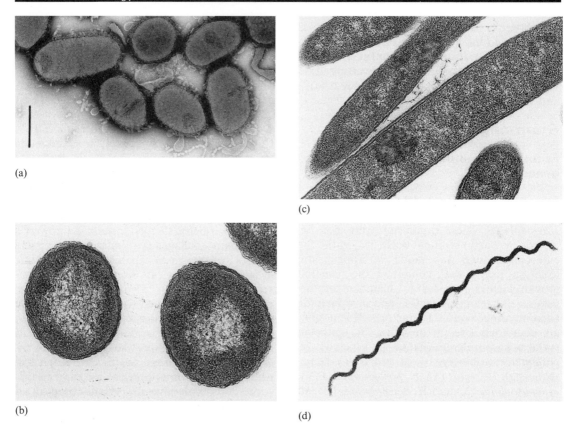

Figure 3.3 Electron micrographs of (a) *Porphyromonas gingivalis*, (b) *Actinobacillus actinomycetemcomitans*, (c) *Fusobacterium nucleatum* and (d) an oral spirochaete. Courtesy of N. Mordan, Eastman Dental Institute

reactive by conventional methods. New species that are at present unculturable in the laboratory have been identified in clinical samples using molecular approaches, e.g. DNA–DNA homology, and 16S rRNA analysis.

The majority of oral anaerobic Gram-negative rods were placed originally in the genus *Bacteroides*. However, taxonomic studies have shown that this genus should have a much narrower definition, with its members restricted to those of the *B. fragilis*-group, which are found predominantly in the gut. Asaccharolytic and saccharolytic oral organisms were placed in the genera *Porphyromonas* and *Prevotella*, respectively. Some organisms from these genera produce colonies with a characteristic brown or black pigment when grown on blood agar. This pigment may act as a defence mechanism helping to protect the cells from the toxic effects of oxygen. These organisms are referred to collectively as black-pigmented anaerobes, and haemin is an essential growth factor. The

primary habitats of members of these new genera can differ. *Porphyromonas gingivalis* (Figure 3.3) is found almost solely at sub-gingival sites (especially in advanced periodontal lesions), although it has also been recovered from the tongue and tonsils. Six serotypes have been recognized based on capsular polysaccharides (K antigens). *P. gingivalis* is highly virulent in experimental infection studies in animals, and produces a range of putative virulence factors associated with tissue destruction and evasion of the host defences. These include highly active proteases, with a specificity for arginine-x bonds and lysine-x bonds, that can degrade host molecules such as immunoglobulins, complement and iron- and haeme-sequestering proteins and glycoproteins, as well as molecules that regulate the host inflammatory response. *P. gingivalis* also produces a haemolysin, collagen-degrading enzymes, cytotoxic metabolites and a capsule (*see* Chapter 7). *P. gingivalis* has fimbriae on its cell surface that mediate adherence to oral epithelial cells, and to saliva-coated tooth surfaces. *Porphyromonas endodontalis* has a more restricted habitat, being mainly recovered from infected root canals. Both *P. endodontalis* and *P. gingivalis* are rarely found in plaque in health, and they may persist in reservoirs on mucosal surfaces, such as the tongue or tonsils. Organisms originally described as *Oribaculum catoniae* have been reclassified as *Porphyromonas catoniae*.

The new definition of *Bacteroides* has meant that many strains have been placed in the genus *Prevotella*. Species within this group are moderately saccharolytic, producing acetic, succinic and other acids from glucose. This new genus includes the pigmented species *P. intermedia*, *P. nigrescens*, *P. melaninogenica*, *P. loescheii*, *P. corporis* (this species is closely related to *P. intermedia*, but is generally isolated from non-oral sites) and some strains of *P. denticola*. In addition, *P. pallens* is a new pigmented species comprising strains previously described as *P. intermedia*/*P. nigrescens*-like organisms (PIN-LO). *P. intermedia* and *P. nigrescens* are difficult to distinguish using simple physiological tests, but DNA homology studies confirmed the existence of two distinct species. Strains of *P. intermedia* usually have greater peptidase activity and are associated more with periodontal disease, while *P. nigrescens* is isolated more often, and in higher numbers, from healthy sites.

The oral non-pigmented species include *P. buccae*, *P. buccalis*, *P. oralis*, *P. oris*, *P. oulora*, *P. veroralis* and *P. zoogleoformans*. Based on genetic approaches, several new species such as *P. dentalis* (this species includes strains formerly classified as *Hallena seregens* and *Mitsuokella dentalis*), *P. tannerae* and *P. enoeca* have been described. The majority of these species can be isolated on occasions from dental plaque, particularly from sub-gingival sites. Some species are associated with disease and increase in numbers and proportions during periodontal disease, and have also been recovered from abscesses (*see* Chapters 7, 8 and 9).

The taxonomic fate of other saccharolytic, non-pigmented species, that no longer fall within the new definition of the genus *Bacteroides,* is uncertain at present, but they will remain with their original epithet until their classification is resolved. These species include '*B. capillosus*' and '*B. forsythus*'; '*B. pneumo-sintes*' is now classified as *Dialister pneumosintes*. Some species have unusual properties; for example, '*B. ureolyticus*' and '*B. forsythus*' can pit the surface of blood agar plates, '*B. ureolyticus*' moves due to an unusual twitching motility but does not possess flagella. These bacterial groups can be distinguished on their patterns of metabolic end products, fermentation profiles and the production of certain constitutive enzymes.

Another major group of obligately anaerobic Gram-negative bacteria belongs to the genus *Fusobacterium*. Cells are characteristically in the form of long filaments (5–25 μm in length; *see* Figure 3.3) and include the following oral species: *F. alocis* and *F. sulci,* from the normal gingival crevice, and *F. periodonticum,* from sites with periodontal disease. The most commonly isolated species, however, is *F. nucleatum,* and several subspecies have been recognized: subsp. *nucleatum*, subsp. *polymorphum* and subsp. *vincentii* (also referred to by some as subsp. *fusiforme*). These subspecies may have different associations with health and disease; *F. nucleatum* subsp. *polymorphum* is most commonly isolated from the normal gingival crevice whereas subsp. *nucleatum* is recovered mainly from periodontal pockets.

Fusobacteria require rich media for growth and are often described as being asaccharolytic, although they can take up carbohydrates for the synthesis of intracellular storage compounds composed of polyglucose. Fusobacteria catabolize amino acids such as aspartate, glutamate, histidine and lysine to provide energy; these can be obtained from the metabolism of peptides if the free amino acids are unavailable. The major end product of metabolism is butyrate together with lower concentrations of other acids (e.g. succinate, acetate, lactate, etc.). *F. nucleatum* is capable of removing sulphur from cysteine and methionine to produce ammonia, butyrate, hydrogen sulphide and methyl mercaptan. The last two compounds are highly odorous, and are implicated in the odour associated with halitosis. Fusobacteria are able to co-aggregate with most other oral bacteria and, consequently, are believed to be an important bridging organism between early and late colonizers during plaque formation (*see* Chapter 5).

Other oral Gram-negative anaerobic and micro-aerophilic bacteria include *Leptotrichia buccalis* (cells have a filamentous morphology with a pointed end), and *Wolinella succinogenes* (an asaccharolytic and formate/fumarate-requiring strain). A number of campylobacter species have been recognized (cells have a spiral morphology) including *Campylobacter concisus*, *C. showae* and *C. sputorum*; in addition, *Wolinella curva* and *W. recta* have now been reclassified as *Campylobacter curvus* and *C. rectus*, respectively, and *Bacteroides gracilis* has become *Campylobacter gracilis*. These strains are not always easily identified by conventional tests and other methods are under investigation, such as whole cell protein profiles. *C. rectus* has been isolated from sites with active periodontal disease, especially in immuno-compromised patients; some strains produce a cytotoxin which shares some sequence homology with the leukotoxin of *A. actinomycetemcomitans*. Some species have flagella and are motile. The *Wolinella* and *Campylobacter* species have a single flagellum, while *Selenomonas sputigena* is a curved to helical bacillus with a tuft of flagella. *Selenomonas noxia*, *S. flueggei*, *S. infelix*, *S. dianae* and *S. artemidis* are new species that have been found in plaque from the human gingival crevice. Another helical or curved Gram-negative oral anaerobe is *Centipeda periodontii*, which has numerous flagella that spiral around the cell. There have been reports of *Helicobacter pylori* in dental plaque; this species is usually isolated from the stomach where it is associated with gastritis, peptic ulcers and possibly gastric cancer. It may be present in the mouth transiently following reflux from the stomach. Some newly described genera include *Johnsonii ignava* and *Cantonella morbi*, which are associated with gingivitis and periodontitis, respectively.

Organisms such as sulphate-reducing bacteria (e.g. *Desulfobacter* and *Desulfovibrio*) and methanogens, which use terminal end products of metabolism, such as hydrogen, CO_2 and organic acids, have been detected in dental plaque. Sulphate-reducing bacteria produce hydrogen sulphide, which can contribute to mouth odour.

Spirochaetes are numerous in sub-gingival plaque and can readily be detected using dark-field or electron microscopy (*see* Figure 3.3). Several morphological types can be distinguished according to cell size and the arrangement of periplasmic flagella (endoflagella). Spirochaetes possess an outer membrane and an inner membrane (which encloses the proto-

plasmic cylinder); the periplasmic flagella lie in the periplasmic space between these two membranes. The periplasmic flagella attach at either pole of the cell by means of a basal hook, and wrap themselves around the helical protoplasmic cylinder. Some of the oral spirochaetes adhere to surfaces in a polar orientation; this type of adhesion results in gross alterations to host cell morphology facilitating penetration into underlying tissues. The numbers of spirochaetes are raised in periodontal disease, but whether they cause disease or merely increase following infection is not clear.

Oral spirochaetes fall within the genus *Treponema* and a number of species have been identified, including *T. denticola*, *T. macrodentium*, *T. oralis*, *T. skoliodontium*, *T. socranskii*, *T. maltophilum*, *T. amylovorum* and *T. vincentii*. The use of culture-independent, molecular approaches, in which 16S rRNA sequences have been compared from clinical samples, is emphasizing the diversity that exists within dental plaque in terms of new species of spirochaete that cannot as yet be grown in the laboratory.

To date, little is known about the physiology of these organisms because of difficulties associated with their laboratory cultivation. *T. denticola* appears to be more proteolytic than other oral spirochaetes, and possesses proline aminopeptidase and an arginine-specific ('trypsin-like') protease; *T. denticola* can also degrade collagen and gelatin. *T. denticola* is asaccharolytic while *T. socranskii* can ferment carbohydrates to acetic, lactic and succinic acids.

Fungi

Fungi form a small part of the oral microflora. The 'perfect fungi' (fungi that divide by sexual reproduction) are rarely isolated from the oral cavity but are occasionally found infecting patients with advanced AIDS. The main perfect fungal species causing oral infection are *Aspergillus*, *Geotrichium* and *Mucor* spp.. The perfect yeast species seen in healthy individuals may be transient rather than resident members of the oral microflora. In contrast, the 'imperfect yeasts' (which divide by asexual reproduction) are commonly found in the mouth (*see* Chapter 11).

The largest proportion of the fungal microflora is made up of *Candida* species. *Candida albicans* is by far the most common species, but a large number of other yeasts have been isolated, including *C. glabrata* (formerly *Torulopsis glabrata*), *C. tropicalis*, *C. krusei*, *C. parapsilosis* and *C. guilliermondi*, as well as *Rhodotorula* and *Saccharomyces* spp.. Estimations of carriage rates of *Candida* spp. in the mouth vary markedly because of the different isolation techniques used (*see* Chapter 11); reported rates range from 2% to 71% of asymptomatic adults. Carriage rates increase, and can approach 100%, in medically compromised patients or those on broad spectrum antibacterial agents.

Candida spp. are distributed evenly throughout the mouth. The most common site of isolation is the dorsum of the tongue, particularly the posterior area near the circumvallate papillae. The isolation of *Candida* is raised by the presence of intra-oral devices such as plastic dentures or orthodontic appliances, particularly in the upper jaw on the fitting surface; indeed, *Candida* spp. attach tenaciously to acrylic. Plaque has also been shown to contain *Candida* spp., but the exact proportion and significance of these yeasts in health and disease is unclear. The mouth may be the source of yeast colonization of the gut, and saliva is the vehicle for the transmission of *Candida* spp. to other areas of the body. Colonization of the mouth by yeasts occurs either at birth or soon afterwards. The carriage rate falls in early childhood and increases during middle and later life for reasons that are as yet unclear.

Mycoplasmas

Mycoplasmas are pleomorphic micro-organisms which possess an outer membrane that is not rigid. They can be grown either on media that are highly enriched with protein and in the presence of carbon dioxide, or in tissue culture. Mycoplasmas have been isolated from saliva (*M. salivarium*, *M. pneumoniae*, *M. hominis*), the oral mucosa (*M. buccale*, *M. orale*, *M. pneumoniae*) and dental plaque (*M. pneumoniae*, *M. buccale*, *M. orale*). Their role at these sites is unclear, and the oral mycoplasmas are not well classified. *M. orale* and *M. salivarium* have been isolated from salivary glands, and it has been postulated that they may have a role in salivary gland hypofunction. *M. salivarium* has been shown to block potassium channels in the outer membranes of salivary gland cells *in vitro*, but whether this occurs *in vivo* has yet to be determined. Estimates of the oral carriage rate of *Mycoplasma* vary from 6% to 32% of the population, but this data is from a limited number of surveys only.

Viruses

Oral viruses have been extensively studied over recent years (*see* Chapter 10), especially since the advent of PCR techniques. It is now no longer necessary to use time-consuming and often unreliable methods of detection of viruses, such as tissue culture or electron microscopy. Indeed, some viruses have only been detected by the use of molecular approaches and have never been grown (e.g. hepatitis G). The reliance on molecular techniques is growing and will lead to more virus species being identified in the future.

The commonest virus detected in the oral cavity is Herpes simplex; both type 1 and type 2 have been isolated from the mouth, but type 1 is the most common. Herpes simplex type 1 is the cause of cold sores. The virus can be detected occasionally in the oral cavity in the absence of cold sores and is, therefore, probably persistent. The virus can also remain latent; it migrates rapidly along the trigeminal nerve to the ganglion where it remains latent until reactivated, e.g. by UV light or stress. Once reactivated, the genome passes back down the peripheral nerve to cause the characteristic cold sores, which rupture to release further virus particles.

Cytomegalovirus is present in most individuals. It has been detected in the saliva of symptomless adults, but its portal of entry into the oral cavity is not clear. Coxsackie virus A2, 4, 5, 6, 8, 9, 10 and 16 have all been detected in saliva and in the oral epithelium. The detection of these viruses has usually been secondary to, or in the primary phase of, an infection of Hand, Foot and Mouth disease or herpangina. A variety of papilloma viruses have been isolated from the oral cavity, usually in association with small warts. These warts have been implicated with oral cancer, and are common in patients with AIDS.

Hepatitis and Human Immunodeficiency Virus (HIV) can be found in the oral cavity, especially in saliva, where their presence poses a significant cross-infection threat. Both groups of viruses are discussed in detail in Chapters 10 and 12. Other viruses found in the oral cavity are measles and mumps, but usually in association with oral lesions.

Protozoa

The diagnosis of protozoal disease in oral tissues still relies primarily on light microscopy of stained specimens, although the use of ribotyping has made species identification more accurate. *Entamoeba gingivalis* is the most common protozoan, and has been isolated from periodontal tissues, particularly in patients who have received radiotherapy and are taking metronidazole. Studies of biopsies of the periodontal tissues from which *E. gingivalis* has been isolated have not demonstrated any invasion by these amoebae into tissues, and its role remains to be elucidated. *Trichomonas tenax*, a flagellated protozoan, has been isolated from the oral cavity of healthy patients; it may cause salivary gland swellings, particularly in the parotid gland. *Giardia lamblia* has also been seen in the oral cavity, but its role and incidence is not known.

Table 3.5 Bacterial genera found in the oral cavity

Gram-positive	Gram-negative
Cocci	
Abiotrophia	*Moraxella*
Enterococcus	*Neisseria*
Peptostreptococcus	*Veillonella*
Streptococcus	
Staphylococcus	
Stomatococcus	
Rods	
Actinomyces	*Actinobacillus*
Bifidobacterium	*(Bacteroides)**
Corynebacterium	*Campylobacter*
Eubacterium	*Cantonella*
Lactobacillus	*Capnocytophaga*
Propionibacterium	*Centipeda*
Pseudoramibacter	*Desulfovibrio*
Rothia	*Desulfobacter*
	Eikenella
	Fusobacterium
	Haemophilus
	Johnsonii
	Leptotrichia
	Porphyromonas
	Prevotella
	Selenomonas
	Simonsiella
	Treponema
	Wolinella

*The genus *Bacteroides* has been redefined. In time, the remaining oral bacteria still placed in this genus will be reclassified.
Mycoplasma are also isolated from the mouth.

Summary

The mouth supports the growth of a wide diversity of micro-organisms including bacteria, yeasts, mycoplasmas, viruses and (on occasions) even protozoa. Bacteria are the predominant components of the resident oral microflora; a list of genera is given in Table 3.5. Many are fastidious in their nutritional requirements and are difficult to grow and identify in the laboratory; many are also obligate anaerobes. Chemotaxonomic methods and molecular approaches have resolved many long-standing problems with the classification of many oral bacteria. The resultant benefits in classification included the finding of closer associations of individual species with sites in health and disease.
The high diversity of the oral microflora reflects the wide range of nutrients available endogenously, the varied types of habitat for colonization, and the opportunity provided by biofilms such as plaque for survival on surfaces. Despite this diversity, many micro-organisms commonly isolated from neighbouring ecosystems, such as the skin and the gut, are not found in the mouth, emphasizing the unique and selective properties of the mouth for microbial colonization.

Bibliography

*Balows, A., Truper, H.G., Dworkin, M. *et al.* (eds) (1991) *The Prokaryotes. A Handbook on the Biology of Bacteria*, 2nd edn, Springer-Verlag, New York.

Beighton, D, Hardie, J.M. and Whiley, R.A. (1991) A scheme for the identification of viridans streptococci. *J. Med. Microbiol.*, **35**, 367–372.

Bolstad, A.I., Jensen, H.B. and Bakken, V. (1996) Taxonomy, biology and periodontal aspects of *Fusobacterium nucleatum*. *Clin. Microbiol. Revs*, **9**, 55–71.

Delwiche, E.A., Pestka, J.J. and Tortorello, M.L. (1985) The Veillonellae: Gram-negative cocci with a unique physiology. *Ann. Revs Microbiol.*, **39**, 175–193.

Murdoch, D.A. (1998) Gram-positive anaerobic cocci. *Clin. Microbiol. Revs*, **11**, 81–120.

Olsen, I. (1993) Recent approaches to the chemotaxonomy of the *Actinobacillus–Haemophilus–Pasteurella* group (family *Pasteurellaceae*). *Oral Microbiol. Immunol.*, **8**, 327–336.

*Parker, M.T. and Duerden, B.I. (eds) (1990) *Topley and Wilson's Principles of Bacteriology, Virology and Immunity,* Volume 2: *Systematic Bacteriology,* Edward Arnold, London.

Paster, B.J., Dewhirst, F.E., Olsen I. and Fraser, G.J. (1994) Phylogeny of *Bacteroides*, *Prevotella* and *Porphyromonas* spp. and related bacteria. *J. Bacteriol.*, **176**, 725–732.

Priest, F.G. and Austin, B. (1993) *Modern Bacterial Taxonomy,* Chapman & Hall, London.

Samaranayake, L.P. and MacFarlane, T.W. (1990) *Oral Candidosis*, Wright, Oxford.

Shah, H.N., Mayrand, D. and Genco, R.J. (eds) (1993) *Biology of the Species, Porphyromonas gingivalis,* CRC Press, Boca Raton, FLA.

Towner, K.J. and Cockayne, A. (1993) *Molecular Methods for Microbial Identification and Typing,* Chapman & Hall, London.

Wade, W.G. (1996) The role of *Eubacterium* species in periodontal disease and other oral infections. *Microb. Ecol. Health Dis.*, **9**, 367–370.

*These volumes contain detailed chapters on the classification, identification, and properties of most of the major groups of bacteria found in the oral cavity, as do Bergey's *Manual of Determinative Bacteriology* and Bergey's *Manual of Systematic Bacteriology*, both published by Williams & Wilkins, Baltimore, MD.

4

Acquisition, adherence, distribution and metabolism of the oral microflora

The foetus in the womb is normally sterile. During delivery the baby comes into contact with the normal microflora of the mother's uterus and vagina, and at birth with the micro-organisms of the atmosphere and of the people in attendance. Despite the widespread possibility of contamination, the mouth of the newborn baby is usually sterile. From the first feeding onwards, however, the mouth is regularly inoculated with micro-organisms and the process of acquisition of the resident oral microflora begins.

Acquisition of the resident oral microflora

Acquisition depends on the successive transmission of micro-organisms to the site of potential colonization. Initially, in the mouth, this is by passive contamination from the mother, from food, milk and water, and from the saliva of individuals in close proximity to the baby. Acquisition of micro-organisms from the birth canal itself may be of only limited significance. Studies on the transmission of candida and lactobacilli from the vagina of the mother to the newborn infant suggest that these organisms do not usually become established initially as part of the resident oral microflora of the newborn, although they may be present transiently. In contrast, the role of saliva in the process of acquisition has been confirmed conclusively. Bacteriocin-typing of strains has enabled the transfer of *S. salivarius*, mutans streptococci

and some other species from mother to child via saliva to be followed. Similarly, comparisons of the DNA fingerprints (genotyping) of a variety of oral bacterial species (using restriction endonuclease mapping techniques) have shown that the same clonal type is found within family groups, and that different patterns are usually observed between such groups. Some bacteria can also be acquired, but less commonly, by young children from other family members, while occasional strains seem to be distinct from any found in close relatives. For example, the genotypes of mutans streptococci found in children appeared identical to those of their mothers in 71% of 34 infant–mother pairs examined. No evidence of father–infant (or father–mother) transmission of mutans streptococci was observed, although transmission between spouses may occur with some periodontal pathogens, such as *P. gingivalis*.

Pioneer community and ecological succession

The mouth is highly selective for micro-organisms, even during the first few days of life. Only a few of the species common to the oral cavity of adults, and even less of the large number of bacteria found in the environment, are able to colonize the mouth of the newborn. The first micro-organisms to colonize are termed **pioneer species**, and collectively they make up the pioneer microbial community. These pioneer species continue to grow and colonize until environmental resistance is encountered. This

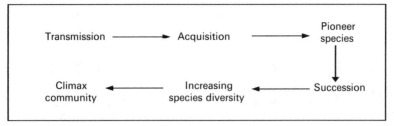

Figure 4.1 Ecological stages in the establishment of a microbial community

can be due to several limiting forces (including physical and chemical factors) which act as barriers to further development. In the oral cavity, physical factors include the shedding of epithelial cells (desquamation), and the shear forces from chewing and saliva flow. Nutrient requirements, Eh, pH, and the antibacterial properties of saliva can act as chemical barriers limiting growth.

One genus or species is usually predominant during the development of the pioneer community. In the mouth, the predominant organisms are streptococci, and in particular *S. salivarius*, *S. mitis* and *S. oralis*. Many of the pioneer species possess IgA_1 protease activity, which may confer an advantage by enabling producer organisms to evade the effects of this key host defence factor. With time, the metabolic activity of the pioneer community modifies the environment providing conditions suitable for colonization by a succession of other populations, by:

- changing the local Eh or pH;
- modifying or exposing new receptors for attachment ('cryptitopes', *see* Chapter 5); or
- generating novel nutrients, for example, as end products of metabolism (lactate, succinate, etc.) or as breakdown products (peptides, haemin, etc.) which can be used as primary nutrients by other organisms as part of a food chain.

In this way the pioneer community can influence the pattern of microbial succession. This involves the progressive development of a pioneer community (containing few species) through several stages in which the number of microbial groups increases. Eventually a stable situation is reached with a high species diversity; this is termed the **climax community** (Figure 4.1). Succession is associated with a change from a site possessing few niches to one

with a multitude of potential niches. A climax community reflects a highly dynamic situation and must not be regarded as a static state.

The oral cavity of the newborn usually contains only epithelial surfaces for colonization. The pioneer populations consist of mainly aerobic and facultatively anaerobic species. In a study of 40 full-term babies, a range of streptococcal species were recovered during the first three days of life, and *S. oralis*, *S. mitis* biovar 1 and *S. salivarius* were the numerically dominant species (Table 4.1). Indeed, *S. salivarius* has been isolated from the mouth of infants as early as 18 hours after birth. The diversity of the streptococcal microflora increased with time, so that all babies were colonized by more than one species of *Streptococcus* by one month of age; *S. salivarius* and *S. mitis* biovar 1 were isolated most commonly and predominated (Table 4.1).

Table 4.1 Streptococcal species isolated from the mucosal surfaces of babies

Streptococcus	Percentage viable count at age		
	1–3 days	2 weeks	1 month
S. oralis	41	24	20
S. mitis biovar 1	30	28	30
S. mitis biovar 2	4	1	1
S. salivarius	10	30	28
S. sanguis	4	3	2
S. anginosus	3	5	5
S. gordonii	1	2	4

The diversity of the pioneer oral community increases during the first few months of life, and several Gram-negative anaerobic species appear. In a study of edentulous infants with a mean age of 3 months (range: 1–7 months), *P. melaninogenica* was the most frequently isolated anaerobe, being recovered from 76% of infants

(Table 4.2). Other commonly isolated bacteria were *F. nucleatum* (67%), *Veillonella* spp. (63%) and non-pigmented *Prevotella* spp. (62%). In contrast, *Capnocytophaga* spp., *P. loescheii* and *P. intermedia* were recovered from 4–23% of infants, while *E. corrodens* and *Wolinella succinogenes* were only found in a single mouth. The number of different anaerobes in the same mouth varied from 0 to 7 species.

Table 4.2   The effect of tooth eruption on the composition of the oral microflora in young children

Bacterium	Percentage isolation frequency at mean age	
	3 months	32 months
Prevotella melaninogenica	76	100
Non-pigmented *Prevotella*	62	100
P. loescheii	14	90
P. intermedia	10	67
P. denticola	ND	71
Fusobacterium nucleatum	67	100
Fusobacterium spp.	ND	71
Selenomonas spp.	ND	43
Capnocytophaga spp.	19	100
Leptotrichia spp.	24	71
Campylobacter spp.	5	43
Eikenella corrodens	5	57
Veillonella spp.	63	63

ND, not detected.

The same infants were followed longitudinally during the eruption of the primary dentition. Gram-negative anaerobic bacteria were isolated more commonly, and a greater diversity of species were recovered from around the gingival margin of the newly erupted teeth (infant mean age = 32 months) (Table 4.2). These findings confirmed that the eruption of teeth has a significant ecological impact on the oral environment, and its resident microflora.

During the first year of life, members of the genera *Neisseria*, *Veillonella*, *Actinomyces*, *Lactobacillus* and *Rothia* are commonly isolated, particularly after tooth eruption. Some of the genera (*Porphyromonas* and *Actinobacillus*) associated with the aetiology of periodontal disease have been cultivated from the plaque of infants aged around 12 months, albeit infrequently and in low numbers (*see* Chapter 5).

The acquisition of some bacteria may occur optimally only at certain ages. Studies of the transmission of mutans streptococci to children have identified a specific **'window of infectivity'** between 19 and 31 months (median age = 26 months). This opens up the possibility of targeting preventive strategies over this critical period to reduce the likelihood of subsequent colonization in the infant.

Allogenic and autogenic succession

The development of a climax community at an oral site can involve examples of both allogenic and autogenic succession. In allogenic succession, factors of non-microbial origin are responsible for an altered pattern of community development. For example, species such as mutans streptococci and *S. sanguis* only appear in the mouth once teeth have erupted, or following the insertion of artificial devices such as acrylic obturators in children with cleft palate. The increase in number and diversity of obligate anaerobes once teeth are present is an example of autogenic succession in which community development is influenced by microbial factors. The metabolism of the aerobic and facultatively anaerobic pioneer species lowers the redox potential in plaque and creates conditions suitable for colonization by strict anaerobes (*see* Chapter 5). Other examples of autogenic succession include the development of food chains and food webs, whereby the metabolic end product of one organism becomes a primary nutrient source for a second:

$$\text{complex substrate} \xrightarrow{\substack{\text{primary} \\ \text{feeder}}} \text{product} \xrightarrow{\substack{\text{secondary} \\ \text{feeder}}} \text{simpler product}$$

A further example is the exposure of new receptors on host macromolecules for bacterial adhesion ('cryptitopes'; *see* Chapter 5).

Methods such as ribotyping (*see* Chapter 3) can differentiate among strains within a species on the basis of genetic variation, thereby allowing specific **clonal types** to be recognized. Relatively few clones are found within species of pathogenic bacteria, and a limited number of these may be responsible for the majority of infections. In contrast, species that comprise the resident human microflora display large numbers of clones; this may be a strategy to help such species evade the host defences. Clones of some species appear to persist for long periods at a site whereas others appear to be transient, and undergo replacement by distinct clones. For example, clonal replacement appears to maintain *S. mitis* biovar 1 in the mouth of neonates; 93 clonal types were detected among 101 strains of *S. mitis* colonizing 40 infants over a one month period. The clonal types that could be isolated were found to vary at different sampling times, suggesting that individual clones did not persist and were replaced by new clones. In a further study of the clonal diversity of *S. mitis* biovar 1, limited sharing of genotypes was found among three members of a particular family under study, and each individual carried between 6 and 13 types. Differences were also found between isolates recovered from the pharyngeal and buccal mucosa of the same individual. The reasons for, and the mechanisms involved in, the persistence of certain clones of some species, but the continual turnover of clones of other species, is not yet understood. Variations in the expression of carbohydrate and protein antigens were found among the different genotypes of *S. mitis* biovar 1 from the family group, suggesting that this 'turnover' might function as an 'immune-evasion' mechanism for this species.

Ageing and the oral microflora

The acquisition of the oral microflora continues with age. Following tooth eruption, the isolation frequency of spirochaetes and black-pigmented anaerobes increases. For example, the latter group of organisms are recovered from 18–40% of children aged 5 years but are found in over 90% of teenagers aged 13–16 years. It has been proposed that the increased prevalence of both bacterial groups during puberty might be due to hormones entering the gingival crevice and acting as a novel nutrient source. The rise in *P. intermedia* in plaque during pregnancy has also been ascribed to elevated hormone levels in serum, and similarly, black-pigmented anaerobes also increase in women taking oral contraceptives. In contrast, spirochaetes were detected by microscopy in the sub-gingival microflora of pre-pubertal Dutch children, implying that hormonal changes cannot be the only factor affecting the prevalence of these fastidious bacteria.

In adults, the resident oral microflora remains relatively stable and coexists in reasonable harmony with the host. This stability (termed **microbial homeostasis**, *see* Chapter 5) is not a passive response to the environment, but is due to a dynamic balance among the members of the resident flora due to numerous inter-bacterial and host–bacterial interactions.

Some variations in the oral microflora have been discerned in later life and can be attributed to both direct and indirect effects of ageing. In the case of the latter, variations can occur if the habitat or environment is severely perturbed. For example, the risk of cancer rises with age, and cytotoxic therapy or myelosuppression combined with the disease itself is associated with the increased carriage of *C. albicans* and non-oral opportunistic pathogens such as enterobacteria (e.g. *Klebsiella* spp., *Escherichia coli*, *Pseudomonas aeruginosa*) and *Staphylococcus aureus*. The wearing of dentures also increases with age and this also promotes colonization by *C. albicans*. Many elderly subjects take a variety of medications, the side-effects of which can reduce the flow of saliva and thereby perturb the normal balance of the resident oral microflora.

Direct age-related changes in the oral microflora have also been detected. Significantly higher proportions and isolation frequencies of lactobacilli and staphylococci (mainly *S. aureus*) in saliva were found in healthy subjects aged 70 years or over while yeasts were isolated more often and in higher numbers from saliva in those aged 80 years or more. It has been proposed that cell-mediated immunity declines with age, but the precise effect of old age on the innate and specific host defences of the mouth is uncertain. Serum IgM antibody titres to selected oral and gut commensal bacteria were lower in elderly subjects. These antibodies represent the initial response by the host to infection, and such a decrease in titre may be one explanation for the increased susceptibility to disease seen in older subjects. Age-related changes in salivary antibodies have also been reported. In general, activities of specific salivary IgG and IgM antibodies decreased in the elderly, whereas specific sIgA antibodies increased with age.

The incidence of oral candidosis is more common in the elderly and this has been attributed not only to the increased likelihood of denture wearing but also to physiological

Table 4.3 Some properties of the oral microflora that contribute to the difficulty in determining its composition

Property	Comment
High species diversity	The oral microflora, and especially dental plaque, consists of a diverse number of microbial species, some of which are present only in low numbers
Surface attachment/co-aggregation	Oral micro-organisms attach firmly to surfaces and to each other, and therefore have to be dispersed without loss of viability
Obligate anaerobes	Many oral bacteria lose their viability if exposed to air for prolonged periods
Fastidious nutrition	Some bacteria are difficult to grow in pure culture and may require specific cofactors etc. for growth. Some groups (e.g. certain spirochaetes) cannot be cultured in the laboratory
Slow growth	The slow growth of some organisms makes enumeration time-consuming (e.g. 14 days)
Identification	The classification of many oral micro-organisms remains unresolved or confused; simple criteria for identification are not always available (particularly for some obligate anaerobes)

changes in the oral mucosa, malnutrition, and to trace element deficiencies. There have been reports of increased isolations of enterobacteria from the oro-pharynx of the elderly, but this seems to be related in many cases to the health of the individual rather than to their age *per se*, with the highest incidences being in the most debilitated individuals. One of the fundamental problems in determining whether the oral microflora changes in old age is that the chronological age of a person does not always equate to their physiological age!

Social habits can perturb the balance of the oral microflora. The regular intake of dietary carbohydrates can lead to the enrichment of aciduric (acid-tolerant) and potentially cariogenic species such as mutans streptococci and lactobacilli. In contrast, mutans streptococci and *S. sanguis* are rarely detected in the mouth when full dentures are not worn, although both groups of bacteria can reappear when these 'hard surfaces' are inserted again. Smoking has been shown to reduce bacterial counts, especially those of *Neisseria* spp., on a variety of oral surfaces. Smoking is also a risk factor for periodontal diseases, and can perturb the sub-gingival environment.

Methods of determining the resident oral microflora

Difficulties associated with determining the composition of oral microbial communities at various sites relate to the removal of the micro-organisms (many of which are of necessity bound tenaciously to a surface or to each other), their transport to the laboratory in a viable state, and then their cultivation, enumeration and identification (Table 4.3; Figure 4.2).

Sample taking

The microflora can vary in composition over relatively small distances. Therefore, large plaque samples, or the pooling of smaller samples from different sites, are of little value because important site differences will be obscured. Consequently, small samples from discrete sites are preferable, but the method of sampling will depend on the site to be studied.

The oral mucosa can be sampled by swabbing, direct impression techniques, or by removing epithelial cells by scraping or scrubbing with a blunt instrument into a container. Data can then be related to a fixed area or to an individual epithelial cell. Saliva can be collected by expectoration into a sterile container; the saliva flow can be at a normal resting rate (i.e. unstimulated) or it can be stimulated by chemical means or by chewing. Although a greater volume is collected by stimulation, such samples will also contain many more organisms that have been dislodged from oral surfaces.

There is no universally accepted way of sampling dental plaque. The accessible smooth surfaces of enamel pose few problems and a range of dental instruments have been used. It is more difficult to remove plaque from approximal surfaces between teeth although dental probes, scalers, dental floss and abrasive strips have been used. Pits and fissures are also difficult to sample and the amount of plaque

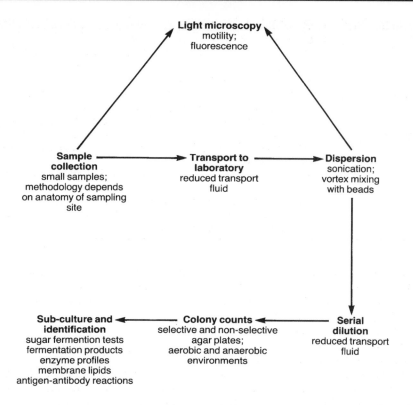

Figure 4.2 Stages in the microbiological analysis of the oral microflora

removed can be dependent on the anatomy of the site; fine probes, wire, blunt hypodermic needles and toothpicks are suitable. Sub-gingival plaque has proved to be the most difficult to sample because of the inaccessibility and anaerobic nature of the site. In disease, the organisms at the base of the pocket, near the advancing front of the lesion, are of most interest (*see* Chapter 7). Ideally, plaque should not be removed from other areas within the pocket so as not to obscure significant relationships between specific bacteria and disease.

A simple approach has been to insert paper points into pockets but the number of firmly adherent organisms removed from the root of the tooth will be small. Samples have also been taken by irrigation of the site and retrieval of the material through syringe needles; however, this method will also remove plaque from the whole depth of the pocket. A sophisticated method employs a broach kept withdrawn in a cannula which is flushed constantly with oxygen-free nitrogen. The broach is used to sample plaque only when the cannula is in position

near the base of the pocket. After sampling, the broach is retracted into the cannula and withdrawn. The most frequent approach has been to use a curette or scaler after the supra-gingival area has been cleared. The scaler tips can be detached and placed immediately in gas-flushed tubes containing reduced (i.e. anaerobic) transport fluid for rapid delivery to the laboratory to preserve the viability of anaerobes. Alternatively, when periodontal surgery is needed, plaque has been removed from extracted teeth or from surfaces exposed when 'gingival flaps' are reflected. It is important to realize, particularly when comparing studies in which different sampling procedures have been used, that the results will, to a certain extent, reflect the method adopted.

Transport and dispersion

All samples should be transported to the laboratory for processing as quickly as possible. Specially designed transport fluids, containing reducing agents to maintain a low redox potential, maintain the viability of fastidious organisms during delivery to the laboratory.

Clumps and aggregates of bacteria must be dispersed efficiently (ideally to single cells) if the specimen is to be diluted and counted accurately. Mere vortex mixing of a sample is inadequate. Mild sonication produces the maximum number of particles from a specimen but it exerts a selective effect by specifically damaging spirochaetes and other Gram-negative bacteria, particularly *Fusobacterium* spp. One of the most efficient methods, particularly for sub-gingival plaque, is to vortex samples with small glass beads in a tube filled with carbon dioxide.

Cultivation

Once dispersed, samples are usually serially diluted in transport fluid and aliquots are spread on to freshly prepared, pre-reduced agar plates. These media are designed to grow either (a) the maximum number of bacteria (e.g. blood agar) or, (b) only a limited number of species (**selective media**) in order to grow minor components of the microflora. For example, the addition of vancomycin to blood agar plates will inhibit most Gram-positive bacteria, while a high sucrose concentration encourages the growth of oral streptococci, and plates with a low pH favour lactobacilli. It should be emphasized that these media are selective and not specific. The identity of the colonies on these plates must be confirmed; colonial appearance or growth on a particular medium should not be regarded as diagnostic. Media have to be incubated for different times and under different atmospheric conditions depending on the bacteria being cultivated. For example, 7–14 days incubation at $37\,^{\circ}C$ in an anaerobic jar or cabinet filled with a gas mix containing $CO_2/H_2/N_2$ will be needed to grow some obligate anaerobes; in contrast, *Neisseria* require only 2 days' incubation in air. Some organisms are capnophilic (CO_2-loving) and grow optimally in 10% CO_2 in air.

Enumeration and identification

Colonies are counted and their concentration in the original sample is determined by compensating for the dilution steps. Representative colonies are sub-cultured to check for purity and for subsequent identification. This process assumes that:

(a) cells of the same micro-organism produce colonies with an identical morphology;

(b) cells of different species produce colonies with distinct morphologies; and

(c) one colony arises from a single cell.

Generally, these assumptions hold true except for (c), as most colonies inevitably arise from small aggregates of cells, emphasizing the importance of efficient dispersion of samples. It is also advisable to take several examples of a particular colony type to ensure that some species are not overlooked due to their appearance being similar to a numerically dominant organism. One strategy to determine the predominant microflora involves identifying 30–50 random colonies, irrespective of their morphology, rather than selecting only those colony types that appear different.

The first level of discrimination usually involves the Gram-staining of sub-cultured colonies; bacteria are then grouped according to whether their cells are Gram-positive or Gram-negative, and are rod- or coccal-shaped. This dictates which tests will be necessary to achieve speciation (*see* Table 3.2). The use of probes (antibody or nucleic acid) on colonies, or directly on plaque samples, is now being used to speed up identification. It is also possible to distinguish between strains of the same species, e.g. by genotyping. Molecular approaches (e.g. the amplification of 16S rRNA gene sequences) enable the identification in clinical specimens of species that are as yet unculturable in the laboratory.

Microscopy

As an alternative to many of the lengthy steps associated with conventional culture techniques (*see* Figure 4.2), the principal morphological groups of bacteria can be determined using light microscopy. Dark-field illumination or phase contrast techniques have been used to quantify the numbers of motile bacteria (including spirochaetes) directly in dental plaque (particularly from sub-gingival sites). Such organisms are related to the severity of some periodontal diseases, and this approach has been used in the clinic to monitor sites undergoing treatment. However, most of the putative pathogens cannot be recognized by morphology alone. To overcome this problem, cells can be identified by reaction with antisera (monoclonal or specific polyclonal) or nucleic acid probes.

Scanning and transmission electron microscopy have proved useful in studying plaque formation, and have also been used to show that bacteria invade gingival tissues in aggressive forms of periodontal disease. Electron dense markers (ferritin, peroxidase, gold granules) conjugated with antibodies can label specific surface antigens on bacteria and facilitate their identification within plaque. Electron microscopy requires samples to be processed before viewing which can distort the structure of plaque. Non-invasive techniques such as confocal laser scanning microscopy are now being used, with and without the use of specific probes (antibody or nucleic acid), to determine the true architecture of plaque and the location of selected bacteria within the biofilm (*see* Chapter 5). Confocal microscopy involves the generation of numerous focused images throughout the depth of an untreated specimen (optical sections); image analysis software is then used to combine these sections and reconstruct the three-dimensional structure of the original specimen. Confocal microscopy has shown that plaque may have a more open structure than previously thought from studies involving electron microscopy.

In situ models

Various model surfaces for microbial colonization have been developed that can be worn in the mouth by volunteers, and subsequently removed from the mouth to facilitate sampling. The microbiology of fissure plaque has been studied using artificial or natural fissures mounted in a crown or in an occlusal filling. Removable pieces of enamel, denture acrylic, Mylar foil, adhesive tape, spray plast or epoxy resin have been placed on natural teeth or dentures in a desired position and have been used for studies of colonization or of the structural development of dental plaque. Removable appliances have the additional advantage that experiments can be performed on the surfaces when out of the mouth that would not be permitted on natural teeth, e.g. the effect of regular sugar applications, or the evaluation of novel antimicrobial agents. Such models can

also be used with confocal laser scanning microscopy for studies of plaque structure and of plaque formation (*see* Chapter 5).

Distribution of the resident oral microflora

The populations making up the resident microbial community of the oral cavity are not distributed uniformly throughout the mouth. The predominant microflora from several different sites in the oral cavity will be compared in the following sections.

Lips and palate

The lips form the border between the skin microflora, which consists predominantly of staphylococci, micrococci and Gram-positive rods (e.g. *Corynebacterium* and *Propionibacterium* spp.), and the mouth, which contains streptococci and many anaerobic Gram-negative species. Facultatively anaerobic streptococci comprise a large part of the microflora on the lips. *S. vestibularis* is recovered most commonly from the 'gutter' between the lower lip and the gums, and occasionally black-pigmented anaerobes and fusobacteria have been detected. *Veillonella* and *Neisseria* have been found, but only in very low numbers (<1% of the total cultivable microflora). *Candida albicans* can colonize damaged lip mucosal surfaces in the corners of the mouth ('angular cheilitis', *see* Chapter 11).

Table 4.4 Predominant microflora of the healthy human palatal mucosa

Micro-organism	Total cultivable microflora (%)	Isolation frequency (%)
Streptococcus	52	100
Actinomyces	15	100
Lactobacillus	1	87
Neisseria	2	93
Veillonella	1	100
Prevotella	4	100
Candida	+[a]	7

[a]Present, but in numbers too low to count.

The microflora of the normal palate can show large variations between subjects, not only in the total colony forming units removed (which may reflect differences in the area sampled and the success in removing organisms) but also in the proportions of the individual species. The majority of the bacteria are streptococci and actinomyces; haemophili, veillonellae and Gram-negative anaerobes are also regularly recovered but at lower levels (Table 4.4). Candida are not regularly isolated from the normal palate although their prevalence does increase if dentures are worn, and the mucosa can become infected with *C. albicans* (denture stomatitis, *see* Chapter 11).

Cheek

Streptococci are the predominant bacteria from the cheek (buccal mucosa), especially members of the *S. mitis*-group (Table 4.5). As with other mucosal surfaces, obligate anaerobes are not regularly isolated and when present they do not constitute a large percentage of the microflora. Spirochaetes and other motile organisms have been observed occasionally (by phase contrast microscopy) attached to the buccal mucosa. Haemophili (especially *H. parainfluenzae*) are commonly isolated in relatively high numbers. The concentration of micro-organisms on the cheek epithelium is similar to that of the palate (5–25 bacteria per cheek epithelial cell). *Simonsiella* spp. are isolated primarily from the cheek cells of humans and animals.

Table 4.5 Proportions of some bacterial populations at different sites in the normal oral cavity

Bacterium	Saliva	Buccal mucosa	Tongue dorsum	Supragingival plaque
S. sanguis	1	6	1	7
S. salivarius	3	3	6	2
S. oralis/S. mitis	21	29	33	23
mutans streptococci	4	< 1	< 1	5
A. naeslundii	2	1	5	5
A. odontolyticus	2	1	7	13
Haemophilus spp.	4	7	15	7
Fusobacterium spp.	1	< 1	< 1	< 1
Black-pigmented anaerobes	< 1	< 1	1	+[a]

[a]Detected on occasions at relatively high levels.

Tongue

The dorsum of the tongue, with its highly papillated surface, has a large surface area and therefore supports a higher bacterial density than other oral mucosal surfaces (100 bacteria per tongue epithelial cell). A relatively diverse microflora is found, including obligately anaerobic species (Table 4.5). Streptococci are the predominant bacteria (approximately 40% of the total cultivable microflora), with *S. salivarius*- and *S. mitis*-group organisms predominating. *Peptostreptococcus* spp. have also been isolated in some studies while *Stomatococcus mucilagenosus* is found almost exclusively on the tongue. Other major groups of bacteria (and their proportions) include *Veillonella* spp. (16%), Gram-positive rods (16%) of which *A. naeslundii* and *A. odontolyticus* are common, and haemophili (15%). Both pigmenting (*P. intermedia*, *P. melaninogenica*) and non-pigmenting anaerobes can be recovered from the tongue and this site is regarded as a potential reservoir (along with the tonsils) for some of the organisms implicated in periodontal diseases. Other organisms, including lactobacilli, yeasts, fusobacteria, spirochaetes and other motile bacteria are isolated in low numbers (< 1% of the total microflora) while *Neisseria* are found in high proportions (20%) on the tongue of infants (age 8–13 months).

Oral malodour is associated with an increased bacterial load, especially in Gram-negative anaerobes (including *Porphyromonas*, *Prevotella* and *Fusobacterium* spp.) on the tongue. The chemical basis of odour is not fully understood, but includes the production of volatile sulphur compounds by the resident microflora; some of the implicated compounds are described later.

Saliva

Although saliva contains up to 10^8 micro-organisms/ml it is not considered to have a resident microflora. The normal rate of swallowing ensures that bacteria cannot be maintained in the mouth by multiplication in saliva. The organisms found are derived from other surfaces by saliva and GCF flow, chewing, and oral hygiene, but the tongue is the major source. Attempts have been made to use the levels of mutans streptococci and/or lactobacilli in saliva as an indicator of the caries susceptibility of an individual, and kits for their culture are commercially available. Subjects with high counts of these potentially cariogenic bacteria are considered to be 'at-risk', and can be targeted for intense oral hygiene and dietary counselling (*see* Chapter 6).

Teeth

The microbial community associated with teeth (dental plaque) varies in composition at each tooth surface due to differences in the local environmental conditions (*see* Chapter 2). For these reasons, plaque is described on the basis of the sampling site by terms such as smooth surface, approximal, fissure, or gingival plaque (Figure 2.2). Similarly, samples taken from above the level of the gum margin are termed 'supra-gingival plaque', while those from below the gum margin are described as 'sub-gingival plaque'. The detailed composition of dental plaque from these sites will be given in Chapter 5. As teeth are non-shedding surfaces, the highest concentrations of micro-organisms are found in stagnant sites which afford protection from removal forces. Dental plaque is an example of a biofilm; bacteria growing in biofilms can display novel properties, including an enhanced resistance to antimicrobial agents. The properties of plaque as a biofilm are discussed in Chapter 5.

Gram-positive rods (mainly *Actinomyces* spp.) are a major group of bacteria in plaque (Table 4.5). Mutans streptococci and members of the *S. mitis*- and *S. anginosus*-groups are found in highest numbers on teeth. These organisms have a strong affinity for hard surfaces, and do not usually appear in the mouth until after tooth eruption. In addition, *S. sanguis* can be isolated from many of the exposed surfaces of teeth such as the smooth surfaces while, in contrast to mucosal surfaces, *S. salivarius* is only a minor component of dental plaque. Haemophili are present in moderate numbers, although the individual species can differ from those found on other oral surfaces. Obligate anaerobes are found in high numbers particularly in the gingival crevice, and oral spirochaetes are almost uniquely associated with this region. Thus, the composition of dental plaque differs both qualitatively and quantitatively from the communities of other oral surfaces.

Factors influencing the distribution of oral micro-organisms

Factors affecting the distribution of the oral microflora include the redox potential at sites (*see* Chapter 2), nutrient availability (e.g. GCF provides novel compounds for the growth of fastidious anaerobes), and the ability to adhere to particular surfaces. Bacteria adhere with considerable specificity not only to particular tissues, but also to the particular tissue of their particular animal host (**tissue tropism**).

Factors involved in adherence of micro-organisms to oral surfaces

Microbial adherence is one of the most active fields of research, not only in oral ecology but also in other aspects of microbiology. As adherence is essential for colonization by pathogenic as well as by commensal micro-organisms, any approach that can successfully interfere with these processes could have far-reaching implications.

The first stage of adherence involves the initial interaction between micro-organism and substrate. It involves the external surfaces of both organism and substrate, and will be influenced by the suspending medium, and can be described in terms of precise physico-chemical interactions of attraction and repulsion (*see* Chapter 5). Subsequently, attachment involves specific molecular interactions between complementary molecules on the microbial and host surface. In general, the bacterial components which function in adherence are termed **'adhesins'** while the host-derived factors are called **'receptors'**. A bacterial cell surface can express multiple adhesins while the host surface can contain several receptors. Bacteria also express receptors for adhesins on other microbial cell types that are used for cell–cell attachment (**co-aggregation**; *see* Chapter 5). Consequently, the molecular interactions by which a given strain attaches to receptors on dissimilar surfaces (e.g. enamel, buccal mucosa, etc.) could be different. The polymers of host and bacterial origin that are involved in adherence are discussed below.

Host receptors
Epithelial cells, especially buccal epithelium, have sialic acid exposed on their surfaces which can interact with adhesins on bacteria, e.g. *S. mitis*. If the sialic acid residue is removed by neuraminidase, then another receptor (a galactosyl residue) can be exposed which is recognized by *Actinomyces* spp. and Gram-negative

bacteria including *F. nucleatum, P. intermedia* and *E. corrodens*. Collagen fibres, which are major structural components of connective tissue, can also act as receptors for certain mutans streptococci (*S. cricetus, S. rattus*) and *P. gingivalis*, while specific domains for the attachment of streptococci can be found on fibronectin.

The major groups of host receptors are found in saliva; these receptors, when adsorbed onto oral mucosal and enamel surfaces, will influence bacterial attachment. The greatest amount of research has been directed towards the receptors found on the enamel surface (the **acquired pellicle**). This pellicle is generally < 1 μm thick and is formed by the selective adsorption of components, mainly from saliva but also from GCF and from secreted bacterial products. Pellicles form on all oral surfaces (hard and soft) and are not identical; the components that adsorb to cementum differ from those on enamel, and both are distinct from those which form on the oral mucosa. These differences are sometimes recognized by the use of different terminologies, e.g., the acquired enamel pellicle or the acquired cementum pellicle, while the pellicle that forms on epithelial surfaces is referred to as the mucus coat. Pellicle forms as soon as a clean surface is exposed to saliva; it takes around 90–120 minutes for the adsorption of molecules to reach a plateau and cease. Pellicles contain proteins, lipids and glycolipids, but little is known of the conformational state of the adsorbed molecules. Once formed, the composition and structure of pellicles will change and be modified.

Within the enamel pellicle, acidic proline-rich proteins and statherin promote the adherence of *A. naeslundii*, some *S. mutans* strains and black-pigmented anaerobes. Amylase, lysozyme, albumin and immunoglobulins, as well as bacterial components, including glucosyltransferases (GTFs) and glucans, have been detected by immunological probes. These adsorbed compounds can act as receptors for oral bacteria. GTFs in the pellicle are still able to function and the glucans produced from sucrose can bind to molecules (glucan-binding proteins) on bacteria, such as mutans streptococci. The polymer synthesized by adsorbed GTF on the tooth surface may have an altered chemical structure to that produced by free-living bacteria.

Bacterial adhesins

Many bacterial adhesins are lectins (carbohydrate-binding proteins) which bind to carbohydrate receptors on a surface. Often these adhesins are associated with surface structures termed fibrils or fimbriae. Fibrils can be distinguished from fimbriae in that they clump together and have no measurable width while fimbriae have a measurable width (3–14 nm) and a variable length up to 20 μm. Some cells possess both fibrils and fimbriae, and sometimes of different types. For example, *S. salivarius* strains has four different classes of fibril, each with a specific length. The 91 nm fibrils are responsible for co-aggregation with *V. parvula* while the 73 nm fibrils are involved with adhesion to buccal epithelial cells. The longest (178 nm) and shortest (63 nm) fibrils have yet to be ascribed a function. Similarly, *A. naeslundii* possesses two types of fimbriae. Type 1 fimbriae mediate the binding of cells to adsorbed proline-rich proteins and to statherin in salivary pellicle on enamel whereas type 2 fimbriae are associated with a galactosyl-binding lectin which mediates attachment to host cells and to other bacteria (co-aggregation). Fibrils on the surface of *P. nigrescens* are shown in Figure 4.3.

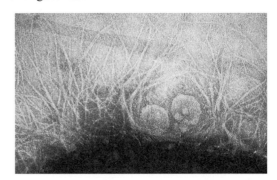

Figure 4.3 Scanning electron micrograph to show fibrils on the cell surface of *P. nigrescens*. Courtesy of Dr D. Devine

A significant adhesin is the antigen I/II family of cell surface-anchored polypeptides found in most oral streptococci. These linear polypeptides are structurally complex, multi-functional adhesins, with multiple receptor binding sites. Discrete regions within these peptides bind to human salivary glycoproteins, other microbial cells ('co-aggregation', *see* Chapter 5), and calcium. Other bacterial adhesins include glucosyltransferases (GTFs); these GTFs can

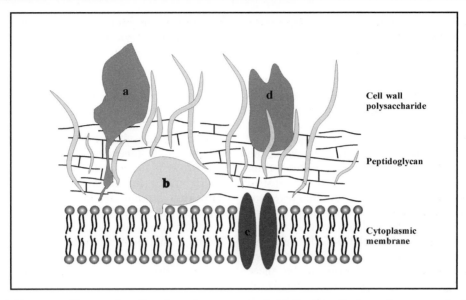

Figure 4.4 Diagram to illustrate the cell surface of a streptococcal cell showing adhesins and receptors associated with adherence, and substrate transport: (*a*) cell wall anchored polypeptide; (*b*) membrane anchored polypeptide; (*c*) transmembrane polypeptide (e.g. in transport of substrates); (*d*) extracellular polypeptide (e.g. GTF)

interact with receptors in pellicle such as blood group reactive proteins or adsorbed dextrans and glucans. The latter can also react with glucan-binding proteins expressed by other streptococci. Many oral Gram-positive bacteria have lipoteichoic acid (LTA), which is composed of sugar phosphates, usually glycerol and ribitol phosphate. LTA has also been shown to interact with blood group reactive substances in pellicle. As antibodies are found in the acquired pellicle, a number of antigens may also act indirectly as 'adhesins'. Similarly, lysozyme in the pellicle can also bind to protein receptors on bacteria.

Some of the adhesins on the streptococcal cell surface are now known to have a lipid tail (i.e. they are lipoproteins), which helps in their retention in the cell membrane. These lipoproteins are similar to the solute binding molecules that function in the ATP-binding-cassette-type (ABC-type) transport systems. These lipoproteins might bind to an immobilized solute (an adsorbed sugar or peptide) within the salivary pellicle or on another bacterial cell surface, and facilitate attachment. Thus, the surface of oral Gram-positive bacteria is a complex mosaic of peptidoglycan, lipoteichoic acid, polysaccharide, proteins and lipoproteins (Figure 4.4), the production of which will be influenced by environmental conditions. The issue as to

whether oral bacteria can detect that they are on a surface (e.g. by the presence of 'touch sensors') remains a topical subject.

Functions of the climax community: colonization resistance

One of the main beneficial functions of the resident microflora at any site is their ability to exclude exogenous organisms by preventing their colonization; such organisms are often pathogenic for the host. This property of exclusion has been termed **colonization resistance**, and the microbial factors that contribute to this property are:

- Competition for receptors for adhesion.
- Competition for essential endogenous nutrients and cofactors.
- Creation of micro-environments that discourage the growth of exogenous species.
- Production of inhibitory substances.

A key mechanism is the production of inhibitors, e.g. the production of hydrogen peroxide by members of the *S. mitis*-group, bacteriocin production by a range of Gram-positive bacteria, especially streptococci, and the formation of acidic end products of metabolism. It has been proposed that strains of *S. salivarius* that produce an inhibitor (termed 'enocin' or 'salivaricin'), and which is active against Lancefield group A streptococci (*S. pyogenes*), can prevent or reduce colonization by this pathogen on mucosal surfaces.

Attempts have been made to enhance the colonization resistance of the resident oral microflora. As the mother is the major source of bacteria (including cariogenic species) in the infant, levels of mutans streptococci have been suppressed in expectant mothers by professional oral hygiene, dietary counselling with, if necessary, treatment with chlorhexidine or fluoride (*see* Chapter 6). The result is that the natural microflora of the infant becomes established in the absence of mutans streptococci. The subsequent colonization by these cariogenic streptococci is therefore delayed, as is the average time for the first caries lesion to form. Other approaches that are still at the laboratory stage are to use pre-emptive colonization with either low virulence mutants of *S. mutans* (e.g. strains deficient in glucosyltransferases, intracellular polysaccharide production, or lactate dehydrogenase activity) or with organisms that are more competitive than wild-type *S. mutans* strains. It is not possible to delete lactate dehydrogenase from *S. mutans*, as such a mutation is lethal. Stable mutants can be produced, however, by introducing an alcohol dehydrogenase gene from an unrelated organism; such mutants of *S. mutans* grow well but produce no detectable lactic acid. In addition, *S. salivarius* (strain TOVE) has been shown to displace virulent strains of *S. mutans* from teeth in experimental animal studies while bacteriocin-producing but avirulent mutants of *S. mutans* have been shown to be able to colonize human teeth in volunteers. Both strains could be candidates as possible effector strains for this type of replacement therapy (*see* Chapter 6).

Host factors also play a role in colonization resistance. The immune and innate host defences will help exclude invading organisms. However, colonization resistance can be impaired by factors that compromise the integrity of the host defences or perturb the resident microflora. Examples include the long-term use of broad spectrum antibiotics or of cytotoxic therapy, but other more subtle mechanisms can apply. Fibronectin has been shown to prevent adherence of *Pseudomonas aeruginosa* to buccal epithelial cells. Levels of fibronectin in seriously ill adults and in infants are lower than those in healthy adults and may account for the higher rates of colonization by Gram-negative bacilli in these subjects.

Metabolism of oral bacteria

The persistence of the resident oral microflora is dependent on their ability to obtain nutrients and grow in the mouth. Nutrients are derived mainly from the metabolism of endogenous substrates present in saliva and GCF. Superimposed on these components are exogenous nutrients which are supplied intermittently via the diet; the most significant of these for the oral microflora are dietary carbohydrates and casein. The concentration of nutrients will affect the growth rate and physiology of the microflora, as will any changes in pH resulting from their metabolism. The fluctuating supply of nutrients and the resultant environmental changes requires the microflora to possess biochemical flexibility. Indeed, the pattern of metabolism is closely related to whether the resident microflora enjoys a pathogenic or commensal relationship with the host.

Carbohydrate metabolism

Most attention has been paid to the metabolism of carbohydrates because of the relationship between dietary sugars, low pH and dental caries (*see* Chapters 2 and 6). The metabolic fate of dietary carbohydrates is illustrated in simplified form in Figure 4.5. Starches, which contain mixtures of amylose and amylopectin, can be broken into their constituent sugars by amylases of salivary and bacterial origin. Some streptococci (e.g. *S. gordonii*, *S. mitis*) are able to bind amylase, which might provide additional metabolic capability. *S. mutans* possesses a spectrum of enzymes capable of degrading dietary starches although, perhaps significantly from a caries standpoint, little acid is made from starch. These enzymes include an extracellular pullanase, which degrades pullulan and debranches amylopectin, as well as an amylase; there is also an extracellular endo-dextranase and an intracellular exo-dextranase.

Milk is the major source of lactose in the diet, while sucrose occupies a key position in bacterial metabolism in the oral cavity. Sucrose

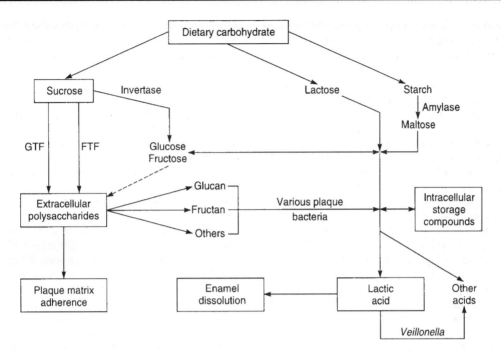

Figure 4.5 Simplified diagram to show the metabolic fate of dietary carbohydrates.
GTF, glucosyltransferase; FTF, fructosyltransferase

is the most widely used sweetening agent and, in many industrialized societies, consumption is approximately 50 kg/person per year. Sucrose can be:

(a) broken down by extracellular bacterial invertases (α-glucosidases) and the resultant glucose and fructose molecules taken up directly by bacteria;

(b) transported intact as the disaccharide or disaccharide phosphate, and cleaved inside the cell by an intracellular invertase or a sucrose phosphate hydrolase; and/or

(c) utilized extracellularly by glycosyltransferases. Glucosyltransferases (GTF) produce both soluble and insoluble glucans (with a release of fructose) which are important in plaque formation and in the consolidation of bacterial attachment to teeth. Fructosyltransferases (FTF) produce fructans (and liberate glucose) which are frequently labile and can be used by other plaque organisms.

Some aspects of the metabolism of carbohy-drates will be considered in more detail in the following sections.

Sugar transport and acid production
All substrates have to be transported across the cytoplasmic membrane and into the bacterial cell if they are to be of value for biomass production or as an energy source. Oral bacteria transport carbohydrates by three known processes:

- the phosphoenolpyruvate-mediated phosphotransferase (PEP-PTS) transport system;
- the multiple sugar metabolism system (Msm); and
- a glucose permease.

The most significant system is the PTS, which is the high affinity sugar transport system for mono- and di-saccharides in acidogenic oral bacteria, especially members of the genera: *Streptococcus*, *Actinomyces* and *Lactobacillus*. The PEP-PTS is a carrier-mediated, group translocation system involving phosphoryl-transfer from PEP via two non-sugar-specific, general cytoplasmic proteins, HPr and enzyme I

(EI), to a sugar-specific, membrane-bound enzyme II complex (EII), that catalyses the transport and phosphorylation of the incoming sugar (Figure 4.6). The phosphate group of EI~P, generated from PEP, is transferred to HPr, forming HPr~P, and then to the EII complex.

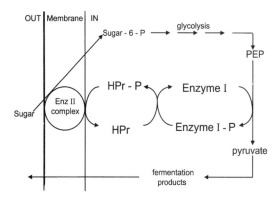

Figure 4.6 Diagrammatic representation of a phosphoenol-pyruvate (PEP)-mediated sugar phosphotransferase (PTS) system. Enzyme I and HPr are cytoplasmic proteins; Enzyme II is a membrane-associated sugar-specific protein that may exist on its own, or as a complex with sugar-specific, cytoplasmic-associated proteins IIA, IIB and IIC

The PTS is constitutive for some sugars, such as glucose, mannose and sucrose, but must be induced for the transport of lactose and sugar alcohols such as mannitol and sorbitol. In all cases, the components induced are those in the EII complex as well as additional enzymes required to convert the substrate to a component of the glycolytic pathway. For example, when *S. mutans* is grown on lactose there is co-induction of the lactose-PTS and phospho-β-galactosidase (the latter enzyme cleaves intracellular lactose-phosphate to galactose-6-phosphate and glucose). Similarly, growth of *S. mutans* on mannitol or sorbitol leads to the induction of distinct PTS systems for these sugar alcohols, although both are rapidly repressed by glucose. The activity of the PTS in oral streptococci is modulated by environmental conditions. It is optimal under conditions of carbohydrate-limitation, neutral pH and slow rates of bacterial growth. In contrast, it is repressed under conditions of excess sugar, low pH and high growth rates. This is significant, because oral steptococci in dental plaque are continually exposed to transitory

conditions of low pH and high sugar concentrations.

Many strains of *S. mutans* possess a second means of transporting sugars into the cell (the multiple sugar metabolism, Msm, transport system). The existence of this system was inferred entirely from the finding of sequence homology of genes cloned from *S. mutans* with known gene products from Gram-negative bacteria. The Msm is analogous to the binding-protein-dependent system that is normally found in Gram-negative bacteria, and is capable of transporting various common sugars, as well as melibiose, raffinose and isomaltosaccharides. The exact role of this system in plaque ecology is unknown, but it might be involved in transporting the breakdown products of extracellular polysaccharide degradation during periods between meals when the supply of more refined dietary mono- and di-saccharides is negligible.

At high sugar concentrations, PTS activity is repressed and sugar transport is augmented by an ATP-dependent glucose permease; this system also functions at high growth rates and at low pH. The sugar is transported into the cell where it is phosphorylated on the inner surface of the membrane. Cells tend to form glycogen under conditions of carbohydrate-excess in order to reduce the toxic intracellular levels of glycolytic intermediates. Organisms with this ability, therefore, are able to cope better than most other oral bacteria with the fluctuating 'feast-and-famine' conditions in the mouth in terms of the availability of dietary sugars.

The resident oral microflora also obtains carbohydrates for biomass and energy from the catabolism of host glycoproteins present in saliva (e.g. mucins) and GCF (e.g. transferrin). Bacteria produce a range of glycosidases that can remove sugars sequentially from the oligosaccharide side chains of these glycoproteins. As no single species possesses the full enzyme complement, bacteria interact synergistically to fully degrade these molecules (*see* Chapter 5). Acid production from these glycoproteins is slow compared to that from exogenous sugars, and would not cause significant enamel demineralization. Strains of *S. oralis* growing in the presence of glycoproteins induce sialidase (neuraminidase) and N-acetylglucosaminidase, which can cleave sialic acid and N-acetyl glucosamine from the oligosaccharide side chains. These sugars are then

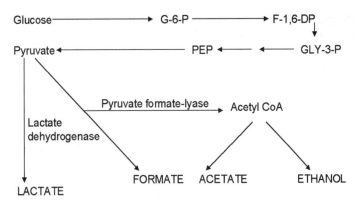

Figure 4.7 Formation of end products of metabolism by mutans streptococci. G-6-P, glucose-6-phosphate; F-1,6-DP, fructose-1,6-diphosphate; GLY-3-P, glyceraldehyde-3-phosphate; PEP, phosphoenolpyruvate

transported inside the cell, and key intracellular enzymes associated with the catabolism of N-acetyl sugars are also induced. Significant concentrations of lactate are not produced from sialic acid metabolism; the main fermentation products are formate and ethanol.

Once sugars have been transported into the bacterial cell, they can be used either in anabolic pathways to generate biomass, or they can be broken down to organic acids (which are excreted) to generate energy. Firstly, sugars are catabolized by glycolysis to pyruvate; the fate of pyruvate will depend on the particular organism and the availability of oxygen. Most oral bacteria metabolize pyruvate anaerobically to organic acids, the pattern of which can be exploited for the identification of some genera (*see* Chapter 3). Oral streptococci, convert pyruvate to lactate by lactate dehydrogenase when sugars are in excess, while formate, acetate and ethanol are the products of metabolism by mutans streptococci and *S. sanguis* (but not *S. salivarius*) under carbohydrate limitation (Figure 4.7). Other bacterial genera produce acetate, butyrate, propionate, and formate as primary products of metabolism.

The mechanism of excretion of lactic acid has been determined in *S. mutans*. Lactate and protons are translocated across the cell membrane as lactic acid in a carrier-mediated, electroneutral process. After the addition of a fermentable substrate to cells, lactate begins to accumulate, and protons are pumped out of the cell by an ATPsynthase (an F_1F_0-ATPase). This generates a transmembrane pH gradient, which can then be used as the driving force to transport lactate as lactic acid out of the cell. Different species produce acid at different rates, and vary in the terminal pH reached, and in their ability to survive under such conditions. Mutans streptococci produce acid at the fastest rates while lactobacilli generate the lowest environmental pH; both groups are also aciduric and can tolerate conditions of acidity that most other oral bacteria would find inhibitory or even lethal; the biochemical mechanisms behind this tolerance are described in the next section.

Variations are found in the profiles of acids found in plaque at different times of the day. Acetic, succinic, propionic, valeric, caproic and butyric acids were found in human and monkey plaque sampled after overnight fasting. These profiles reflect heterofermentation and amino acid catabolism. Following exposure to sucrose, the concentration of volatile acids fell while lactic acid became the predominant fermentation product. Such a switch in metabolism would encourage demineralization.

Acid tolerance

Although many of the saccharolytic bacteria found in dental plaque can generate a low terminal pH from sugar metabolism, few species can survive such conditions for prolonged periods. Glycolysis can continue at pH values that are too low to support growth. One of the prime distinguishing features of cariogenic bacteria such as mutans streptococci and lactobacilli is their ability to tolerate low pH stress.

Microbial survival in acidic environments depends on the ability of a cell to maintain intracellular pH homeostasis. The mechanisms by which *S. mutans* achieves this include:

(a) proton extrusion via membrane-associated, proton-translocating ATP-synthase (H^+/ATPase); and
(b) acid end product efflux (*see above*).

These mechanisms ensure that the intracellular pH remains higher (i.e. more alkaline) than that of the external environment when the pH falls due to the formation of acidic end products of metabolism. In addition, acid tolerant organisms such as mutans streptococci and lactobacilli have higher levels of ATP-synthase activity, and the pH optimum for activity is lower than for less tolerant species such as *S. sanguis* or *A. naeslundii*.

It has been shown that *S. mutans* undergoes a specific alteration in its physiology in order to survive in an acidic environment. The factors involved in this acid tolerance response are:

- increase in glycolytic activity;
- shift to lower pH optimum for glucose transport, glycolysis and proton impermeability;
- decrease in activity of specific components of the PTS sugar transport system;
- increased activity of the H^+/ATP synthase;
- increased capacity to maintain transmembrane pH gradients at lower pH values;
- shift to homo-fermentative metabolism;
- synthesis of stress response proteins;

and this metabolic strategy gives *S. mutans* a competitive advantage at low pH over organisms associated with sound enamel, such as *S. sanguis*, that lack this response. Other species cope with the stress of a low environmental pH by up-regulating genes involved in base production. For example, urease gene expression by *S. salivarius* is enhanced significantly at low pH, while the arginine deiminase system (which degrades arginine to ornithine, CO_2 and ammonia) of *S. sanguis* is active at pH values (pH 4.0) lower than it can grow (pH 5.2) or carry out glycolysis.

Polysaccharide production
Bacteria in the mouth are subjected to continual cycles of 'feast and famine' with respect to dietary carbohydrates. As a consequence, the resident microflora has developed strategies to store these carbohydrates during their brief

exposure to these energy sources. This is both to avoid the lethal effects of the build up of intracellular glycolytic intermediates, and to provide a source of carbon and energy for the subsequent periods of 'famine'. The most common strategy is to store these carbohydrates as intracellular polysaccharides (IPS), and many species of oral streptococci can synthesize polymers that resemble glycogen (1,4-α-glucan), although other polymers might also be formed. IPS production may act as a virulence factor for *S. mutans* since mutants defective in the production of storage compounds produced fewer caries lesions in an animal model than the parent strain.

Many species of oral bacteria are also able to synthesize extracellular polysaccharides (EPS) from carbohydrates, especially from sucrose (Table 4.6). The polysaccharides can be soluble or insoluble; the former are more labile and can be metabolized by other bacteria, while the latter make a major contribution to the structural integrity of dental plaque and can consolidate the attachment of bacteria in plaque. Sucrose has a unique property as a substrate in that the bond between the glucose and fructose moieties has sufficient energy on cleavage to support the synthesis of polysaccharides. The polysaccharides formed are either glucans or fructans, and are synthesized by glucosyltransferases (GTF), and fructosyltransferases (FTF), respectively:

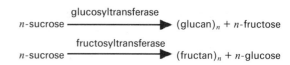

GTFs can be divided into four groups depending on whether they produce a soluble dextran (GTF-S synthesize predominantly α, 1-6 linked glucan) or an insoluble glucan (GTF-I synthesize predominantly α, 1-3 polymers), and whether or not they require a dextran primer for activity. *S. mutans* possesses three GTFs (encoded for by *gtfB*, *gtfC* and *gtfD* genes) which synthesize α1,3- and α1,6-linked glucan polymers. In *S. mutans*, the *gtfB* and *gtfC* genes encode for enzymes that produce water insoluble glucans, consisting primarily of α, 1-3 linkages, which contribute to cell adhesion and plaque formation and structure, and are also essential for the initiation of caries on smooth

Table 4.6 Extracellular polysaccharide-producing bacterial populations found in the oral cavity

Population	Carbohydrate substrate	Type of polymer (with predominant linkages[a])
Streptococcus mutans	Sucrose	Water-insoluble and soluble glucans α-1,3; α 1,3 + 1,6-; α, 1-6
	Sucrose	Fructan β, 2-1
Streptococcus sanguis[b]	Sucrose	Water-insoluble glucan α-1,3- + α-1,6-
	Sucrose	Water-soluble glucan (dextran) α-1,6
Streptococcus salivarius[c]	Sucrose	Fructan (levan) β-2,6
Actinomyces naeslundii	Sucrose	Fructan (levan) β-2,6
	—[d]	Heteropolysaccharide (60% N-acetyl glucosamine)
Lactobacillus sp.	—[d]	Glucan
		Heteropolysaccharide
Eubacterium spp.	—[d]	Heteropolysaccharide (predominantly acetate)
		Homopolysaccharide (D-glycero-D-galacto-heptose)
Rothia dentocariosa	Glucose	Heteropolysaccharide
	Sucrose	Levan
Micrococcus mucilagenosus	—[d]	Heteropolysaccharide (hexoses, hexosamines, amino acids)
Neisseria sp.	Sucrose	Glycogen-like

[a]Where known.
[b]Some strains produce a fructan.
[c]Some strains produce a glucan.
[d]No specific substrate required.

surfaces of teeth in animal models. In contrast, the *gtfD* gene encodes a primer-dependent enzyme responsible for the formation of glucan, predominantly with α,1-6 linked glucose units, that is much more water soluble. The basic structure of some glucans is shown in Figure 4.8.

S. mutans has a single FTF (produced by the *ftf* gene) which catalyses the incorporation of the fructose component of sucrose into a fructan polymer with an inulin-type structure (β,2-1 linked fructose units). Fructans are not involved in adhesion, nor do they remain for long in plaque. These polymers may act more as extracellular carbohydrate storage compounds in plaque biofilms, being broken down to fructose (which can be transported by the PTS for glycolysis) by fructan hydrolases produced by a range of oral bacteria.

Other streptococci possess different numbers of GTF genes. Four GTF activities have been detected in *S. sobrinus*; these include a primer-dependent GTF-I which synthesizes a glucan composed predominantly (79–93%) of α,1-3 linked glucose residues. There are two gene products which produce polymers with mixed α,1-3 and α,1-6 linked glucose molecules (previously, such products were considered to be synthesized only as a result of the concerted action of a mixture of GTF-S and GTF-I enzymes). Finally, there is a primer-independent GTF-S producing a linear glucan composed predominantly of α,1-6 residues. *S. salivarius* also produces four GTFs, although their properties differ from those described for *S. sobrinus*. In contrast, *S. gordonii* possesses only a single GTF, although this can form both soluble and insoluble glucan depending on the prevailing environmental conditions. At present, little is known about the products produced by *S. sanguis* or *S. oralis*, although they probably only synthesize one enzyme. *S. salivarius* also produces a fructan, but in contrast to that of *S. mutans*, it is a levan with a characteristic β,2-6 linkage (*see* Table 4.6). The FTF of *S. salivarius* is cell associated, whereas those of most other organisms are secreted.

Other species that produce EPS are listed in Table 4.6. The hetero-polysaccharides can have a complex composition; for example, the polymer produced by a strain of *A. naeslundii* contains *N*-acetyl glucosamine (62%), galactose (7%), glucose (4%), uronic acids (3%) and small amounts of glycerol, rhamnose, arabinose and xylose. Some of these homo- and hetero-polysaccharides can be metabolized by other oral bacteria.

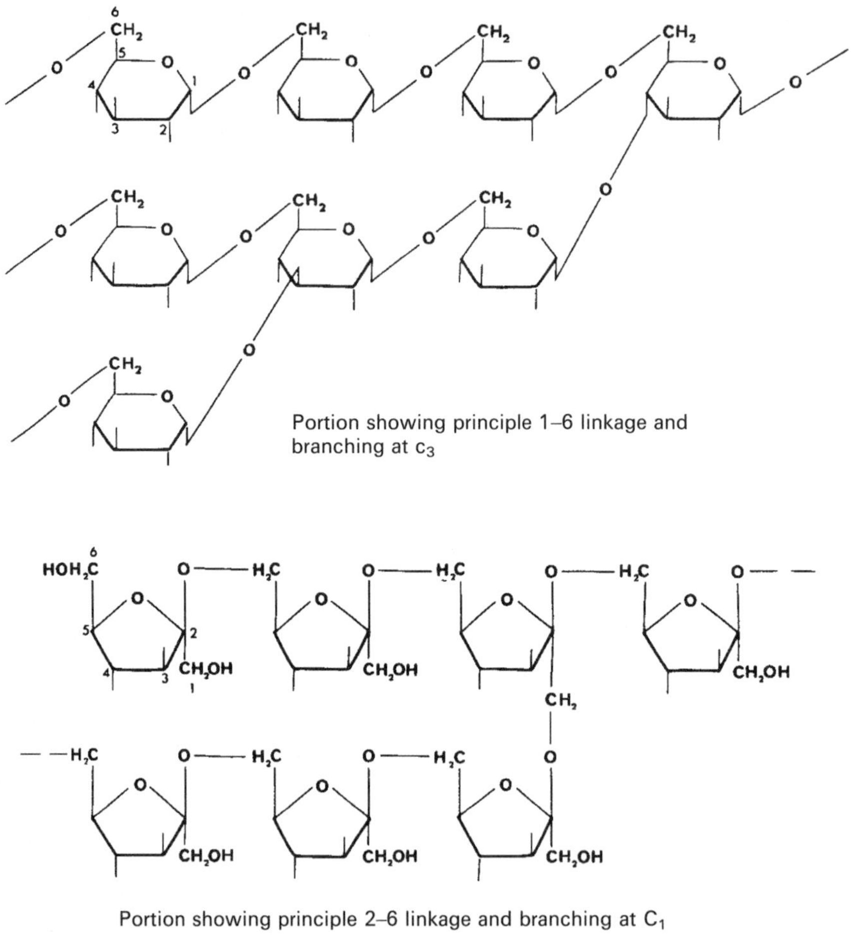

Portion showing principle 1–6 linkage and branching at c_3

Portion showing principle 2–6 linkage and branching at C_1

Figure 4.8 Structure of part of a glucan chain (*top*), showing α,1-6,- and α, 1-3,- linkages, and of part of a typical fructan

Nitrogen metabolism

In contrast to the large amount of data on the metabolism of carbohydrates, much less is known about the metabolism of nitrogenous compounds by oral bacteria. This situation is beginning to change with the appreciation of the role of salivary proteins/glycoproteins as primary nutrient sources in the mouth, and the significance of proteases in the aetiology of periodontal diseases.

Apart from casein, there is little evidence that dietary proteins are utilized to any great extent. Casein can be incorporated into dental plaque and degraded. *S. sanguis* has been shown to have both endo- and exopeptidase (amino- and carboxy-terminal) activity that can cleave proteins such as casein into a range of peptide fragments. Exopeptidase activity is mainly cell-associated and up-regulated at high pH, whereas endopeptidase activity is extracellular and optimal at neutral pH. *S. sanguis* can rapidly release arginine from C-terminal peptides, converting the released arginine to energy (and carbamyl phosphate) via the arginine deiminase pathway. Other oral bacteria have different preferences for individual amino acids; for example, *S. mutans* and *A. naeslundii* preferentially utilize cysteine and asparagine, respectively. Urea is present in relatively high concentrations (200 mg/litre) in saliva. Some oral species possess urease activity (e.g. *A. naeslundii* and *S. salivarius*) and can convert urea to carbon dioxide and ammonia. At acidic pH, decarboxylation of amino acids would yield carbon dioxide and amines, while at high pH, deamination would produce ammonia and keto acids, which can be converted to acetic, propionic, and possibly iso- and n-butyric acids. For example, some periodontal pathogens can convert histidine, glutamine or arginine to acetate and butyrate. In this way, amino acid metabolism is an important mechanism whereby oral micro-organisms counter the extremes of pH caused by the catabolism of carbohydrates and urea.

Essential amino acids can be obtained from the environment or synthesized by the cell. Ammonia can be converted into a number of amino acids, for example:

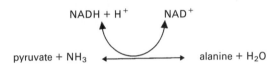

Further transamination reactions can provide other essential amino acids. Deamination reactions also take place which generate NH_3 and the corresponding keto acid; these reactions are important in controlling pH in plaque. There is also evidence for the Stickland reaction occurring in dental plaque. This involves the coupled oxidation–reduction of suitable pairs of amino acids, and is a mechanism whereby various biochemical processes can be balanced in plaque.

Little is known at present about the mechanisms of transport of amino acids and peptides in oral bacteria. In *S. mutans*, glutamate and aspartate are taken up by a primary transport system driven by ATP hydrolysis, whereas branched-chain amino acids (such as leucine) are taken up by an energized membrane (proton motive force)-driven carrier system. Essential amino acids can also be derived from the metabolism of peptides either inside or outside of the cell. It has been demonstrated recently that both *S. mutans* and *S. sanguis* can transport tri-peptides (with an 'X-proline-Y' structure), that are degraded intracellularly by cytoplasmic dipeptidyl peptidases, and then by an enzyme that breaks down X-proline dipeptides. This process is energetically very favourable for the cells because all of the amino acids present in the peptide are obtained for the same energy cost as the transport of a single amino acid.

Salivary peptides can modulate the metabolic activity of oral bacteria. A peptide (termed sialin) with the structure glycine-glycine-lysine-arginine can enhance the glycolytic activity of plaque bacteria and give rise to a significant pH-rise effect in the laboratory and may, therefore, reduce the risk of caries development. Enhanced glycolysis leads to rapid clearance of sugars from the mouth, while base production both neutralizes the acids formed and raises the pH.

Many of the micro-organisms from the periodontal pocket are asaccharolytic (i.e. do not gain energy from the conversion of sugars to acidic fermentation products) but proteolytic, and depend for their growth on their ability to utilize the nutrients provided by GCF. During inflammation, many novel nutrients (e.g. haemoglobin, transferrin, haemopexin, haptoglobin, etc.) are provided by the host, and this can lead to the enrichment of highly proteolytic periodontopathogens such as *P. gingivalis*. These host molecules can be degraded to provide peptides and amino acids, as well as haeme, which is an essential co-factor for black-pigmented anaerobes. Often peptides are transported in preference to amino acids for bioenergetic reasons; such peptides are then broken down within the cell by intracellular peptidases. The mechanism of peptide transport in periodontal bacteria has not been studied in detail; in other bacteria, multi-component ATP-binding systems and ion motive force-driven systems have been described that provide distinct transport systems for di-, tri and oligopeptides. Different species appear to use particular amino acids for different purposes. For example, although both *P. gingivalis* and *F. nucleatum* utilize glutamate, it was used in biosynthetic reactions by the former species and in catabolic pathways to generate energy by the latter; *F. nucleatum* can also obtain energy from histidine, serine and lysine.

In addition to obtaining essential nutrients from GCF, many sub-gingival organisms are also able to degrade structural proteins and glycoproteins associated with the pocket epithelium. The production of enzymes such as chondroitin sulphatase, hyaluronidase and collagenase, therefore, contributes to tissue damage and pocket formation. *P. gingivalis* produces two major extracellular proteases, both encoded as polyproteins containing proteinase and adhesin domains; one of these proteases (gingipain R) is an arginine-specific, thiol-activated cysteine protease (previously described as a 'trypsin-like' protease), while the other (gingipain K) is a lysine-specific, thiol-activated cysteine protease. Both proteinases have C-terminal adhesin domains that are involved in attachment to host proteins. Perhaps surprisingly, considering the major proteolytic activity of gingipain R, mutants lacking this activity are still able to grow on complex substrates, suggesting that the primary role of this enzyme may not be in generating peptides for energy and growth. Other studies suggest that this protease is more important in virulence by deregulating the host inflammatory response (*see* Chapter 7). Therefore, other endo- and exopeptidase activities must be involved in generating peptides for the growth of this organism. Recently, gingipain K has been found essential for growth, liberating haeme from haemoglobin.

The pH optima of some of these enzymes are at neutral or slightly alkaline pH, which corresponds to that of the periodontal pocket. A small change in environmental pH can markedly alter the enzyme activity profile of some bacteria. In *P. gingivalis*, a rise in culture pH from 7.0 to 8.0 led to a change in the ratio of arginine-specific protease activity to collagen breakdown activity from 1:1 to 8:1. These enzymes are potential virulence factors, and are discussed in more detail in Chapter 7.

Synergistic interactions occur in the breakdown of these molecules, and associations may occur between organisms with complementary patterns of enzyme activity (*see* Chapter 5). It has been proposed that the endopeptidase activity of *P. gingivalis* could provide appropriate peptides from the catabolism of host molecules for the growth of *F. nucleatum*. This could be one explanation why these two species are frequently found together in periodontal pockets. The concept of plaque behaving as a microbial community in the breakdown of complex host molecules is developed further in the next chapter.

Collectively, these findings emphasize the significance of nitrogen metabolism in oral microbial ecology. Host and bacterial proteases are associated directly and indirectly with tissue destruction in periodontal disease, while it has been argued that caries results not so much from an over-production of acid but more from a deficiency in base production by plaque bacteria.

Oxygen metabolism

The mouth is an overtly aerobic environment and yet the majority of bacteria are either facultatively anaerobic or obligately anaerobic, especially in dental plaque. Early colonizers are more tolerant of the toxic effects of oxygen metabolism, especially with respect to hydrogen peroxide and hypothiocyanite, than later colonizers. The latter may depend on inter-species metabolic interactions within the biofilm structure of plaque in order to cope with oxygen and toxic radicals. This may be why plaque shows vertical stratification in terms of its structure (*see* Chapter 5).

All plaque bacteria, including obligate anaerobes, are able to metabolize oxygen, albeit at different rates. Aerobic bacteria (such as *Neisseria* spp.) may use cytochrome-containing electron transport chains for oxygen reduction and coupled ATP synthesis. In contrast, facultatively anaerobic lactic acid producing species have a flavin-containing NADH oxidase and NADH peroxidase; similarly, even *T. denticola* (which is considered to be highly anaerobic), possesses NADH oxidases and NADH peroxidases, enabling it to scavenge low levels of oxygen in the sub-gingival environment. Some of these reactions are illustrated below:

$$O_2^- + O_2^- + 2H^+ \xrightarrow{\text{superoxide dismutase}} H_2O_2 + O_2$$

$$2 H_2O_2 \xrightarrow{\text{catalase}} 2 H_2O + O_2$$

$$NADH + H^+ + H_2O_2 \xrightarrow{\text{NADH peroxidase}} NAD^+ + H_2O$$

$$2NADH + 2H^+ + 2O_2 \xrightarrow{\text{NADH oxidase}} 2NAD^+ + 2H_2O$$

Although oxygen itself is not toxic, the production of oxygen metabolites can be, and so oral bacteria possess molecular defence mechanisms to prevent or reduce oxidative damage. These mechanisms involve the production of catalase, peroxidases and superoxide dismutase (*see above*). Thus, oral organisms as metabolically diverse as mutans streptococci and *P. gingivalis* produce protective enzymes; mutans strepto- cocci produce superoxide dismutase, NADH peroxidase and glutathione reductase, while *P. gingivalis* has a superoxide dismutase. In addi- tion, the black, iron porphyrin pigment of *P. gingivalis* can bind and detoxify low levels of oxygen including reactive oxidants generated by neutrophils.

Oral malodour (halitosis)

Oral malodour is a relatively common condi- tion in the adult population. In some indivi- duals, halitosis does not necessarily correlate with poor oral hygiene, while in others it is associated with periodontal diseases, particu- larly acute necrotizing ulcerative gingivitis (ANUG, *see* Chapter 7). The metabolism of bacteria located on the tongue accounts for the majority of the malodorous compounds found in mouth air. High odour subjects generally have a higher total bacterial load on the tongue, and higher numbers of Gram-negative anae- robes, including members of the genera *Por- phyromonas*, *Prevotella*, *Fusobacterium* and *Treponema*.

Malodour production is strongly implicated with high proteolytic activity and the produc- tion of volatile sulphur compounds. The pre- dominant sulphur compounds are hydrogen sulphide, H_2S, and methyl mercaptan (CH_3SH), with smaller concentrations of di- methyl sulphide, $(CH_3)_2S$, and dimethyl di- sulphide, $(CH_3S)_2$. Hydrogen sulphide is gen- erated principally by the action of L-cysteine dehydro-sulphatase on L-cysteine, while methyl mercaptan is produced by the oxidation of L- methionine. *Fusobacterium* spp. and *P. micros* are able to form high concentrations of hydro- gen sulphide from glutathione (a tripeptide: L- δ-glutamyl-L-cysteinylglycine), which is found in most tissue cells and the periodontal pocket. Treatment of periodontal disease usually results in the resolution of halitosis; tongue scraping to reduce the microbial load at this site can also be effective.

Metabolism and inhibitors

Antimicrobial agents are used extensively in toothpastes and mouthrinses to help maintain dental plaque at levels compatible with oral health. Although they are often selected on the basis of a broad spectrum of antimicrobial

activity, they frequently function in the mouth at sub-lethal concentrations and interfere with carbohydrate and nitrogen metabolism (*see* Chapters 6 and 7; Figure 6.5).

Two of the most widely used inhibitors in dentistry can affect sugar transport by the PEP- PTS system of oral bacteria. While the primary caries-preventive action of fluoride is due to its effect on promoting remineralization and in- creasing the acid resistance of enamel (*see* Chapter 6), fluoride at low concentrations is known to decrease the rate of sugar uptake and acid production by plaque bacteria (*see* Figure 6.5). Fluoride has also been reported to reduce EPS production, and to inhibit the synthesis but not the breakdown of IPS. Fluoride inhibits enolase which converts 2-phosphoglycerate to phosphenolpyruvate. This leads to glycolysis being inhibited directly and sugar transport being affected indirectly by a reduction in the availability of PEP for the PTS. Fluoride also inhibits the ATP-synthase, and so interferes with the control of the intracellular pH, as well as metallo-enzymes (e.g., phosphatases and phosphorylases) and oxidative enzymes such as catalase and peroxidase, and this may affect the redox balance within plaque.

The fluoride sensitivity of metabolism is pH- dependent, with the greatest inhibition occur- ring under acidic conditions. This is because at low pH fluoride exists as H^+F^- which is lipophilic and more easily able to penetrate membranes (*see* Figure 6.5). The intracellular pH is relatively alkaline; therefore, once inside the cell, H^+F^- would dissociate and F^- would inhibit various enzymes as described above, while protons would acidify the cytoplasm and so tend to reduce:

(a) the activity of glycolytic enzymes with a pH optimum around neutrality;
(b) the transmembrane pH gradient (and hence pmf-driven uptake and secretion processes);
(c) the aciduricity of cells, by interfering with the membrane-bound ATP- synthase, which helps regulate intracel- lular pH.

Chlorhexidine is widely used as a mouthwash to reduce plaque and prevent or treat gingivitis. It has a broad spectrum of antimicrobial activity but at sub-lethal levels it can affect many functions associated with the bacterial membrane (*see* Figure 6.5). For example, it can

(a) abolish the activity of sugar transport by the PTS, (b) inhibit the ATP-synthase and affect the maintenance of ion gradients in streptococci, (c) interfere with arginine uptake by *S. sanguis,* and (d) inhibit the arginine-specific protease (gingipain) of *P. gingivalis.* Pyrophosphates (used in toothpastes designed to control calculus) can also inhibit the activity of the ATP-synthase.

Summary

Although the mouth is sterile at birth, the acquisition of the resident oral microflora begins within the first few hours of life. The biological properties of the mouth make it highly selective in terms of the types of micro-organisms able to colonize. Few of the species found in the mouths of adults and even fewer of the organisms of the general environment are able to establish successfully. Acquisition of the resident microflora follows a pattern of ecological succession: relatively few organisms (pioneer species) are able to colonize, but their presence enables other species to establish; this process eventually leads to a climax community with a high species diversity. Many species are acquired from the mother by transmission via saliva. For some species, there may be a relatively short time for their optimal colonization during the development of the oral microflora ('window of infectivity'). The development of a climax community in the mouth can involve both allogenic (non-microbial influenced) and autogenic (microbial influenced) succession.

The composition of the resident microflora varies at different sites around the mouth, with each site having a relatively characteristic microbial community. Mutans streptococci and S. sanguis have preferences for hard surfaces for colonization, whereas species such as S. salivarius are recovered predominantly from the oral mucosa. The tongue has the highest microbial load per area of oral mucosal surface, and can act as a reservoir for some Gram-negative anaerobes implicated in periodontal diseases.

The distribution of micro-organisms is related to their ability to adhere at a site, as well as to their nutritional and environmental requirements (pH and redox potential) being satisfied. Bacteria adhere by specific molecular interactions between adhesins located on their cell surface and receptors found in the acquired pellicle and mucus coat on enamel and mucosal surfaces, respectively. The bacterial adhesins can be structurally complex, with multiple binding sites.

In order to cope with the fluctuating nutritional conditions in the mouth, the resident oral microflora is biochemically flexible. The primary source of nutrients is the endogenous supply of host proteins and glycoproteins from saliva and GCF. Specific molecular strategies enable acidogenic bacteria to tolerate conditions of low pH that are inhibitory to other species. Some disaccharides can be metabolized extracellularly into constituent sugars (for transport) or into extracellular polysaccharides (involved in attachment or used as extracellular storage compounds). The extracellular glucans and fructans are synthesized by glucosyl- and fructosyltransferases, respectively.

The metabolism of nitrogen compounds involves the production of exo- and endopeptidases; nitrogen metabolism can lead to base production which will help regulate environmental pH. The catabolism of complex host molecules involves interactions among bacteria with complementary patterns of enzyme activity to ensure their complete breakdown. Anaerobes are found commonly at many sites in the mouth. These bacteria survive oxygen exposure by interacting with oxygen-consuming species, and by the possession of specific enzyme systems to scavenge oxygen and toxic radicals.

Halitosis involves the production of increased levels of malodorous compounds (such as hydrogen sulphide and methyl mercaptan) by proteolytic anaerobic bacteria; many of these organisms are located on the tongue. The metabolism of oral micro-organisms is sensitive to many of the inhibitors used in preventive dentistry.

Bibliography

Bowden, G.H.W. and Hamilton, I.R. (1998) Survival of oral bacteria. *Crit. Revs Oral Biol. Med.,* **9,** 54–85.

Carlsson, J. and Hamilton, I.R. (1994) Metabolic activity of oral bacteria. In *Textbook of Clinical Cariology,* 2nd edn (A. Thylstrup and O. Fejerskov, eds), Munksgaard,

Caufield, P.W., Cutter, G.R. and Dasanayake, A.P. (1993) Initial acquisition of mutans streptococci by infants: evidence for a discrete window of infectivity. *J. Dent. Res.,* **72,** 37–45.

Colby, S.M. and Russell, R.R.B. (1997) Sugar metabolism by mutans streptococci. *J. Appl. Microbiol. Symp. Suppl.,* **83,** 80S–88S.

Dashper, S.G. and Reynolds, E.C. (1992) pH regulation by *Streptococcus mutans. J. Dent. Res.,* **71,** 1159–1165.

Handley, P.S. (1990) Structure, composition and functions of surface structures on oral bacteria. *Biofouling, 2*, 239–264.

Hartley, M.G., El-Maaytah, M.A., McKenzie, C. and Greenman, J. (1996) The tongue microbiota of low odour and malodorous individuals. *Microb. Ecol. Health Dis., 9*, 215–223.

Jenkinson, H.F. and Lamont, R.J. (1997) Streptococcal adhesion and colonization. *Crit. Revs Oral Biol. Med., 8*, 175–200.

Könönen, E., Asikainen, S., Saarela, M. *et al.* (1994) The oral Gram-negative anaerobic microflora in young children: longitudinal changes from edentulous to dentate mouth. *Oral Microbiol. Immunol., 9*, 136–141.

Marquis, R.E. (1995) Oxygen metabolism, oxidative stress and acid-base physiology of dental plaque biofilms. *J. Indust. Microbiol., 15*, 198–207.

Milnes, A.R., Bowden, G.H., Gates, D. and Tate, R. (1993) Predominant cultivable microorganisms on the tongue of preschool children. *Microb. Ecol. Health Dis., 6*, 229–235.

Pearce, C., Bowden, G.H., Evans, M. *et al.* (1995) Identification of pioneer viridans streptococci in the oral cavity of human neonates. *J. Med. Microbiol., 42*, 67–72.

Percival, R.S., Challacombe, S.J. and Marsh, P.D. (1991) Age-related microbiological changes in the salivary and plaque microflora of healthy adults. *J. Med. Microbiol., 35*, 5–11.

Smith, D.J., Anderson, J.M., King, W.F., van Houte, J. and Taubman, M.A. (1993) Oral streptococcal colonization of infants. *Oral Microbiol. Immunol., 8*, 1–4.

Theilade, E. (1990) Factors controlling the microflora of the healthy mouth. In *Human Microbial Ecology* (M.J. Hill and P.D. Marsh, eds), CRC Press, Boca Raton, FLA, pp. 1–56.

Vadeboncoeur, C. and Pelletier, M. (1997) The phospho-enolpyruvate:sugar phosphotransferase system of oral streptococci and its role in the control of sugar metabolism. *FEMS Microbiol. Revs, 19*, 187–207.

Whittaker, C.J., Klier, C.M. and Kolenbrander, P.E. (1996) Mechanisms of adhesion by oral bacteria. *Ann. Rev. Microbiol., 50*, 513–552.

5

Dental plaque

Dental plaque is a general term for the complex microbial community found on the tooth surface, embedded in a matrix of polymers of bacterial and salivary origin. Plaque that becomes calcified is referred to as calculus or tartar. The presence of plaque in the mouth can readily be demonstrated by rinsing with a disclosing solution such as erythrosin. The majority of plaque is found associated with the protected and stagnant regions of the tooth surface such as fissures, approximal regions and the gingival crevice (*see* Figure 2.2). Plaque is found naturally on the tooth surface, and forms part of the host defences by excluding exogenous (and often pathogenic) species. On occasions, however, plaque can accumulate beyond levels compatible with oral health, and this can lead to shifts in the composition of the microflora and predispose sites to disease (*see* Chapters 6, 7 and 8).

Dental plaque and microbial biofilms

Studies of a range of distinct ecosytems have shown that the vast majority of micro-organisms exist in nature associated with a surface. The term '**biofilm**' is used to describe communities of micro-organisms attached to a surface; such microbes are usually spatially organized into a three-dimensional structure and are enclosed in a matrix of extracellular material derived both from the cells themselves and from the environment. If (a) biofilm microbes were simply planktonic (liquid-phase) cells that had adhered to a surface, and (b) the properties of microbial communities were merely the sum of those of the constitutive populations, then interest in such issues would have had limited scientific impact. However, research over recent years has revealed that cells growing as biofilms have unique properties, some of which have great clinical significance (Table 5.1). For example, it has been established that biofilms can be up to 1000 times more resistant to antimicrobial agents than the same cells growing in liquid culture, whilst adhesion can trigger the de-repression of certain genes, giving attached cells a novel phenotype.

Table 5.1 General properties of a biofilm

General properties
Protection from host defences and predators
Protection from desiccation
Protection from antimicrobial agents
• Surface-associated phenotype[a]
• Slow growth rate
• Poor penetration
• Inactivation/neutralization
Novel gene expression and phenotype[a]
Persistence in flowing systems
Spatial and environmental heterogeneity
Spatial organization facilitating metabolic interactions
Elevated concentration of nutrients

[a]One consequence of altered gene expression can also be an increased resistance to antimicrobial agents.

Originally, biofilms were considered to be dense, compressed accumulations of cells. A major recent advance in the study of biofilms has come from the application of novel techniques which enable biofilms to be studied *in situ* without any processing of samples which could distort their structure. An example has been the use of confocal scanning laser microscopy (CSLM) to study biofilm architecture without chemical fixation or embedding techniques. Optical thin sections can be generated throughout the depth of the biofilm, and these can be combined using imaging software to generate three-dimensional images. In addition, the location of specific organisms can be visualized with immunological or nucleic acid probes, while other molecular probes can indicate the vitality and metabolic activity of cells. CSLM can also be used in combination with 'reporter gene technology' to identify genes that are expressed only within a biofilm. This technology involves the insertion of a marker into the bacterial chromosome downstream of a promoter so that a recognizable 'signal' (e.g. fluorescence) is produced when the gene is activated.

The application of these modern approaches to microbial ecology has shown that biofilms that develop in low nutrient environments, especially those from aquatic habitats, have a more open structure than had been predicted previously by electron microscopy. For example, void spaces and water channels, which would enable potentially growth-limiting factors such as nutrients and oxygen to penetrate more extensively, have been observed in environmental biofilms. In addition, micro-electrodes and chemical probes have shown that considerable gradients in key factors (pH, redox potential, etc.) can occur over relatively short distances (a few microns, i.e. a few cell diameters) within biofilms. This produces spatial and temporal heterogeneity within the biofilm enabling fastidious bacteria to survive in apparently hostile or incompatible environments (Table 5.1).

In a biofilm, the properties of an organism may be affected in more than one way. The attachment of cells to a surface may cause a direct effect, perhaps by triggering 'touch sensors' on the cell surface. Adhesion to surfaces has been shown to specifically induce the expression of certain genes, e.g. those involved in exopolysaccharide (alginate) synthesis by *Pseudomonas aeruginosa*. In addition, the growth environment within the biofilm may differ significantly from planktonic culture with respect to key factors. This may result in altered gene expression, and hence an altered phenotype, as an indirect effect of growth in a biofilm. Likewise, organisms may be growing more slowly, e.g. due to a particular nutrient limitation or an unfavourable pH, and this will also affect the properties of a cell. Often, it is difficult to resolve whether any observed phenotypic changes are due to the direct or indirect effects of being in a biofilm. For most practical purposes, the reasons for any phenotypic alteration are less important than the biological significance of the change itself.

A substantial body of evidence has proved that biofilm bacteria are phenotypically distinct from planktonic cells. One particularly important aspect of this is an elevated resistance of biofilm cells to antimicrobial agents. An extreme example was the finding that *Pseudomonas aeruginosa* growing on urinary catheter material was 500–1000 times more resistant to tobramycin than the same cells from liquid culture. Conventionally, the sensitivity of bacteria to antimicrobial agents is determined on cells grown in liquid culture by the measurement of the minimum inhibitory concentration (MIC) or minimum bactericidal concentration (MBC). Given the decreased sensitivity of an organism on a surface to antimicrobial agents, it has been argued that it would be more appropriate to determine the 'biofilm inhibitory concentration (BIC)' and 'biofilm killing concentration (BKC)'. As yet, however, these proposals have not been widely accepted, and there are no generally agreed methods by which these concentrations could be determined.

The increased resistance of biofilms to antimicrobial agents may be due to the age and structure of the biofilm, and to the chemical properties of the agent. In addition, attachment may induce (or de-repress) genes that are not normally expressed during growth in liquid culture. Such genes may alter the phenotype of cells in such a way as to make them more resistant. In addition, biofilms contain extracellular polymers (sometimes described as a **matrix** or **glycocalyx**); these can form a thick, continuous, hydrated, charged layer around a cell. Such a matrix could hinder the access of certain antimicrobial agents, perhaps by a combination of ionic interactions or by molecular sieving effects ('exclusion hypothesis'). The binding of positively charged antibiotics (e.g. aminoglycosides) can occur, although such effects may be minimal for less charged anti-

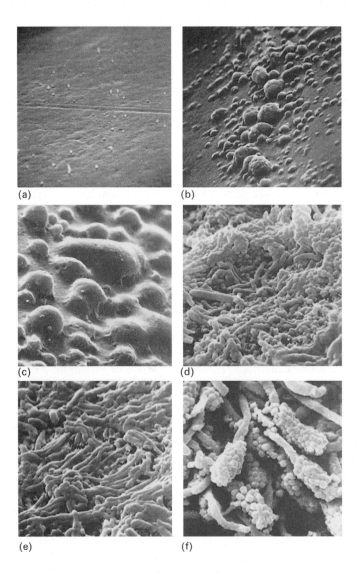

(a)   (b)   (c)   (d)   (e)   (f)

Figure 5.1 Development of dental plaque on a clean enamel surface. Coccal bacteria attach to the enamel pellicle as pioneer species (*a*) and multiply to form micro-colonies (*b*) eventually resulting in confluent growth (a biofilm) embedded in a matrix of extracellular polymers of bacterial and salivary origin (*c*). With time, the diversity of the microflora increases, and rod and filament-shaped bacteria colonize (*d* and *e*). In the climax community, many unusual associations between different bacterial populations can be seen, including 'corn-cob' formations (*f*). (Original magnification approx. ×1150) Published with permission of Dr A. Saxton

biotics such as tobramycin. Exopolymers can also bind, and therefore concentrate, extracellular enzymes, such as β-lactamases, that are capable of degrading or inactivating some antimicrobials. Generally, bacteria grow slowly in biofilms, either because of nutrient limitation or to unfavourable conditions, and the phenotype of these cells is often inherently more resistant to antimicrobial agents.

Dental plaque was probably the first biofilm to have been studied in terms of either its microbial composition or its sensitivity to antimicrobial agents. In the seventeenth century, Antonie van Leeuwenhoek pioneered the approach of studying biofilms by direct microscopic observation when he reported on the diversity and high numbers of 'animalcules' present in scrapings taken from around human teeth. He also conducted early studies on the novel properties of surface-grown cells when he failed to kill plaque bacteria *in situ* on his teeth by prolonged rinsing with wine-vinegar; in contrast, the organisms were 'killed' if they were first removed from his molars and mixed with vinegar in his laboratory.

The following sections describe the key features of dental plaque, with particular emphasis on properties that relate to its biofilm structure. Another dentally relevant biofilm develops on the tubing associated with dental unit water supply systems (DUWS); this will be discussed in detail in a later chapter, but some of the principles governing their formation and properties will be similar to those described below for dental plaque.

Development of dental plaque

Bacteria rarely come into contact with clean enamel. As soon as a tooth surface is cleaned, salivary glycoproteins are adsorbed forming a surface conditioning film which is termed the acquired enamel pellicle (*see* Chapter 4) (Figure 5.1). Pellicle shows local variations in chemical composition and this can influence the pattern of microbial deposition. Large numbers of bacteria (up to 10^8 CFU/ml) are found in saliva and, unless swallowed, any of these organisms are likely to come into contact with a tooth surface. Indeed, the colonization of many oral populations is related directly to their concentration in saliva.

Coccal bacteria are adsorbed onto the pellicle-coated enamel within two hours of cleaning. These pioneer species include *Neisseria* and streptococci, predominantly members of the *S. mitis*-group (e.g. *S. sanguis*, *S. oralis* and *S. mitis*) (Table 5.2). *Actinomyces* spp. are also commonly isolated after 2 hours, as are haemophili, but obligately anaerobic species are detected only rarely at this stage and usually occur in low numbers. These pioneer populations multiply, forming micro-colonies which become embedded in bacterial extracellular slimes and polysaccharides together with addi-

tional layers of adsorbed salivary proteins and glycoproteins (Figure 5.1*a* and *b*).

Table 5.2 Proportions of bacteria in developing supragingival plaque

Bacterium	Time of plaque development (h)		
	2	24	48
S. sanguis	8	12	29
S. oralis	20	21	12
mutans streptococci	3	2	4
S. salivarius	<1	<1	<1
A. naeslundii	6	7	5
A. odontolyticus	2	3	6
Haemophilus spp.	11	18	21
Capnocytophaga spp.	<1	<1	<1
Fusobacterium spp.	<1	<1	<1
Black-pigmented anaerobes	0	<0.01	<0.01

Growth of individual micro-colonies eventually results in the development of a confluent film of micro-organisms (Figure 5.1*c–e*). Growth rates of bacteria are fastest during this early period, with doubling times ranging from 1 to 3 hours. Studies with gnotobiotic rats have shown that individual species vary in their doubling times (t_d); *S. mutans* and *A. naeslundii* had t_d of 1.4 and 2.7 hours, respectively. In human plaque, the gross microbial generation times were less than 60 minutes during the first 4 hours of plaque formation, but this increased to between 13 and 15 hours in more mature biofilms (aged 24–72 hours). The proportions of the *S. mitis*-group increase during the first 48 hours of plaque formation. The majority of isolates are *S. sanguis* and *S. mitis*; fewer *S. gordonii* are recovered during these early stages. Many of these early colonizers produce IgA1 proteases, which may enable them to evade the effects of sIgA.

As plaque develops into a biofilm so the metabolism of the pioneer species creates conditions suitable for colonization by bacteria with more demanding atmospheric requirements. Oxygen is consumed by the aerobic and facultatively anaerobic species and replaced with carbon dioxide and other gases generated as end products of microbial metabolism. Gradually the Eh is lowered, which favours the growth of obligately anaerobic species. Additional nutrients also become available due to the metabolism of the pioneer species,

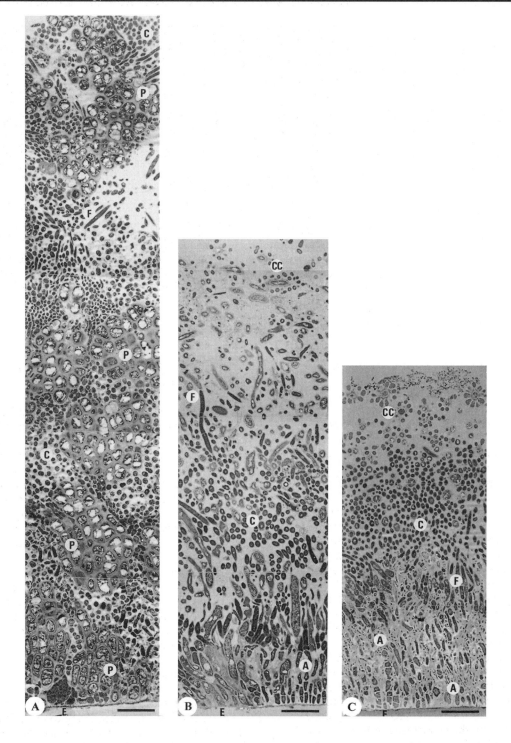

Figure 5.2 Ultrastructure of 2-week-old dental plaque from three individuals with different patterns of microbial colonization (A–C). C, Gram-positive coccal bacteria; F, Gram-negative filamentous bacteria; CC, corn-cob formations; P, large, irregular shaped bacteria; E, space remaining after demineralization of enamel. Bar = 5 μm. (Published with permission of B. Nyved, O. Fejerskov and Munksgaard)

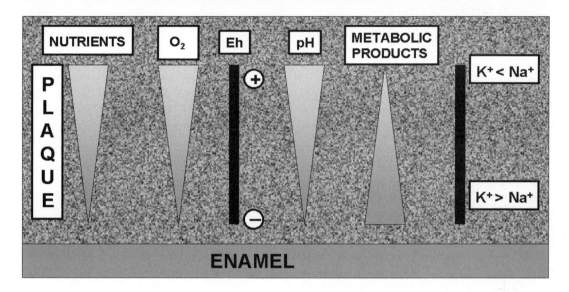

Figure 5.3 Schematic representation of the development of gradients in dental plaque

and the diversity of the microflora increases both in terms of the morphological types (Figure 5.1 *d–f*) and in the actual numbers of species.

The predominant bacteria colonizing the root surfaces (using an *in situ* appliance model) were streptococci, particularly *S. oralis*, *S. mitis* and *S. sanguis*; the proportions of *S. salivarius* decreased with time. The few Gram-positive rods recovered during the early stages are mainly *Actinomyces* spp. *Stomatococcus mucilagenosus* was found to be an early plaque colonizer in some people but not others. *Propionibacterium* spp., *Rothia dentocariosa* and haemophili are found occasionally, and Gram-negative cocci (*Neisseria* and *Veillonella* spp.) make up a small fraction (approximately 2%) of the total cultivable microflora. Figure 5.2 shows a pallisading structure of dental plaque from a root surface.

If plaque is allowed to accumulate undisturbed (as happens at stagnant sites) then there is a shift in the proportions of the bacteria within the biofilm. After 7 days, streptococci remain the dominant group of organisms but by 14 days, they constitute only around 15% of the cultivable microflora, and anaerobic rods and filaments predominate. The composition of the climax community varies depending on the site; the predominant bacteria will be described in a later section.

Structure and organization of dental plaque

The accumulation of plaque on teeth will be a result of the balance between adhesion, growth and removal of micro-organisms. The development of plaque in terms of mass will continue until a critical size is reached. Shear forces will then limit any further expansion, although structural development and re-organization take place continually. Electron microscopy has demonstrated both pallisaded regions (where filaments and cocci are aligned in parallel at right-angles to the enamel surface) and micro-colonies (presumably of single populations). In mature plaque, organisms have been seen in direct contact with the enamel due to enzymatic attack on the pellicle. Electron microscopy has also confirmed the presence of an inter-bacterial matrix of polysaccharide; this may function as a carbohydrate reserve and contribute towards the structure of the biofilm by facilitating the formation of channels.

Many bacterial associations can be observed, in which cocci are arranged along the length of filamentous organisms. Such associations are described as 'corn-cob' and 'test tube brush' formations (Figure 5.1*f*). The components of the 'corn-cob' will be described later.

As discussed earlier, the preparation of samples for electron microscopy may distort and compress the natural structure of biofilms. CSLM has recently been used to study the architecture of dental plaque that had developed on *in situ* devices (containing removable enamel surfaces) placed in the mouth. Dental plaque on these surfaces had a more open structure than previously thought. Channels have been seen consistently in these samples, similar to those observed in biofilms from environmental habitats.

Gradients extending over short distances will exist in plaque for many of the parameters (physical and chemical) influencing microbial growth and survival. Sites close together may be vastly different in the concentration of key nutrients, pH, Eh and concentrations of toxic products of metabolism (Figure 5.3). Such vertical and horizontal stratifications will cause local environmental heterogeneity resulting in a mosaic of micro-environments (and hence microhabitats). Each microhabitat potentially could support the growth of a different microbial community. Similarly, organisms residing in apparently the same general environment might be growing under quite dissimilar conditions and, therefore, exhibiting a different phenotype. Thus, when studying plaque, it is essential to take small samples from defined areas.

Mechanisms of dental plaque formation

The development of a biofilm such as dental plaque can be sub-divided arbitrarily into several stages. As a bacterium approaches a surface a number of specific and non-specific interactions will occur between the substratum and the cell which will determine whether attachment and colonization will take place. Distinct stages in plaque formation include:

1 Adsorption of host and bacterial molecules to the tooth surface to form a conditioning film (the acquired pellicle) (*see* Chapter 4).
2 Transport of micro-organisms to the pellicle-coated tooth surface.
3 Long-range physico-chemical interactions between the microbial cell surface and the pellicle-coated tooth. The interplay of van der Waals attractive forces and electrostatic repulsion can produce a weak area of net attraction that facilitates reversible adhesion.
4 Short-range interactions involving specific, stereo-chemical interactions between adhesins on the microbial cell surface and receptors in the acquired pellicle; these interactions usually result in irreversible adhesion.
5 The co-aggregation (or co-adhesion) of micro-organisms to already attached cells; this stage results in an increased diversity of the plaque microflora.
6 The multiplication of the attached organisms to produce confluent growth and a biofilm. Extracellular polymer synthesis also occurs, and
7 The detachment of cells from the biofilm into the planktonic phase (usually saliva), facilitating colonization of fresh sites.

These stages are shown schematically in Figure 5.4, and will be described below. It should be remembered that the seven phases distinguished above are only arbitrary and the attachment, growth, removal and reattachment of bacteria is a continuous and dynamic process, and a microbial biofilm such as plaque will undergo continuous reorganization.

Pellicle formation, microbial transport to the host surface and long-range physico-chemical forces

Micro-organisms are transported passively to the tooth surface by the flow of saliva; only a few oral bacterial species are motile. Organisms do not colonize clean enamel but interact with specific molecules of host (predominantly) and bacterial origin present in the acquired pellicle (*see* Chapter 4). As the cell approaches the pellicle-coated surface, long range physico-chemical forces operate. Micro-organisms are negatively charged due to the molecules on their cell surface, while acidic proteins present in the acquired pellicle would also produce a net negative charge. The Derjaguin and Landau and the Verwey and Overbeek (DLVO) theory has been used to describe the interaction between an inert particle (as a micro-organism might be envisaged at large separation distances) and a substratum. This theory states that the total interactive energy, V_T, of two smooth particles is determined solely by the sum of the van der Waals attractive energy (V_A)

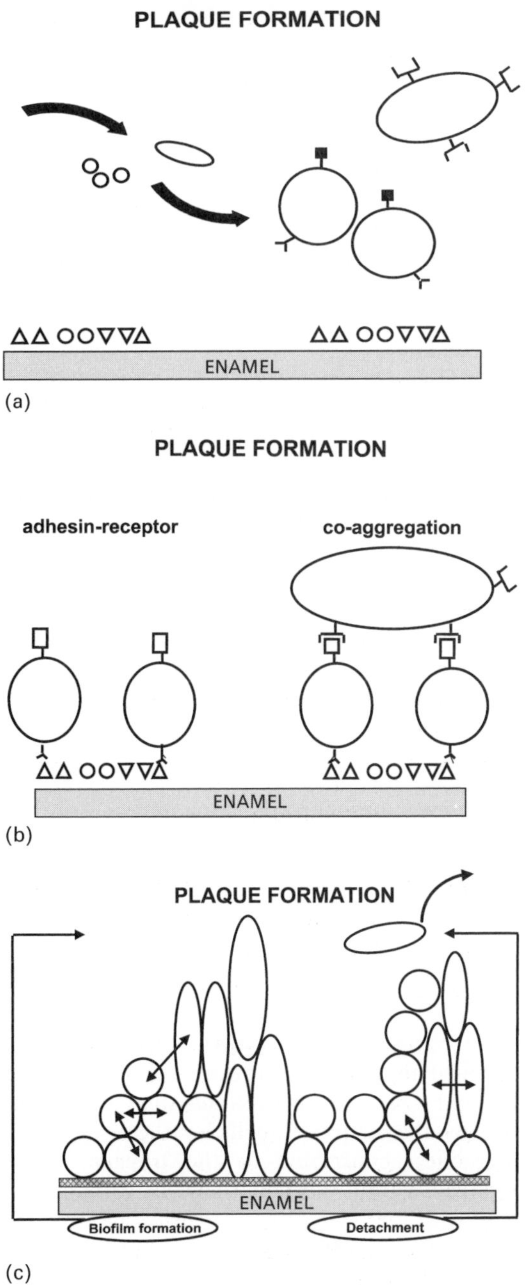

PLAQUE FORMATION

(a)

PLAQUE FORMATION

adhesin-receptor   co-aggregation

(b)

PLAQUE FORMATION

Biofilm formation   Detachment

(c)

Figure 5.4 Schematic representation of the different stages in the formation of dental plaque: (*a*) bacteria are transported passively to the tooth surface where they may be held reversibly by weak electrostatic forces of attraction; (*b*) attachment becomes irreversible by specific stereochemical molecular interactions between adhesins on the bacterium and receptors in the acquired pellicle, before; (*c*) growth results in biofilm formation, facilitating interbacterial interactions. Eventually, detachment can occur, sometimes as a result of the degradation by bacteria of their adhesins

and the usually repulsive, electrostatic energy (V_R). Particles in aqueous suspension and surfaces in contact with aqueous solutions can acquire a charge due to, for example, the preferential adsorption of ions from solution or the ionization of certain groups attached to the particle or surface. The charge on a surface in solution is always exactly balanced by an equivalent number of counter ions. Thus, the charge of a surface and the corresponding counter ion charge in solution form an electrical double layer the size of which is inversely proportional to the ionic strength of the environment. As a particle approaches a surface, therefore, it experiences a weak van der Waals attraction induced by the fluctuating dipoles within the molecules of the two approaching surfaces. This attraction increases as the particle moves closer to the substratum. However, if the surfaces continue to approach each other a repulsive force is encountered due to the overlap of the electrical double layers.

Curves can be plotted which show the variation of the total interactive energy, V_T, of a particle and a surface with the separation distance, *h* (Figure 5.5, see overleaf). A net attraction can occur at two values of *h*; these are referred to as the primary minimum (*h* very small) and the secondary minimum (*h* = 10–20 nm) and are separated by a repulsive maximum. The reversible nature of bacterial deposition suggests that the primary minimum is not usually encountered while the high ionic strength of saliva will increase the likelihood of oral bacteria experiencing a secondary minimum. Bacteria captured by a surface in this way are in equilibrium with the remaining organisms in the suspending medium, while the number of captured cells will be dependent on the concentration of bacteria in suspension and on the depth of the secondary minimum.

The pattern of deposition could also be influenced by the type of interface from which the bacteria deposit. In many systems, bacteria adhere from a solid–liquid interface such as when a surface is immersed in a suspension of micro-organisms. In the mouth, however, a solid–liquid–air (s–l–a) interface is common which could be static but is more likely to be moving due to the continuous drainage of saliva over oral tissues. Oral bacteria and polymeric material in saliva preferentially adsorb at the s–l–a interface, and so the movement of these interfaces over the teeth

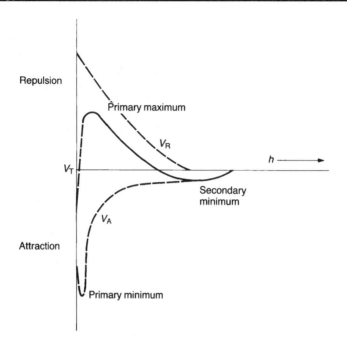

Figure 5.5 Diagram illustrating the DLVO theory. The total interactive energy, V_T, between a particle and a surface is shown with respect to the separation distance, h. The total interaction curve is obtained by the summation of an attraction curve, V_A, and a repulsion curve, V_R

may be important in the formation of dental plaque.

At separation distances of between 10 and 20 nm, organisms may be held irreversibly in a weak secondary minimum. With time, this interaction may become irreversible due to adhesins on the cell surface becoming involved in specific short-range interactions. For this to occur, water films must be removed from between the interacting surfaces. A major role of cell hydrophobicity and hydrophobic cell surface components is their dehydrating effect on this water film enabling the surfaces to get closer so that short range interactions can occur. A direct relationship between the degree of cell surface hydrophobicity and the adhesion of oral bacteria to saliva-coated surfaces has been demonstrated.

The binding of bacteria to saliva-coated hydroxyapatite beads has been used as a model of oral bacterial adhesion. Such binding is saturable and reversible, and can be described by the Langmuir adsorption isotherm. Analysis of such isotherms suggests a 'two-site' model involving high- and low-affinity binding sites. Such models have also shown how saliva can modulate bacterial attachment. The binding of

S. sanguis and certain *Actinomyces* spp. to hydroxyapatite was enhanced by a salivary pellicle, whilst attachment of other species (e.g. *S. mutans, S. salivarius*) was reduced.

Molecular interactions between adhesins and receptors

Short range forces involve specific stereochemical interactions between components on the microbial cell surface (**adhesins**) and **receptors** in the acquired pellicle; these types of interaction contribute to the **tropism** of an organism with a particular surface or habitat.

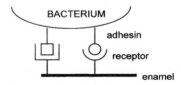

Several examples of these molecular interactions have been characterized (Table 5.3). In addition, adhesins on *S. gordonii* can bind to α-amylase, while *A. naeslundii* and *F. nucleatum* interact with statherin. *S. mutans* (but not *S. sobrinus*), *P. gingivalis*, *P. loescheii* and

P. melaninogenica adhere preferentially to hydroxyapatite treated with proline-rich proteins (PRPs), although different regions of the acidic PRPs bind to particular organisms. Colonization by *S. sobrinus* appears to involve sucrose-mediated mechanisms, such as the interaction of glucans with receptors (including glucan binding proteins).

Table 5.3 Some examples of host–bacterial interactions involved in adhesion

Bacterium	Adhesin	Receptor
Streptococcus spp.	Antigen 1/11	Salivary agglutinin
Streptococcus spp.	LTA	Blood group reactive glycoproteins
mutans streptococci	Glucan binding protein	Glucan
S. parasanguis	35 kDa lipoprotein	Fibrin, pellicle
A. naeslundii	Type 1 fimbriae	Proline-rich proteins
P. gingivalis	150 kDa protein	Fibrinogen
P. loescheii	70 kDa lectin	Galactose
F. nucleatum	42 kDa protein	Co-aggregation with *P. gingivalis*

Some adhesion mechanisms involve lectin-like bacterial proteins interacting with carbohydrates, or oligosaccharides, in glycoproteins adsorbed to the tooth surface. Thus, *S. sanguis* can bind to terminal sialic acid residues in adsorbed salivary glycoproteins, while *S. oralis* expresses either a galactose-binding lectin or a lectin that interacts with a trisaccharide structure containing sialic acid, galactose and *N*-acetylgalactosamine.

Actinomyces spp. have two antigenically and functionally distinct types of fimbriae; type 1 fimbriae mediate bacterial adherence to PRPs and to statherin (i.e. a protein–protein interaction), whereas type 2 fimbriae are associated with a lactose sensitive mechanism (i.e. a lectin-like activity) involving the adherence of cells to already attached bacteria (**co-aggregation**, *see below*) or to buccal epithelial cells.

A number of proteins in the cell walls of streptococci have been identified as adhesins. A high molecular weight protein from *S. mutans* (termed antigen I/II, B, P1 or Pac), interacts with salivary agglutinins. Antibody directed against this surface molecule blocked adhesion of *S. mutans* to saliva-coated surfaces. Similar proteins have been found on other streptococci, with one segment being highly conserved. The large size of some of the bacterial cell wall proteins mean that they may be involved in more than one function. For example, a protein of *S. gordonii* can interact both with salivary proteins and with *A. naeslundii* (co-aggregation). Some of the other adhesins found on *S. sanguis* and *S. gordonii* are now known to be lipoproteins (*see* Chapter 4).

Streptococci probably rely on multiple adhesins to bind to saliva-coated surfaces, e.g. *S. sanguis* can adhere via lectin-like, hydrophobic and/or specific protein (adhesin) interactions. Such adhesins can be expressed simultaneously on more than one macromolecule, while a single adhesin may contain more than one adhesive domain or epitope. For example, *S. sanguis* can express a 150 kDa protein that possesses two distinct adhesive epitopes. *S. gordonii* possesses more than one adhesin enabling it to bind to at least three distinct receptors: (a) acidic proline-rich proteins, (b) salivary agglutinins and (c) salivary amylase. These adhesins may include cell surface proteins of 20–36 kDa or 82–87 kDa (the size can vary with the strain) which bind to amylase, and a 162 kDa sialic acid-binding lectin for the proline-rich proteins and the agglutinins.

A critical factor in plaque formation centres around the site at which the specific interactions between bacterial adhesins and host receptors takes place. The host-derived receptors reside on molecules that are not only adsorbed to the tooth surface but which are also freely accessible in solution in saliva. Some of these molecules are designed to aggregate bacteria in solution, thereby facilitating their removal from the mouth by swallowing (*see* Chapter 2). For plaque formation to proceed, however, it is implicit that all bacteria are not aggregated in saliva before they reach the tooth surface. A novel mechanism may function to overcome this problem. It was found that although *A. naeslundii* could bind to the acidic proline-rich peptides when the latter were bound to a surface, cells did not interact with this protein in solution. It has been proposed that hidden molecular segments of PRPs become exposed, as a result of conformational changes, only when the protein is adsorbed to hydroxyapatite.

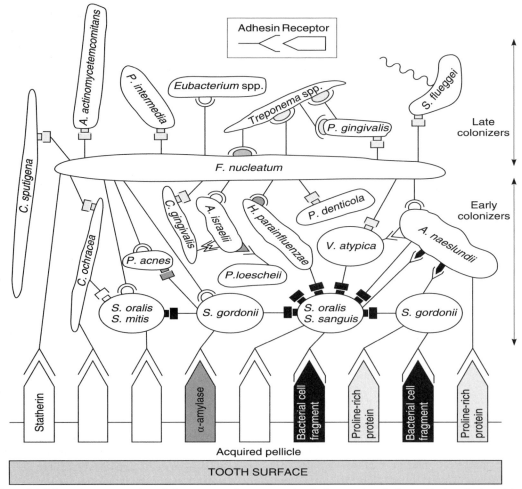

Figure 5.6 Schematic representation of the patterns of co-aggregation in human dental plaque. Early colonizers bind to receptors in the acquired pellicle; subsequently, other early and later colonizers bind to these already attached cells (co-aggregation). Adhesins (symbols with stems) are cell components that are heat- or protease-sensitive; the receptor (complementary symbol) is insensitive to either treatment. Identical symbols do not imply identical molecules. The symbols with rectangular shapes represent lactose-inhibitable co-aggregations. (Reproduced from Kolenbrander and London, 1993, with permission American Society for Microbiology)

Such hidden receptors for bacterial adhesins have been termed **'cryptitopes'**. In this way, a selective mechanism for facilitating natural plaque formation has evolved by which the host can promote the attachment of specific bacteria without compromising this process in the planktonic phase.

Adhesins which recognize cryptitopes in surface-associated molecules would provide a strong selective advantage for any micro-organism which colonizes a mucosal or tooth surface. Another example of a cryptitope involving conformational change is the binding of members of the *S. mitis*-group to fibronectin when complexed to collagen but not to

fibronectin in solution. It has been suggested that this might be a mechanism whereby certain oral streptococci are able to colonize damaged heart valves in endocarditis. A different type of cryptitope involves the recognition of galacto-syl-binding lectins by oral bacteria. Epithelial cells and the acquired enamel pellicle have mucins with oligosaccharide side chains with a terminal sialic acid. Bacteria such as *A. naeslundii* synthesize neuraminidase which cleaves the sialic acid exposing the penultimate galactosyl sugar residue. Many oral bacteria possess galactosyl-binding lectins including *A. naeslundii*, *L. buccalis*, *F. nucleatum*, *E. corro-dens* and *P. intermedia*, and would benefit from the exposure of these cryptitopes. Similarly, the binding of *P. gingivalis* is greater to epithelial cells that have been mildly treated with trypsin. Some periodontopathogens, including *P. gingivalis,* produce proteases with an arginine specificity that may create appropriate cryptitopes for their colonization.

Co-aggregation

Co-aggregation (or co-adhesion) is the cell-to-cell recognition of genetically distinct partner cell types, and has been observed with isolates representing 18 bacterial genera from the mouth (Figure 5.6). Early plaque accumulation is facilitated by intrageneric co-aggregation among streptococci and among actinomyces, as well as by intergeneric co-aggregation between streptococci and actinomyces. The subsequent development of dental plaque will involve further intergeneric co-aggregation between other genera and the primary colonizers. For example, co-aggregation can occur between:

Gram-positive species:
e.g. *S. sanguis* and *Actinomyces* spp.,
or *S. mitis*   *C. matruchotii,* or *P. acnes*

Gram-negative species:
e.g. *P. melaninogenica* and *F. nucleatum*

Gram-positive and Gram-negative species:
e.g.
Streptococcus spp. and *Prevotella* spp.,
or *Actinomyces* spp.   *Capnocytophaga* spp.,
                        F. nucleatum, E. corrodens,
                        Veillonella spp. or *P. gingivalis*

Co-aggregation often involves lectins; these carbohydrate-binding proteins interact with the complementary carbohydrate-containing receptor on another cell. Thus, the lectin-mediated interaction between streptococci and actinomyces can be blocked by adding galactose or lactose, or by treating the receptor with a protease. The process of co-aggregation can also lead to the development of the 'corn-cob' structures (*see* Figure 5.1*f*). 'Corn-cobs' can be formed between 'tufted-fibril' streptococci (*see* Chapters 3 and 4) and *C. matruchotii*; similar associations have also been found between *Eubacterium* and *Veillonella* spp.

Detailed studies of the co-aggregation between *A. naeslundii* and *S. sanguis* or *S. mitis* have identified three types of interaction. One involves a lectin on the fimbriae of the Gram-positive rod and a receptor on the streptococcus; the interaction is inhibited by galactose or lactose, and by heat or protease treatment of the *Actinomyces* but not of the streptococcus. The second type of interaction involves a heat- or protease-sensitive lectin on the streptococcus binding to 'treatment-resistant' receptors on the *Actinomyces*, while the third involves labile components on both cell types.

Fusobacteria have been found to co-aggregate with the widest range of bacterial genera although, curiously, they do not co-aggregate with each other. Early colonizers of plaque co-aggregate extensively with *F. nucleatum*, while late colonizers such as *Selenomonas flueggei* or *Eubacterium* spp. do not co-aggregate with early colonizers but do co-aggregate with *F. nucleatum*. It has been proposed that fusobacteria act as a bridge between early and late colonizing bacteria (Figure 5.6).

Lectin-mediated co-aggregation may be an important mechanism in the structural organization of microbial communities such as dental plaque. The development of food-chains including those between streptococci and veillonellae, and the formation of the 'corn-cob' structures might be facilitated by co-aggregation. Likewise, the persistence and survival of obligately anaerobic bacteria in an essentially aerobic habitat has been shown to be enhanced by the presence of oxygen-consuming species with which the anaerobes are able to co-aggregate.

Multiplication, polymer synthesis and biofilm formation

Once the pioneer bacteria have attached, then growth and micro-colony formation will occur. The early colonizers include members of the *S. mitis*-group; the production of an IgA_1 protease by *S. sanguis* and *S. oralis* may enable these bacteria to survive and proliferate during the early stages of plaque formation. These early colonizers possess extensive glycosidase activity which will enable them to use salivary glycoproteins for growth. In addition, salivary molecules will continue to be adsorbed on to bacteria already attached to the tooth surface and, therefore, several of the adhesive mechanisms described above will continue to operate. As stated earlier, the growth rate of bacteria within plaque will change as the biofilm matures. Measurements made in humans have shown that mean doubling times of < 60 minutes during the first 4 hours of plaque formation increase to between 12 and 15 hours after 24–72 hours.

Another important phase in the development of plaque is the synthesis of extracellular polymers by adherent bacteria. In particular, the synthesis of water-insoluble mutan by *S. mutans* will make a significant contribution to the structural integrity of plaque, and may help create and maintain channels within plaque. Glucosyltransferases (GTF) are responsible for the synthesis of a range of soluble and insoluble glucans (*see* Chapter 4). GTFs can be secreted, and adsorb onto other bacteria or onto the tooth surface to form part of the acquired pellicle. In both situations, the GTFs can remain functional and contribute to plaque formation. The structure of the glucan produced by adsorbed GTF may differ to that synthesized by the enzyme in solution. Fructans produced by FTFs are short-lived in plaque, and act as extracellular storage compounds for use by other plaque bacteria.

Plaque development involves the growth of the attached bacteria to produce a biofilm. Research on surface-associated growth of micro-organisms from other habitats suggests that the physiology of bacteria in plaque might be different from that predicted from studies of the organisms in liquid cultures. Gene expression may be altered on a surface. Expression of GTF genes, but not the gene for FTF activity, was up-regulated several-fold when *S. mutans* was attached to saliva-coated hydroxyapatite; such effects were more apparent in older than younger biofilms. Similarly, lactic acid production by some oral streptococci was enhanced by surfaces. The initial rate of growth of bacteria on a surface from a variety of habitats has also been shown to be faster compared to the same cells growing in liquid culture. This may be because there is an increased concentration of nutrients at an interface between a surface and a liquid. Another explanation is based on the hypothesis that energy-conserving and energy-sharing interactions between bacterial cells would be more likely to occur on a surface, particularly in a biofilm. Studies of ecosystems as diverse as the gastrointestinal tract and marine sediments have recovered bacteria able to utilize end products of metabolism such as lactate in close association with lactate-producers.

Research of other habitats has provided evidence of cell density dependent growth (quorum sensing), whereby individual cells are able to communicate with, and respond to, neighbouring cells by means of diffusible effector molecules (bacterial 'hormones', e.g. the homoserine lactones of Gram-negative or peptides in Gram-positive bacteria). The rate of growth is increased when a critical number of organisms are 'sensed'. There has been a report of a type of quorum sensing occurring during plaque development; when a critical cell density $(2–6 \times 10^6$ cell/mm^2) was reached, the growth rate of cells attached to an intra-oral surface was enhanced, before being reduced when higher cell densities are reached.

The sensitivity of surface-associated oral micro-organisms to a range of antibiotics and disinfectants is reduced compared to the same organisms in solution. Older biofilms of *S. sanguis* were less susceptible to chlorhexidine than younger biofilms; the biofilm killing concentration for the former being 200 μg/ml compared with 50 μg/ml for the latter. Diverse mixed cultures of oral bacteria when grown as a biofilm were unaffected when exposed to concentrations of chlorhexidine equivalent to MIC values of the component species. Ten-fold higher concentrations were needed to demonstrate some effectiveness, but even at these levels, some species were not inhibited.

Detachment from surfaces

Bacteria can detach themselves from a surface, or from within the biofilm, so as to be able to colonize elsewhere. An enzyme synthesized by *S. mutans* was shown to be able to liberate surface proteins from its own cell surface and thereby detach itself from a mono-species biofilm. Similarly, a protease produced by *P. loescheii* could hydrolyse its own fimbrial-associated adhesin which was responsible for co-aggregation with *S. oralis* as well as binding to host molecules such as fibrin.

The final outcome of these phases is the development of a complex, multi-species, spatially and functionally organized biofilm. The diversity of potential mechanisms for adherence together with the molecular heterogeneity of the microbial and host surface will mean that biofilm formation involves multiple interactions.

Bacterial composition of the climax community of dental plaque from different sites

Environmental conditions on a tooth are not uniform; different surfaces vary in their degree of protection from oral removal forces and in the source of nutrients. These differences will be reflected in the composition of the microbial community, particularly at sites so obviously distinct as the gingival crevice, approximal regions, smooth surfaces, and pits and fissures.

Fissure plaque

The microbiology of fissure plaque has been determined using either 'artificial fissures' implanted in occlusal surfaces of pre-existing restorations, or by sampling 'natural' fissures. The microflora is mainly Gram-positive and is dominated by streptococci, especially extracellular polysaccharide-producing species. In one study, no obligately anaerobic Gram-negative rods were found, while others have recovered anaerobes including *Veillonella*, and *Propionibacterium* spp. in low numbers (Table 5.4). *Neisseria* spp. and *Haemophilus parainfluenzae* have also been isolated on occasions. A striking feature of the microflora is the wide range of numbers and types of bacteria in the different fissures (1×10^6 to 33×10^6 CFU per fissure) (Table 5.4), suggesting that the ecology of individual fissures might vary. The simpler community found in fissures compared to other enamel surfaces probably reflects a more severe environment, perhaps with a relatively limited range of nutrients. Saliva will be of significance as a nutrient source compared to the gingival crevice. The distribution of bacteria within a fissure has not been studied, although it has been claimed that lactobacilli and mutans streptococci preferentially inhabit the lower depths of a fissure. Environmental conditions at the base of the fissure will certainly be very different in terms of nutrient availability, pH, buffering effects of saliva, etc. than areas nearer the plaque surface (Figure 5.7).

Approximal plaque

The main organisms isolated from approximal plaque are shown in Table 5.5. Although streptococci are present in high numbers, these sites are frequently dominated by Gram-positive rods, particularly *Actinomyces* spp. The more reduced nature of this site compared to that of fissures can be gauged from the higher recovery of obligately anaerobic organisms although spirochaetes are not commonly found. Again, the range and percentage isolation frequency of most bacteria is high, suggesting that each site represents a distinct ecosystem.

Table 5.4 The predominant cultivable microflora of 10 occlusal fissures in adults

Bacterium	Median % of total cultivable microflora	Range	Isolation frequency (%)
Streptococcus	45	8–86	100
Staphylococcus	9	0–23	80
Actinomyces	18	0–46	80
Propionibacterium	1	0–8	50
Eubacterium	0	0–27	10
Lactobacillus	0	0–29	20
Veillonella	3	0–44	60
Individual species			
mutans streptococci	25	0–86	70
S. sanguis-group	1	0–15	50
S. oralis-group	0	0–13	30
S. anginosus-group	0	0–3	10
A. naeslundii	3	0–44	70
L. casei	0	0–10	10
L. plantarum	0	0–29	10

Gingival crevice plaque

The gingival crevice is an obviously distinct microbial habitat, influenced both by the anatomy of the site and the flow and properties of GCF. This is reflected in the higher species diversity at this site, although the total numbers of bacteria can be low (10^3–10^6 CFU/crevice). In contrast to the microflora of fissures and approximal surfaces, higher levels of obligately anaerobic bacteria can be found, many of which are Gram-negative (Table 5.6). Indeed, spirochaetes and anaerobic streptococci are isolated almost exclusively from this site (Figure 5.8). Many organisms are asaccharolytic but proteolytic, and derive their energy from the hydrolysis of host proteins and peptides and from the catabolism of amino acids found in GCF. In disease, the gingival crevice enlarges to become a periodontal pocket (*see* Figure 2.1)

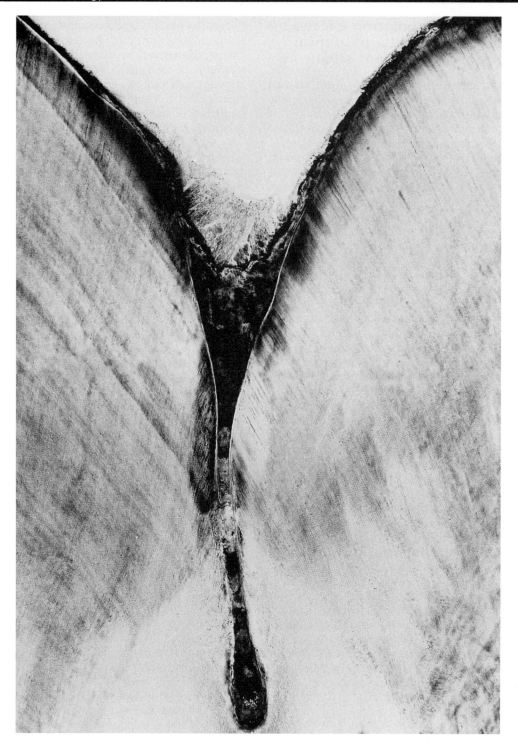

Figure 5.7 Dental plaque in a fissure on the occlusal surface of a molar. (Original magnification approx. ×100; courtesy K.M. Pang)

Table 5.5 The predominant cultivable microflora of approximal plaque

Bacterium	Median % of total cultivable microflora	Range	Isolation frequency (%)
Streptococcus	23	0.4–70	100
Gram-positive rods (predominantly *Actinomyces*)	42	4–81	100
Gram-negative rods (predominantly *Prevotella*)	8	0–66	93
Neisseria	2	0–44	76
Veillonella	13	0–59	93
Fusobacterium	0.4	0–5	55
Lactobacillus	0.5	0–2	24
Rothia	0.4	0–6	36
Individual species			
mutans streptococci	2	0–23	66
S. sanguis	6	0–64	86
S. salivarius	1	0–7	54
S. anginosus-group	0.5	0–33	45
A. israelii	17	0–78	72
A. naeslundii	19	0–74	97

and the flow of GCF increases. The diversity of the microflora increases still further and will be described in more detail in Chapter 7. Among the genera and species associated with the healthy gingival crevice are members of the *S. mitis*-group and *S. anginosus*-group; in addition, Gram-positive rods such as *Actinomyces meyeri*, *A. odontolyticus*, *A. naeslundii*, *A.*

georgiae and *Rothia dentocariosa* can also be found. The most commonly isolated black-pigmented anaerobe in the healthy gingival crevice is *P. melaninogenica* while *P. nigrescens* has also been recovered on occasions; *P. gingivalis* is rarely isolated from healthy sites. Fusobacteria are among the commonest anaerobes found in the healthy gingival crevice.

Denture plaque

The microflora of denture plaque from healthy sites (i.e. with no sign of denture stomatitis, *see* Chapter 8) is highly variable as can be deduced from the wide ranges in viable counts obtained for individual bacteria shown in Table 5.7. Clear differences are also apparent between the fitting and the exposed surfaces of the denture. In the relatively stagnant area on the denture-fitting surface, plaque tends to be more acidogenic, thereby favouring streptococci (especially mutans streptococci) and sometimes *Candida* spp. In edentulous subjects, dentures become the primary habitat for mutans streptococci and members of the *S. sanguis*-group. Denture plaque can harbour obligate anaerobes including *A. israelii* and low proportions of Gram-negative rods. Interestingly, *Staphylococcus aureus* has been regularly isolated from denture plaque (Table 5.7); it is also found commonly in the mucosa of patients with denture stomatitis (*see* Chapter 11).

Table 5.6 The predominant cultivable microflora of the healthy gingival crevice

Bacterium	Mean % of total cultivable microflora	Range	Isolation frequency (%)
Gram-positive facultatively anaerobic cocci (predominantly *Streptococcus*)	40	2–73	100
Gram-positive obligately anaerobic cocci (predominantly *Peptostreptococcus*)	1	0–6	14
Gram-positive facultatively anaerobic rods (predominantly *Actinomyces*)	35	10–63	100
Gram-positive anaerobic rods	10	0–37	86
Gam-negative facultatively anaerobic cocci (predominantly *Neisseria*)	0.3	0–2	14
Gram-negative obligately anaerobic cocci (predominantly *Veillonella*)	2	0–5	57
Gram-negative obligately negative facultatively anaerobic rods	ND	ND	ND
Gram-negative obligately rods	13	8–20	100

Samples were taken from the gingival crevice of seven adult humans.
ND, not detected.

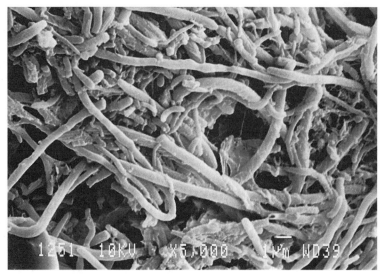

Figure 5.8 Scanning electron micrograph of sub-gingival plaque, showing rods, curved rods, filaments and spiral-shaped cells. (Original magnification approx. ×5000; courtesy K.M. Pang)

Table 5.7 The predominant cultivable microflora of denture plaque

Micro-organism	Viable count (%) Median	Range	Isolation frequency (%)
Streptococcus	41	0–81	88
mutans streptococci	< 1	0–48	50
S. sanguis-group	1	0–4	63
S. oralis-group	2	0–30	75
S. anginosus-group	2	0–51	63
S. salivarius	0	0–41	38
Staphylococcus	8	1–13	100
S. aureus	6	0–13	88
'*S. epidermidis*'	0	0–7	13
Gram-positive rods	33	1–74	100
Actinomyces	21	0–54	88
A. israelii	3	0–47	63
A. naeslundii	3	0–48	63
A. odontolyticus	0	0–48	25
Propionibacterium	< 1	0–5	50
Veillonella	8	3–20	100
Gram-negative rods	0	0–6	38
Yeasts	0.002	0–0.5	63

Dental plaque from animals

There is interest in the microbial composition of dental plaque from animals for two main reasons: (a) to study the influence of widely different diets and life-styles on the microflora, and (b) to determine the similarity between the microflora of an animal with that of humans to ascertain their relevance as a model of human oral diseases. At the genus level, the plaque microflora is similar among animals representing such diverse dietary groups as insectivores, herbivores and carnivores. This again emphasizes the significance of endogenous nutrients in maintaining the stability and diversity of the resident microflora. Thus, *Actinomyces, Streptococcus, Neisseria, Veillonella* and *Fusobacterium* are widely distributed in both zoo and non-zoo primates and other animals, and can, therefore, be genuinely considered as autochthonous members of dental plaque (*see* Chapter 4). Following recent taxonomic studies, differences between isolates from man and animals have emerged at the species level. For example, *S. rattus* and *S. macacae* are isolated exclusively from rodents and primates, respectively, whereas different species of mutans streptococci are found in humans.

Plaque fluid

Plaque fluid is the free aqueous phase of plaque, and can be separated from the microbial components by centrifugation. Plaque fluid has a different composition from both saliva and GCF. In particular, the protein content of plaque fluid is higher than that of saliva, as are the concentrations of several important ions including sodium, potassium, magnesium and fluoride. Likewise, the levels of albumin, lactoferrin and lysozyme are greater in plaque fluid than saliva, although this trend is reversed for amylase (Table 2.2). A number of enzymes of both bacterial and host (e.g. from polymorphs) origin can be detected in plaque fluid. Specific host defence factors are also found in plaque fluid; sIgA is present at the same concentration as in whole saliva whereas IgG and complement are at higher levels, and are probably derived from GCF. Fluoride binds to plaque components, but is also found free in plaque fluid. Bound fluoride can be released from these components because fluoride concentrations increase in plaque fluid when the pH falls during the bacterial metabolism of fermentable carbohydrates. Acidic products of metabolism are retained in plaque fluid, and shifts in their profile from a hetero- to a homofermentative pattern can be observed following the intake of dietary sugars. The ratio of K^+/Na^+ is higher in plaque fluid, and this can enhance acid production and GTF secretion by oral streptococci.

Calculus

Calculus, or tartar, is the term used to describe calcified dental plaque. It consists of intra- and extracellular deposits of mineral, including apatite, brushite and whitlockite, as well as protein and carbohydrate. Mineral growth can occur around any bacteria; areas of mineral growth can then coalesce to form calculus which may become covered by an unmineralized layer of bacteria. Calculus can occur both supragingivally (especially near the salivary ducts) and sub-gingivally, where it may act as an additional retentive area for plaque accumulation, thereby increasing the likelihood of gingivitis and other forms of periodontal disease. Calculus can be porous leading to the retention of bacterial antigens and the stimulation of bone resorption by toxins from periodontal pathogens. Over 80% of adults have calculus, and its prevalence increases with age. An elevated calcium ion concentration in saliva may predispose some individuals to be high calculus formers. Once formed, huge removal forces are required to detach calculus; this removal takes up a disproportionate amount of clinical time during routine visits by patients to the dentist. Consequently, a number of dental

products are now formulated to restrict calculus formation. These products contain pyrophosphates, zinc salts, or polyphosphonates to inhibit mineralization by slowing crystal growth and reducing coalescence. These agents may provide some antimicrobial benefit by inhibiting the ATP-synthase of oral bacteria; this enzyme is important in the control of intracellular pH in bacterial cells.

Microbial interactions in dental plaque

In a biofilm such as dental plaque, microorganisms are in close proximity with one another and interact as a consequence. These interactions can be beneficial to one or more of the interacting populations, while others can be antagonistic (Table 5.8). Microbial metabolism within plaque will produce localized gradients in factors affecting the growth of other species, ranging from the depletion of essential nutrients with the simultaneous accumulation of toxic or inhibitory by-products (*see* Figure 5.3), to the consumption of oxygen enabling the growth of obligate anaerobes. These gradients lead to the development of vertical and horizontal stratifications within the plaque biofilm, which enables organisms with widely differing requirements to grow, and ensures the coexistence of species that would be incompatible with one another in a homogeneous habitat.

Table 5.8 Factors involved in microbial interactions in dental plaque

Beneficial	Antagonistic
Enzyme complementation	Bacteriocins
Food chains (food webs)	Hydrogen peroxide
Co-aggregation	Organic acids
	Low pH
	Nutrient competition

Synergistic interactions

Although competition for nutrients will be one of the primary ecological determinants dictating the prevalence of species in dental plaque, bacteria also have to collaborate in order to breakdown the complex endogenous substrates. Salivary proteins and glycoproteins are the

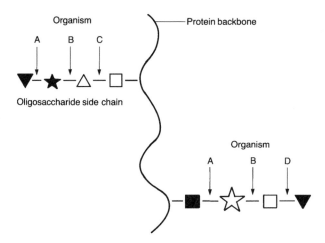

Figure 5.9 Bacterial cooperation in the degradation of host glycoproteins (enzyme complementation). For example, organisms A and D are able to cleave the terminal sugar of the oligosaccharide side chain, which enables organism B to cleave the penultimate residue, etc.

major sources of nitrogen and carbon in plaque. Individual species of oral bacteria possess different but overlapping patterns of glycosidase and protease activity, so that the concerted action of several species is necessary for the complete degradation of host molecules (Figure 5.9, and *see* Figure 5.11). For example, the growth of some organisms will be dependent on others for the removal of the terminal carbohydrate from the oligosaccharide side chain of a glycoprotein to expose subsequent sugars.

Microbial cooperation in the breakdown of host macromolecules was observed when subgingival bacteria were grown on human serum (used to mimic GCF). Shifts in the microbial composition of the consortia occurred at different stages of glycoprotein breakdown. Initially, carbohydrate side chains were removed by organisms with complementary glycosidase activities, including *S. oralis*, *E. saburreum* and *Prevotella* spp. This was followed by the hydrolysis of the protein core by anaerobes such as *P. intermedia*, *P. oralis*, *F. nucleatum*, and to a lesser extent, *Eubacterium* spp.; some amino acid fermentation occurred and the remaining carbohydrate side chains were metabolized leading to the emergence of *Veillonella* spp. A final phase was characterized by progressive protein degradation and extensive amino acid fermentation; the predominant species included *Peptostreptococcus micros* and *E. brachy*. Significantly, individual species grew only poorly in pure culture in serum. A consequence of these interactions is that different species avoid direct competition for individual nutrients, and hence are able to coexist. This type of interaction is an example of protocooperation or mutualism, whereby there is benefit to all participants that are involved in the interaction.

Bacterial polymers are also targets for degradation. Some types of extracellular polysaccharide (*see* Table 4.6) can be metabolized by other bacteria in the absence of exogenous (dietary) carbohydrates. The fructan of *S. salivarius* and other streptococci, and the glycogen-like polymer of *Neisseria*, are particularly labile, and only low levels of fructan are detected in plaque. In addition, mutans streptococci, members of the *S. mitis*-group, *S. salivarius*, *A. israelii*, *Capnocytophaga* spp. and *Fusobacterium* spp. possess exo- and/or endo-hydrolytic activity and metabolize streptococcal glucans.

Another type of nutritional interaction is when the products of metabolism of one organism (primary feeder) become the main source of nutrients for another (secondary feeder). For example, lactate produced from the metabolism of dietary carbohydrates by a range of other species can be utilized by *Veillonella* spp. and converted to weaker acids. In this way, *Veillonella* spp. could reduce the cariogenic potential of other plaque bacteria. Evidence to support this hypothesis came from

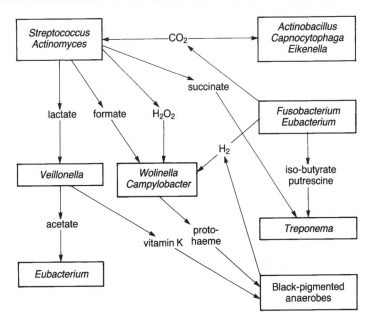

Figure 5.10 Some potential nutritional interactions (food chains) between plaque bacteria

gnotobiotic animal studies. Fewer carious lesions were obtained in rats inoculated with either *S. mutans* or *S. sanguis* and *Veillonella* than in animals mono-infected with either of the streptococci:

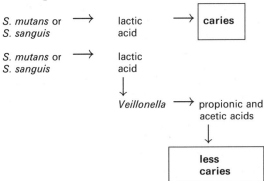

Strains of *Neisseria*, *Corynebacterium* and *Eubacterium* are also able to metabolize lactate.

Other nutritional interactions between oral bacteria have been described in the laboratory. Under anaerobic conditions, a strain of *S. mutans* required *p*-aminobenzoic acid for growth, and this could be supplied by *S. sanguis*. Oral spirochaetes can be dependent on the production of iso-butyrate and putrescine or spermine by fusobacteria, and on succinate produced by various Gram-positive

rods. Similarly, *Fusobacterium* and *Prevotella* species provide hydrogen and formate for the growth of *Wolinella* spp., while the metabolism of some black-pigmented anaerobes is dependent on the synthesis of vitamin K by other bacteria in the gingival crevice. As can be deduced from this evidence, a complex array of interbacterial nutritional interactions can take place in plaque, with the growth of some species being dependent on the metabolism of other organisms. Indeed the diversity of the plaque microflora is due, in part, to (a) the development of such food chains and food webs (Figure 5.10) and (b) the lack of a single nutrient limiting the growth of all bacterial species. Bacterial survive by adopting, where possible, alternative metabolic strategies in order to avoid direct competition. Another beneficial interaction among plaque bacteria is co-aggregation which can aid colonization of surfaces and also facilitate metabolic interactions between mutually dependent strains.

Antagonistic interactions

Antagonism is also a major contributing factor in the determination of the composition of microbial ecosystems such as dental plaque. The production of antagonistic compounds (such as bacteriocins or bacteriocin-like substances (BLIS)) can give an organism a competitive advantage when interacting with other microbes. Bacteriocins are relatively high molecular weight proteins that are encoded by a plasmid; the producer strains are resistant to the action of the bacteriocins they produce. Bacteriocins are produced by most species of oral streptococci (e.g. mutacin by *S. mutans* and sanguicin by *S. sanguis*), as well as by *C. matruchotii*, black-pigmented anaerobes, and *A. actinomycetemcomitans*. In contrast, *Actinomyces* species are not generally bacteriocinogenic. Although bacteriocins are usually limited in their spectrum of activity, many of the streptococcal bacteriocins are broad spectrum, inhibiting species belonging to several Gram-positive genera including *Actinomyces* spp. A strain of *S. sanguis* was active not only against most Gram-positive species but also against Gram-negative bacteria including *Capnocytophaga* and *Prevotella* species. In gnotobiotic animal studies, only bacteriocin-producing strains of *S. mutans* could become established, with the degree of colonization being proportional to the level of *in vitro* activity. Interestingly, even bacteriocin-producing strains of *S. mutans* had difficulty in colonizing when the rat microflora became conventionalized, and hence more complex in composition. The likely explanation for this colonization resistance was that all of the available niches within the microbial community were now occupied.

Other inhibitory factors produced by plaque bacteria include organic acids, hydrogen peroxide and enzymes. The production of hydrogen peroxide by members of the *S. mitis*-group has been proposed as a mechanism whereby the numbers of periodontopathic bacteria are reduced in plaque to levels at which they are incapable of initiating disease. Some periodontal pathogens (e.g. *A. actinomycetemcomitans*) produce factors inhibitory to oral streptococci, so that certain periodontal diseases (*see* Chapter 7) might result from an ecological imbalance between dynamically interacting groups of bacteria. The low pH generated from carbohydrate metabolism is also inhibitory to many plaque species, particularly Gram-negative organisms. The production of antagonistic factors will not necessarily lead to the complete exclusion of sensitive species. As discussed previously, the presence of distinct micro-habitats within a biofilm such as plaque enables bacteria to survive that would

be incompatible with one another in a homogeneous environment. Also, where there is competition for nutrients, the production of inhibitory factors might be a mechanism whereby less-competitive species can persist (negative feed-back).

Bacterial metabolism will also be a mechanism whereby exogenous (allochthonous) species are prevented from colonizing the oral cavity. For example, some *S. salivarius* strains can produce an inhibitor (enocin or salivaricin) active against Lancefield group A streptococci. Bacteriocin-producing strains may prevent colonization of the mouth by this pathogen in a manner similar to that proposed for streptococci in the pharynx. It has been claimed that *S. salivarius* is more frequently isolated from the throats of children who do not become colonized following exposure to group A streptococci than from those who do become infected. Thus, microbial interactions will play a major role in determining both the final composition and the pattern of development of the plaque microflora.

Dental plaque as a microbial community

Numerous studies have shown that oral bacteria do not behave randomly during the development of dental plaque. Plaque forms in an organized manner via physico-chemical and specific inter-molecular adhesin-receptor interactions, followed later by inter-bacterial co-aggregation. These interactions produce a spectrum of ecological niches (metabolic functions, *see* Chapter 1) enabling the survival and growth of fastidious species by:

(a) the synergistic catabolism of complex host macromolecules so that substrates can be utilized that would be recalcitrant to degradation by individual species;

(b) modulation of local environmental conditions (pH, oxygen tension, redox potential etc.), enabling the growth of obligate anaerobes in an overtly aerobic habitat, and of pH-sensitive bacteria during periods of low pH; and (c) efficient nutrient and energy cycling via cross-feeding and food webs.

Great metabolic diversity exists within the plaque microflora, ranging from organisms capable of cleaving complex host polymers into smaller units, to sulphate reducing bacteria and methanogens that gain energy from the utilization of simple end products of metabolism (Figure 5.11). In such a microbial community, the metabolic efficiency of the whole is greater than that of the sum of the individual species, since substrate utilization involves both the concerted and sequential catabolism of these complex molecules. Growth of such a community as a biofilm confers additional benefits since cells are protected from the host defences, antimicrobial agents and from other hostile factors. In addition, the closely coupled physical and metabolic interactions leave few niches

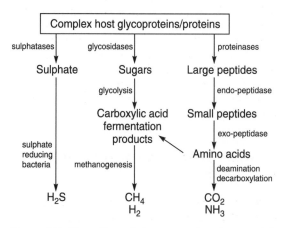

Figure 5.11 Illustration of the concerted and sequential breakdown of complex host substrates by communities of oral bacteria with complementary enzyme activities

unfilled, thereby reducing the likelihood of colonization by exogenous microbes, and contributes to the natural microbial stability of the flora of plaque (microbial homeostasis; *see below*).

Microbial homeostasis in dental plaque

In spite of its microbial diversity, the composition of dental plaque at any site is characterized by a remarkable degree of stability or balance among the component species. This stability is maintained in spite of the host defences, and despite the regular exposure of the plaque community to a variety of modest environmental stresses. These stresses include diet, the regular challenge by exogenous species, the use of dentifrices and mouthwashes containing antimicrobial agents, and changes in saliva flow and hormone levels (Figure 5.12). The ability to maintain community stability in a variable environment has been termed **microbial homeostasis.** This stability stems not from any metabolic indifference among the components of the microflora but results rather from a balance of dynamic microbial interactions, including synergism and antagonism. When the environment is perturbed, self-regulatory mechanisms (homeostatic reactions) come into force to restore the original balance. An essential component of such mechanisms is negative feedback, whereby a change in one or

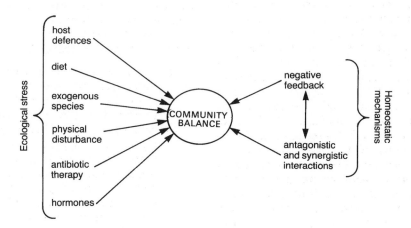

Figure 5.12 Factors involved in the maintenance of microbial homeostasis in the mouth

more organisms results in a response by others to oppose or neutralize such a change. There is a tendency for homeostasis to be greater in microbial communities with a higher species diversity.

Table 5.9 Factors responsible for the breakdown of microbial homeostasis

Immunological factors	Non-immunological factors
sIgA-deficiency	Xerostomia
Neutrophil dysfunction	Antibiotics
Chemotherapy-induced myelosuppression	Dietary carbohydrates/ low pH
Infection-induced myelo- suppression (e.g. AIDS)	Increased GCF flow
	Oral contraceptives

Despite the microbial diversity of dental plaque, homeostasis does break down on occasions. The main causes for this can be divided into either (a) deficiencies in the immune response, or (b) other (non-immune) factors (Table 5.9). The host defences, together with the resident microflora, serve to maintain microbial homeostasis in plaque (and on other oral surfaces), and together they act synergistically to prevent colonization by exogenous species and the invasion of host tissues by opportunistic pathogens. The remainder of this book will be devoted to describing the consequences of the breakdown of microbial homeostasis in the mouth, and describe the aetiology of the major oral diseases.

Summary

Dental plaque is a microbial biofilm with a high species diversity, embedded in polymers of salivary and bacterial origin, found on the tooth surface. The development of dental plaque is an example of autogenic succession whereby microbial factors influence the pattern of the development of the microflora. The formation of dental plaque can be divided arbitrarily into a number of distinct stages. These include the adsorption of host and bacterial molecules to form the acquired pellicle, transport of bacteria to the pellicle-coated tooth surface, a reversible phase involving van der Waals attractive forces and electrostatic repulsion, an irreversible phase involving specific inter-molecular interactions between bacterial adhesins and host receptors, co-aggregation of bacteria to already attached organisms and cell division leading to confluent growth and biofilm formation. The properties of bacteria in a biofilm can be different from those of planktonically grown cells. Gene expression can be altered on a surface, and cells in biofilms are more resistant to antimicrobial agents.

The pioneer species that form the plaque biofilm include members of the S. mitis-group, haemophili and Neisseria spp.; many of the streptococci produce an IgA protease. The composition of the climax community of plaque shows variations at different sites on the tooth surface due to differences in their biological properties. The microbial community of fissures is less diverse than that of approximal sites and the gingival crevice. Obligate anaerobic bacteria form a significant part of the microflora from these latter two sites, so special precautions are necessary when sampling and processing plaque from these areas in order to maintain the viability of these micro-organisms.

The balance of the microflora at a site remains reasonably stable unless severely perturbed by an environmental stress. Such a stable microflora is also able to prevent exogenous species from colonizing. This stability (termed microbial homeostasis) is due to a dynamic balance of microbial interactions, including synergism and antagonism. Synergistic interactions include co-aggregation, the development of food-chains and the concerted degradation of complex host and bacterial polymers. Antagonism can be due to the production of bacteriocins, hydrogen peroxide, enzymes, organic acids and low pH. The spatial heterogeneity of a biofilm such as plaque can lead to the coexistence of species that would be incompatible with one another in a homogeneous environment. Dental plaque functions as a true microbial community; the interactions of the component species results in a metabolic efficiency and diversity that is greater than the sum of its constituent species.

Bibliography

Babaahmady, K.G., Marsh, P.D., Challacombe, S.J. and Newman, H.N. (1997) Variations in the predominant cultivable microflora of dental plaque at defined sub-sites on approximal tooth surfaces in children. *Archs Oral Biol.*, **42**, 101–111.

Costerton, J.W., Lewandowski, Z., Caldwell, D.E., Korber, D.R. and Lappin-Scott, H.M. (1995) Microbial biofilms. *Ann. Rev. Microbiol.*, **49**, 711–745.

Edgar, W.M. and Higham, S.M. (1990) Plaque fluid as a bacterial milieu. *J. Dent. Res.*, **69**, 1332–1336.

Gibbons, R.J. (1989) Bacterial adhesion to oral tissues: a model for infectious diseases. *J. Dent. Res.*, **68**, 750–760.

Kolenbrander, P.E. and London, J. (1993) Adhere today, here tomorrow: oral bacterial adherence. *J. Bacteriol.*, **175**, 3247–3252.

Listgarten, M.A. (1994) The structure of dental plaque. *Periodontol. 2000*, **5**, 52–65.

Marsh, P.D. (1989) Host defences and microbial homeostasis: role of microbial interactions. *J. Dent. Res.*, **68**, 1567–1575.

Marsh, P.D. (1995) Dental plaque. In *Microbial Biofilms* (H.M. Lappin-Scott and J.W. Costerton, eds), Cambridge University Press, Cambridge, pp. 282–300.

Milnes, A.R., Bowden, G.H., Gates, D. and Tate, R. (1993) Normal microbiota on the teeth of preschool children. *Microb. Ecol. Health Dis.*, **6**, 213–227.

Novak, M.J. (ed.) (1997) Biofilms on oral surfaces: implications for health and disease. *Adv. Dent. Res.*, **11**, 4–196.

Nyvad, B. and Kilian, M. (1987) Microbiology of the early colonization of human enamel and root surfaces *in vivo*. *Scand. J. Dent. Res.*, **95**, 369–380.

Slots, J. (1977) Microflora of the healthy gingival sulcus in man. *Scand. J. Dent. Res.*, **85**, 247–254.

Theilade, E., Fejerskov, O., Karring, T. and Theilade, J. (1982) Predominant cultivable microflora of human dental fissure plaque. *Infect. Immun.*, **36**, 977–982.

White, D.J. (1997) Dental calculus: recent insights into occurrence, formation, prevention, removal and oral health effects of supragingival and subgingival deposits. *Eur. J. Oral Sci.*, **105**, 508–522.

Wilson, M. (1996) Susceptibility of oral bacterial biofilms to antimicrobial agents. *J. Med. Microbiol.*, **44**, 79–87.

6

Dental caries

In industrialized societies, caries affects the vast majority of individuals. Caries of enamel surfaces is particularly common up to the age of 20 years, whereas, in later life, root surface caries is an increasing problem due to gingival recession exposing the vulnerable cementum to microbial colonization. Dental caries can be defined as the localized destruction of the tissues of the tooth by bacterial fermentation of dietary carbohydrates. Cavities begin as small demineralized areas below the surface of the enamel; once enamel has been affected, caries can progress through the dentine and into the pulp. Demineralization of the enamel is caused by acids, particularly lactic acid, produced from the microbial fermentation of dietary carbohydrates. Lesion formation involves dissolution of the enamel and the transport of the calcium and phosphate ions away into the surrounding environment. The initial stages of caries are reversible and remineralization can occur, particularly in the presence of fluoride.

Relationship of plaque bacteria to disease: general principles

Preventive and curative regimens for caries, periodontal disease and other plaque-mediated diseases would be more precise if the particular micro-organism(s) causing the disease was known. Historically, for any microbe to be considered responsible for a given condition, Koch's postulates were applied:

1 The microbe should be found in all cases of the disease with a distribution corresponding to the observed lesions.

2 The microbe should be grown on artificial media for several subcultures.

3 A pure subculture should produce the disease in a susceptible animal.

To these three postulates was added:

4 A high antibody titre to the microbe should be detected during infection; this may provide protection on subsequent reinfection.

Despite extensive sampling of plaque in health and disease, together with data from studies using gnotobiotic and germ-free animal experiments, no single microbe has been found which completely satisfies Koch's postulates for plaque-mediated diseases. The groups of organisms associated with disease will be described later in this chapter and in Chapter 7; these 'pathogens', however, can often be detected at healthy sites, albeit in lower numbers. Thus, another version of Koch's postulates has had to be devised to explain the role of individual bacteria from plaque in caries or one of the periodontal diseases:

1 A microbe should be present in sufficient numbers to initiate disease.

2 The microbe should generate high levels of specific antibodies.

3 The microbe should produce relevant virulence factors.

4 The microbe should cause disease in an appropriate animal model.

5 Elimination of the microbe should result in clinical improvement.

There have been two main schools of thought on the role of plaque bacteria in the aetiology of caries and periodontal diseases. The **'specific plaque hypothesis'** proposed that, out of the diverse collection of organisms comprising the resident plaque microflora, only a few species are actively involved in disease. This proposal has been valuable because it focused efforts on controlling disease by targeting preventative measures and treatment against a limited number of organisms. In contrast, the **'non-specific plaque hypothesis'** considered that disease is the outcome of the overall activity of the total plaque microflora. In this way, a heterogeneous mixture of micro-organisms could play a role in disease. In some respects, the arguments about the relative merits of these hypotheses may be about semantics, since plaque-mediated diseases are essentially mixed culture (polymicrobial) infections, but in which only certain (perhaps specific!) species are able to predominate. The arguments then centre around the definitions of the terms specific and non-specific. If not actually specific, then the diseases certainly show evidence of specificity. Recently, an alternative hypothesis has been proposed (the **'ecological plaque hypothesis'**) which reconciles the key elements of the earlier two hypotheses. In brief, the ecological plaque hypothesis proposed that the organisms associated with disease may also be present at sound sites, but at levels too low to be clinically relevant. Disease is a result of a shift in the balance of the resident microflora due to a change in local environmental conditions, e.g. repeated conditions of low pH in plaque following frequent sugar intake favours the growth of species that cause caries. These theories will be discussed later in more detail.

Evidence for caries as an infectious disease

In his famous Chemico-Parasitic Theory, Miller (1890) suggested that oral bacteria converted dietary carbohydrates into acid, which solubilized the calcium phosphate of the enamel to produce a caries lesion. Although Clarke isolated an organism (which he called *Streptococcus mutans*) from a human caries lesion in 1924, definitive proof for the causative role of bacteria came only in the 1950s and 1960s following experiments with germ-free animals.

Pioneer experiments showed that germ-free rats developed caries when infected with bacteria described as enterococci. Evidence for the transmissibility of caries came from studies on hamsters. Caries-inactive animals had no caries even when fed a highly cariogenic (i.e. sucrose-rich) diet. Caries only developed in these animals when they were caged with or ate the faecal pellets of a group of caries-active hamsters. Further proof came when streptococci, isolated from caries lesions in rodents, caused rampant decay when inoculated into the oral cavity of previously caries-inactive hamsters, while animals treated with appropriate antibiotics did not develop caries. The importance of diet became apparent when the colonization and production of caries by most streptococcal populations occurred only in the presence of sucrose.

Mutans streptococci can cause caries of smooth surfaces, as well as in pits and fissures, in hamsters, gerbils, rats and monkeys fed on cariogenic diets, and are the most cariogenic group of bacteria found. Other bacteria, including members of the *S. mitis*-, *S. anginosus*-, and *S. salivarius*-groups, *E. faecalis*, *A. naeslundii*, *A. viscosus* and lactobacilli, can also produce caries under conducive conditions in some animals, although the lesions are usually restricted to fissures. The key role of mutans streptococci in dental caries has also been demonstrated during vaccination studies. Immunization of rodents or primates with whole cells or specific antigens of *S. mutans* and *S. sobrinus* reduced the number of these organisms in plaque and decreased the number of caries lesions when compared with control animals.

Aetiology of human enamel caries

Unlike the studies of animals, any relationship between particular oral bacteria and caries in humans must be derived by indirect means. Patients on long-term broad-spectrum antibiotic therapy frequently exhibit a reduced caries experience, while epidemiological surveys of different human populations have found a strong association between mutans streptococci and caries.

Natural history of dental caries

Cavitation is the final stage of enamel caries (Figure 6.1); it is preceded by a clinically detectable small lesion, known as a 'white spot', and before that by sub-surface demineralization, which can only be detected by histological techniques (Figure 6.2). Not all white-spot lesions progress to cavitation; in some studies only about half of these early lesions penetrated the dentine after 3–4 years. White-spot lesions do not just arrest, but can even remineralize, a process that is enhanced by fluoride. Enamel caries often occurs in teeth shortly after eruption (hence, its association with young people), and some teeth and surfaces are more vulnerable than others. The prevalence of caries is highest on the occlusal surfaces of first and second molars, and lowest on the lingual surfaces of mandibular teeth. The risk to approximal surfaces is intermediate to those described above. Some individuals are more caries prone than others, and this may be related to their diet (e.g. frequency of sugar intake), saliva flow (e.g. flow is severely reduced in xerostomia patients), and exposure to fluoride.

Implications for the design of studies of the aetiology of caries

The ability of lesions to de- and remineralize at different rates can complicate the interpretation of clinical studies. In **cross-sectional surveys**, pre-determined surfaces in a population are sampled at a single time point, and the plaque microflora is related to the caries status of the site at that time. However, it cannot be determined for certain whether the species that are isolated at the time of lesion diagnosis caused the decay or arose because of it. Only 'associations' can be derived from these latter study designs, but they have the advantage that large numbers of sites/people can be analysed, and different patient groups, age groups, tooth surfaces etc. can be compared. Likewise, it cannot be determined whether the lesion, at the time of sampling, was progressing, arrested, or healing, and each phase may have a different microflora. In order to overcome these difficulties, **longitudinal studies** have been designed in which initially clinically sound sites are sampled at regular intervals over a set time period. Surfaces are selected on the basis of previous epidemiological surveys from which it can be predicted that a statistically suitable number of sites should decay within the time span of the

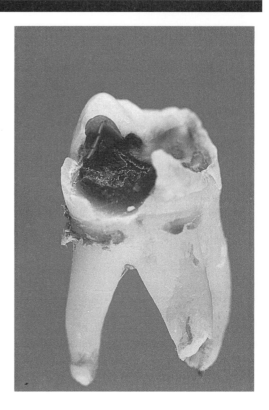

Figure 6.1 Extensive cavitation

study. The microflora can then be compared: (a) before and after the diagnosis of a lesion, and (b) between those surfaces that decayed and those that remained caries-free throughout the study, so that true cause-and-effect relationships can be established. A disadvantage of this approach is that, for practical reasons, only a limited number of individuals can be followed.

Superimposed on the problems of study design outlined above, are those associated with the microbiological analysis of plaque (*see* Chapter 4). The plaque microflora is diverse, and disease is not due to exogenous species, which would be easy to identify, but to changes in the relative proportions of members of the resident microflora. There are wide inter-subject variations in the composition of the plaque microflora (*see* Chapter 5), so that when data is averaged from numerous individuals, clear associations between bacteria and disease can be obscured. Despite these problems of study design and methodology, much progress has been made, and the major findings will now be discussed.

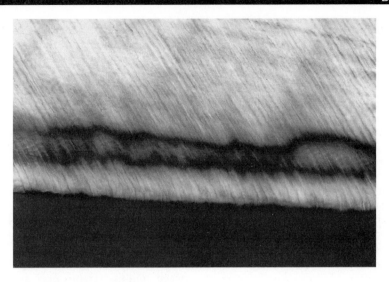

Figure 6.2 Sub-surface demineralization of enamel

Microbiology of enamel caries

Smooth surface caries

Buccal and lingual smooth surfaces are easy to clean and generally suffer from decay only rarely. However, they are easy to study for experimental purposes, both in terms of clinical diagnosis and in plaque sampling. Higher proportions (10–100-fold) of mutans streptococci are found on white-spot lesions on smooth surfaces compared with adjacent sound enamel. As stated earlier, such an association does not prove a causal relationship and the actual proportions of mutans streptococci are often low. Suspensions of plaque from white-spot lesions produce a lower pH minimum and a faster rate of pH-fall than plaque from sound enamel.

Approximal surface caries

A problem with studies of approximal sites is that early lesions cannot be diagnosed accurately, and plaque samples are inevitably removed from the whole interproximal area, including that overlying sound enamel as well as that from areas undergoing demineralization. The microflora can vary markedly at different sites around the contact area between teeth, irrespective of whether a lesion is developing, so that specific associations can be obscured. As a consequence, data concerning the specificity of particular species and caries initiation has been more equivocal at approximal sites than at other surfaces.

Early cross-sectional studies found a positive correlation between elevated levels of mutans streptococci and lesion development; the likelihood of caries rises with increased levels of mutans streptococci in plaque. Many of these studies, however, are limited in scope, and only monitor a small number of micro-organisms, and sometimes only mutans streptococci. In order to combat this, a major longitudinal study was carried out in the mid-1970s on English schoolchildren, aged 11–15 years, in which all of the predominant plaque microflora was characterized, but no unique association between any organism and caries initiation was found. Mutans streptococci could be found in high numbers prior to demineralization at a number of sites, but lesions also appeared to develop in the apparent absence of this group of bacteria on occasions. Mutans streptococci could also be present at other sites in equally high numbers for the duration of the study without any evidence of caries. This may relate to differences in the ecology at various sites. Both the isolation frequency and proportions of mutans streptococci increased after, rather than before, the radiographic detection of a lesion, especially in those lesions that progressed deeper into the enamel, suggesting that shifts in the composition of the microflora might occur as the lesion progresses through the tooth.

Analogous findings were found in a study of Dutch army recruits, aged 18–20 years. Mutans streptococci were isolated from 40% and 86% of sites from caries-free and caries-active recruits, respectively. Interestingly, marked differences in the distribution of individual species were found in these recruits; *S. mutans* strains were isolated from both groups whereas *S. sobrinus* was recovered almost exclusively from caries-active recruits. The prevalence of the combined species of mutans streptococci also showed a direct but not unique correlation with the progression of a lesion into the dentine (Table 6.1). Again, relatively high proportions of mutans streptococci persisted at tooth surfaces without caries progression while caries could also develop in their apparent absence.

Table 6.1 Prevalence of mutans streptococci at approximal tooth surfaces with and without caries progression

	Total number of tooth surfaces	Prevalence of mutans streptococci[a] 0%	0–5%	> 5%
Caries progression	14	1[b]	3	10
No caries progression	41	21	17	3

[a]Prevalence of mutans streptococci is expressed as their percentage of the total cultivable microflora.
[b]Number of tooth surfaces.

Fissure caries

Fissures on occlusal surfaces (*see* Figures 2.2 and 5.7) are the most caries-prone sites. Caries can develop rapidly on these surfaces, and it is at these sites that the strongest association between mutans streptococci and dental decay has been found. In one cross-sectional study, 71% of carious fissures had viable counts of mutans streptococci greater than 10% of the total cultivable plaque microflora, whereas 70% of the fissures that were caries-free at the time of sampling had no detectable mutans streptococci. An inverse relationship between mutans streptococci and *S. sanguis* is frequently observed. In a longitudinal study of North American children, the proportions of mutans streptococci, *S. sanguis*, and lactobacilli were monitored before and at the time of caries development in occlusal fissures. The subjects were divided into several groups (defined in

Table 6.3 below) according to their previous caries experience and to their caries activity during the study. The proportions of mutans streptococci increased significantly at the time of diagnosis of most lesions. However, mutans streptococci were only a minor component of the plaque from five fissures which became carious. Counts of lactobacilli were significantly higher at these sites and, it was concluded, that these were responsible for lesion formation. Furthermore, in a group who remained caries-free during the study, but who had a previous high caries experience (HCI group, Table 6.2), mutans streptococci comprised, on average, approximately 8% of the total cultivable microflora over a 12-month period. Thus, although there was a strong correlation between mutans streptococci and fissure decay, lesions could also develop in the absence of this group of bacteria, and they could persist in moderately high numbers at apparently caries-free sites.

A major prospective study of young Swiss children (7–8 years) specifically examined the question as to whether colonization by mutans streptococci was a risk factor for caries in fissures (and on smooth surfaces). Both fissures and smooth surfaces of first permanent pre-molars that suffered demineralization without cavitation were heavily colonized with mutans streptococci (10^4–10^5 cfu/ml of sample) around 12–18 months prior to the clinical diagnosis of the lesion. The proportions of mutans streptococci appeared to markedly increase 6–9 months prior to lesion detection to reach 11–18% and 10–12% of the total streptococcal microflora of fissures and smooth surfaces, respectively. This study demonstrated that colonization and an increase in proportions of mutans streptococci preceded lesion formation by about 6 months. As with other studies of caries, however, several sites had high counts of mutans streptococci (> 20% of the total streptococcal count) but no evidence of caries. Larger lesions (with cavitation) were found only at a relatively few sites. In five out of six carious fissures, the median count of mutans streptococci rose from 10^2 to $> 10^4$ cfu/ml sample around 12 months prior to lesion detection; this represented a final mean proportion of 18% of the total streptococcal count. The remaining carious fissure had no detectable mutans streptococci at any time during the study, again illustrating that species other than

Table 6.2 Percentage viable count of mutans streptococci, *S. sanguis* and lactobacilli in occlusal fissure plaque of children participating in a longitudinal study relating plaque microflora to caries initiation

Carious state of tooth	No. of teeth	Viable count (%)		
		mutans streptococci	*S. sanguis*	Lactobacilli
Carious				
LCA	5	0.1	4.6	4.0
HCA	37	24.6	7.8	1.0
Caries-free				
CF	24	2.0	12.8	0.3
LCI	31	1.6	20.6	0
HCI	24	8.3	6.4	0.2
LCA	6	0	7.0	0
HCA	68	7.2	12.3	0.4

LCA   Caries diagnosed at target site during study, but with a previously low experience of caries.
HCA   Caries diagnosed at target site during study, but with a previously high experience of caries.
CF   Caries-free.
LCI   Caries inactive (no new lesions developed during the study) but with a previously low experience of caries.
HCI   Caries inactive (no new lesions developed during the study) but with a previously high experience of caries.

mutans streptococci can play a role in lesion formation. An additional feature of the design of this study was that some sites were recognized that developed a lesion and then remineralized. Some of these sites had levels of mutans streptococci greater than 20% of the streptococcal microflora, and yet the lesion remineralized within 12 months. During this period, the levels of mutans streptococci fell markedly between 6–9 months prior to the diagnosis of the reversal. This study provides convincing data on the role of mutans streptococci in the initiation of dental caries.

Rampant caries

Rampant caries can occur in particular subgroups of people who are especially prone to decay, such as xerostomic patients, who have a markedly reduced salivary flow rate due to radiation treatment for head and neck cancer, those with Sjögren's syndrome, or due to medication. These patients also generally consume soft diets, with a high sucrose content, and may often suck 'candies' to relieve their symptoms. Longitudinal studies of patients undergoing radiation treatment showed large increases in the numbers and proportions of mutans streptococci and lactobacilli in plaque and saliva. Other species, associated with sound enamel, such as *S. sanguis*, *Neisseria* spp. and Gram-negative anaerobes, decreased during this period.

'Nursing-bottle' caries is the extensive and rapid decay of the maxillary anterior teeth associated with the prolonged and frequent feeding of young infants with bottles or pacifiers containing formulas with a high concentration of fermentable carbohydrate. Plaque bacteria receive an almost continuous provision of substrates from which they can make acid. Such prolonged conditions of low pH are conducive, and indeed, selective for mutans streptococci and lactobacilli, and proportions of mutans streptococci in plaque can reach > 50% of the microflora. Children with nursing caries can be colonized by more ribotypes of *S. mutans* than those who are caries-free; this may relate to the increased frequency of sugar consumption in these children. Lactobacilli (including *L. fermentum* and *L. plantarum*) are also prevalent in plaque from this type of caries.

Early (sub-surface) demineralization

As discussed earlier, a problem with many studies of caries is that diagnosis of a lesion has to rely on relatively insensitive techniques such as radiographs or tactile criteria. By the time a lesion can be reliably diagnosed in this way, it is relatively well-advanced, and the bacteria associated with the established lesion may not be the same as those responsible for its initiation. In order to circumvent these problems, some studies have examined the integrity of enamel

Table 6.3 Prevalence and isolation frequency of some bacteria recovered from progressive and non-progressive incipient caries lesions in young schoolchildren

Bacterium	Progressive lesion		Non-progressive lesion	
	Viable count (%)	Isolation frequency (%)	Viable count(%)	Isolation frequency (%)
mutans streptococci	10	100	3	75
S. mitis-group	10	100	14	100
A. naeslundii	29	100	33	100
A. odontolyticus	<1	50	0	0
Lactobacillus spp.	<1	75	0	0
Veillonella spp.	11	100	9	100

from teeth that were being extracted for orthodontic purposes. Very small samples of plaque could be taken from discrete sites around the contact area on approximal surfaces; demineralization could be determined by sensitive histological criteria using polarized light microscopy or microradiography (Figure 6.2). Orthodontic bands have been used on these teeth as an *in vivo* model system to create artificially a protected area for plaque accumulation. Surprisingly, wide differences in demineralization rates were found; demineralization occurred after <2 days of plaque accumulation in some to >14 days in others. Lactobacilli, *S. mutans* and *A. naeslundii* were detected more commonly at day 14 than at day 1. Demineralization was more common in the presence of *S. mutans*, although demineralization also occurred in 24% of sites from which *S. mutans* could not be isolated.

Similar trends were found in another study; the proportions of mutans streptococci and *A. naeslundii* were found to be statistically higher at sites with demineralization. Very early stages of demineralization were also associated with increases in *A. odontolyticus*; in contrast, lactobacilli were only isolated from the later stages of demineralization. Again, mutans streptococci could not be detected from 37% of sites with pronounced demineralization. It should be borne in mind, however, that this type of study suffers from the problem discussed earlier that it is not possible to ascertain whether the demineralization was active, arrested or even repairing at the time of sampling. Collectively, however, these two studies emphasize the role of mutans streptococci in early demineralization; they also point to a potential role for *Actinomyces* spp., with lactobacilli

becoming prevalent only at the later stages of lesion formation.

Lesion progression

Indirect evidence from many of the preceding sections suggests that bacterial succession may occur during the development of a caries lesion, and that the microflora responsible for initiation may differ from that causing progression. During a 12-month longitudinal study of the plaque microflora of small incipient approximal lesions in deciduous molar teeth of schoolchildren (aged 4–9 years), some of the lesions progressed while others did not. Differences were found in the plaque microflora at the start of the study from lesions which ultimately progressed and those that were arrested. Lactobacilli and *A. odontolyticus* were isolated in low numbers (<1% of the total microflora), but only from lesions which eventually progressed, and were never isolated from non-progressive lesions, or from sound enamel. Other positive associations with caries progression were found with mutans streptococci. (Table 6.3). These findings could find clinical application in that the detection of lactobacilli or *A. odontolyticus* at incipient lesions might indicate a site with a high-risk of cavitation. Such sites could warrant the topical application of agents to either encourage remineralization (e.g. fluoride) or to disrupt the ecology of the microflora (e.g. antimicrobial agents).

Recurrent (secondary) caries

Caries can re-occur beneath and around previous restorations, and treatment of this accounts for a large proportion of the restorative needs of the adult population. Recurrent caries can result from the penetration of micro-organisms around the margins of poorly fitting (leaky) restorations or due to the incomplete removal of bacteria from infected dentine when the initial lesion was originally restored. Secondary dentinal involvement is of particular concern because it can be difficult to diagnose non-invasively, and it poses the threat of pulpal inflammation and infection (*see below*).

Mutans streptococci have been isolated in high numbers from recurrent caries while a more diverse microflora has been isolated when dentine is affected (*see below*). Interestingly, the type of restoration may influence the development of the microflora and affect recurrent caries. Conventional amalgam is being replaced on occasions by new materials including glass ionomer cement. This material may leach fluoride and silver ions into the immediate environment, and exert an antibacterial effect. Plaque removed from approximal sites restored with glass ionomer cement had lower levels of mutans streptococci than those restored with amalgam.

Value of microbiological tests in the prediction of caries activity

Microbiological tests have been used in an attempt to predict sites or individuals at risk of caries. These usually involve the estimation of the numbers of mutans streptococci in either plaque or saliva samples by plate counts in the laboratory, or by semi-quantitative, commercially available, chairside tests. Although a strong positive correlation has been found between levels of mutans streptococci and caries experience on a group or population level, the association is less apparent for individuals. This is perhaps not surprising given that caries is a multi-factorial disease (*see* Figure 1.1), and clinical studies indicate that the relationship between mutans streptococci and caries is not absolute.

Probably the best predictor of future caries is the current caries status of the individual. In such cases, patients with a high incidence of caries can be assumed to have not only the relevant microflora but also the additional factors (cariogenic diet, impaired saliva flow etc.) conducive to lesion formation. In such patients, microbiological tests based on counts of mutans streptococci can give a high positive predictive value, while in other subjects the positive prediction is only around 40–50%. Generally, the absence of mutans streptococci is a stronger indicator of low caries risk than is the presence of these bacteria for high risk.

The most valuable use of salivary microbiological tests could be in young children (e.g. under the age of 4 years), because this could identify infants at risk of subsequent disease. Such tests would also be useful in monitoring high-risk patients, such as those wearing orthodontic bands, and also xerostomic patients. The tests can also be used in a secondary role to monitor patient compliance in terms of dietary control, or in motivating patients by giving them tangible evidence of events in their own mouth.

Microbiology of root surface caries

The reduction in enamel caries in industrialized societies has resulted in large proportions of the public retaining their teeth into later life. In old age, however, gingival recession occurs and exposes the susceptible cementum surface of the root to microbial colonization; root surfaces can also become exposed due to mechanical injury or to periodontal surgery (e.g. following scaling and root planing, *see* Chapter 7). These cementum surfaces are especially vulnerable to demineralization by plaque acids. The prevalence of root surface caries increases with age; approximately 60% of individuals aged 60 years or older now have root caries or fillings.

Experimental animal studies

Direct evidence for the role of oral micro-organisms in root surface caries came from animal studies in the 1960s in which filamentous bacteria were found to invade the root surfaces of hamsters and produce caries. Human isolates of *A. naeslundii* were then shown to cause root surface caries (and periodontal disease) in gnotobiotic rats and hamsters, as were pure cultures of mutans streptococci, *S. mitis*-group, and *S. anginosus*-group bacteria.

Human studies

Early studies were designed around the findings from the first animal experiments, and focused

Table 6.4 Mean percentage viable counts (and percentage isolation frequencies in parentheses) of some plaque bacteria from root surfaces, with and without caries

Bacterium	Sound root surface	Root surface caries	
		Initial (soft)	Advanced (hard)
mutans streptococci	2 (84)	29 (92)	8 (92)
S. sanguis	19 (96)	11 (97)	22 (85)
A. naeslundii	12 (90)	11 (85)	13 (96)

on the role of Gram-positive filamentous bacteria, especially *Actinomyces* spp., in root surface caries. Among the organisms isolated from lesions were *Rothia dentocariosa*, *A. naeslundii* and *A. odontolyticus*; in some studies, mutans streptococci were also reported to be significant components of the microflora.

Subsequent studies have tended to find stronger associations between mutans streptococci and lactobacilli with root surface caries. In a major longitudinal survey in Canada, although no direct correlation between specific bacteria and root caries was found, the presence of mutans streptococci and lactobacilli on root surfaces were predictive for the subsequent development of a lesion. Other studies have attempted to sub-divide the lesions into initial (or 'soft') and advanced (or 'hard'). Several groups reported higher proportions (often around 30% of the total cultivable microflora) of mutans streptococci at the initial lesion (Table 6.4), sometimes in association with lactobacilli. Lactobacilli have occasionally been found at arrested (hard, black-coloured) lesions.

Model systems have been developed using *in situ* devices to study the microflora of actively progressing root surface caries lesions. Elderly subjects (mean age: 70 years) volunteered to carry defined root surface specimens from human molars on their partial dentures for 3 months. After this period, the predominant plaque microflora was determined and the integrity of the experimental root surface was measured by highly sensitive techniques (quantitative microradiography). Although the composition of the microflora showed distinct individual differences, plaque samples from surfaces showing the highest loss of mineral were dominated either by (a) *A. naeslundii*, or (b) a combination of mutans streptococci and lactobacilli (*L. casei* and *L. brevis*). Plaque from root surfaces with less pronounced mineral loss harboured a more complex microflora includ-

ing *Actinomyces* spp., mutans streptococci, *S. mitis* biovar 1, *Veillonella* spp., Gram-negative rods and low numbers of lactobacilli.

The recent application of more sophisticated approaches to sampling plaque has given new insights into the relationship between the composition of the microflora and lesion development. For example, marked variations were found when the microflora from superficial plaque from root lesions requiring restoration was compared with that of the underlying, carious dentine. Although the numbers of bacteria were lower in the infected dentine, the proportions of lactobacilli and pleomorphic Gram-positive rods were significantly higher, suggesting a role for these bacteria in the destruction of the dentine.

In a separate study, a novel procedure was used to sample plaque from highly defined sites; a specially designed device lifted plaque from discrete areas, which was then sucked immediately into reduced transport fluid. The caries status of these precise sampling sites was then assessed by a variety of techniques including contact microradiography, and light and electron microscopy. In this way, the surface directly beneath the plaque that had been sampled could be reliably classified as being a sound, active or arrested carious root lesion. Regardless of the degree of mineralization, the microflora from these root surfaces was more diverse than had previously been reported, and resembled that associated with gingivitis (*see* Chapter 7). On all surfaces, *Actinomyces* were the predominant group of bacteria, especially *A. naeslundii*, *A. odontolyticus* and *A. gerencseriae*. Surprisingly, and in contrast to other studies, mutans streptococci and lactobacilli were relatively uncommon and comprised only a small proportion of the microflora. Arrested lesions had significantly lower numbers of bacteria than either sound surfaces or active lesions. Gram-negative species formed around 50% of the microflora on sound and active

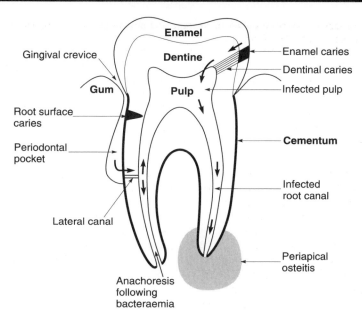

Figure 6.3 Progression of infections affecting the tooth and its supporting structures

carious surfaces, with *Prevotella* spp. (particularly *P. nigrescens*) being highly prevalent. Other Gram-negative bacteria, including *Capnocytophaga* spp., '*B. ureolyticus*', *P. buccae*, *Campylobacter* spp. and *L. buccalis* were preferentially isolated from plaque overlying active lesions. This may be because a number of these species are sufficiently saccharolytic to demineralize cementum and dentine, while others are proteolytic, and could hydrolyse the dentine collagen matrix. The data from this study suggested a polymicrobial aetiology for caries initiation on root surfaces. Collectively, the data suggest that bacterial succession also occurs during the development of root surface lesions.

Bacterial invasion of dentine and root canals

Dentine can be invaded by:

(a) direct progression of an enamel caries lesion;

(b) from caries of the root surface;

(c) from a periodontal pocket via lateral or accessory canals (Figure 6.3);

(d) as a result of fracture or trauma during operative procedures; or

(e) as a result of secondary, or recurrent caries.

Scaling and root planing can predispose some root surfaces to bacterial invasion by exposing dentine tubules; in addition, bacteria may lodge in injured pulp following a transient bacteraemia (anachoresis) (Figure 6.3).

The microbial community from the advancing front of a dentinal lesion is diverse and contains many facultatively and obligately anaerobic bacteria belonging to the genera *Actinomyces*, *Bifidobacterium*, *Eubacterium*, *Lactobacillus*, *Peptostreptococcus*, *Propionibacterium* and *Rothia*. Gram-negative bacteria such as *Prevotella*, *Porphyromonas*, *Fusobacterium* spp. can also be isolated but they are generally present only in low numbers. Streptococci are recovered less frequently, but when mutans streptococci have been isolated they can be one of the predominant members of the community. In a cross-sectional study of dentine infected as a result of secondary (recurrent) caries, a wide range of bacteria were recovered from lesions of comparable severity. Although streptococci were commonly isolated, no single species was specifically associated with recurrent dentinal caries.

The microflora found in the dentine and pulp of periodontally diseased human teeth was also diverse and may be derived predominantly from the subgingival area. Both Gram-positive and Gram-negative species were identified (Table 6.5); some were more prevalent in the dentine

Table 6.5 Prevalence of some bacteria invading the dentine and pulp of periodontally diseased teeth

Bacterium	Mean % viable count[a]		Isolation frequency (%)	
	Dentine[b]	Pulp	Dentine[b]	Pulp
S. sanguis	46	56	28	7
S. intermedius	10	56	3	2
Peptostreptococcus spp.	2	0	2	0
A. naeslundii	57	61	24	13
A. odontolyticus	40	2	11	3
Bifidobacterium spp.	18	0	3	0
Eubacterium spp.	54	66	3	7
Lactobacillus spp.	1	0	2	0
P. propionicus	21	0	2	0
Propionibacterium spp.	36	22	23	2
Clostridium spp.	37	0	12	0
Veillonella spp.	29	34	7	8
Black-pigmented anaerobes	8	20	13	7
Capnocytophaga spp.	19	3	20	7
F. nucleatum	32	37	15	5
S. sputigena	0	11	0	2
E. corrodens	2	0	2	0

[a]Mean value in positive sample.
[b]Mean value for inner, middle and outer layers of dentine

(e.g. *A. odontolyticus*), some predominated in the pulp (e.g. black-pigmented anaerobes), while others were found equally at both sites (e.g. *Veillonella* spp., and *F. nucleatum*). Little is known about the nutritional sources at these sites, but both saccharolytic and asaccharolytic species appear to flourish. Dentine collagen is denatured and modified during the caries process, and becomes more susceptible to breakdown by non-specific proteases, and this explains the presence of both acidogenic and proteolytic bacteria.

Once bacteria are in the pulp, inflammation can occur which may result eventually in necrosis of the root canal. A further consequence is that micro-organisms can invade and destroy tissue surrounding the apex of the root, producing a spreading or localized infection (periapical osteitis; Figure 6.3). A diverse mixed culture of bacteria can be cultured, including black-pigmented anaerobes (*P. intermedia, P. melaninogenica*), *Porphyromonas endodontalis* and *Porphyromonas* (formerly *Mitsuokella*) *dentalis, C. sputorum, Eubacterium* spp. and *Peptostreptococcus* spp.. Some of these species (*P. endodontalis, P. dentalis*) are found almost exclusively in infected root canals and abscesses of endodontal origin. Another study of necrotic

pulps found *Propionibacterium*, *Eubacterium* and *Fusobacterium* spp. to be the predominant bacteria, with *Bifidobacterium, Lactobacillus, Actinomyces* and *Veillonella* spp. as minor components. Certain bacterial combinations are associated with endodontic clinical symptoms, e.g. *P. melaninogenica* and *Peptostreptococcus micros* were linked with pain.

The treatment of infections of the root canal (endodontics) involves the removal of infected and dead tissue both mechanically and by irrigation, sometimes accompanied by treatment with antimicrobial agents to reduce the microbial community to a level where the cavity can be restored effectively.

Pathogenic determinants of cariogenic bacteria

Much attention has been paid to the identification of determinants of pathogenicity of cariogenic bacteria such as mutans streptococci and lactobacilli (Table 6.6). The optimum approach for unequivocally identifying a virulence factor is to isolate a mutant defective in the specific property under consideration. Originally, relevant strains were isolated as either spontaneous

Table 6.6 Characteristics of mutans streptococci that contribute to their cariogenicity

Property	Comment
Sugar transport	High and low affinity transport systems operate over a wide range of conditions to ensure substrate uptake, even under extreme conditions, e.g. low pH
Acid production	An efficient glycolytic pathway rapidly produces low terminal pH values in plaque
Aciduricity	Cells have specific biochemical attributes that enable them to survive, metabolize and grow at low pH values
Extracellular polysaccharide (EPS) production	EPS contributes to the plaque matrix, consolidates attachment of cells, and may localize acidic fermentation products
Intracellular polysaccharide (IPS) production	IPS utilization allows acid production to continue in the absence of dietary sugars

Table 6.7 The use of mutants of mutans streptococci to determine traits linked to cariogenicity

Trait	Property of mutant	Effect on cariogenicity[a]
Glucosyltransferase[b]	Decreased colonization and plaque formation	Reduced
Fructosyltransferase	Loss of extracellular fructan	None
Fructanase	No breakdown of extracellular fructan	None
IPS production	No intracellular glycogen	Reduced
Antigen 1/11	Decreased ability to adhere	None
Enzyme II (PTS)	Decreased sucrose transport	None
Lactic dehydrogenase	No lactic acid production	Reduced
'Aciduricity'[c]	Reduced tolerance of low pH	Reduced

[a]If a mutation did not lead to a reduction in caries, it does not necessarily mean that the trait is not important in cariogenicity. It may reflect the fact that the particular trait is not essential for caries in an animal model; also, mutans streptococci often have more than one mechanism for a particular function.
[b]Mutations in *gtf*B and C led to a reduction in cariogenicity, but not in *gtf*D.
[c]This mutant was not fully characterized.

mutants or following treatment with chemical mutagens. Although much valuable data was derived from the study of these strains, it was not possible to precisely define the nature of the mutation; the possibility of multiple defects could not be discounted. The development of molecular biology as a discipline has enabled the construction of defined mutants defective only in a single gene. Such mutants can be tested in animal model systems, so that direct relationships between a particular trait and cariogenicity can be demonstrated (Table 6.7).

Sucrose has been shown to have a specific role in caries aetiology. Consequently, mutants defective in various aspects of sucrose metabolism have been compared in terms of their relative cariogenicity. Early studies showed that strains of *S. mutans* defective in insoluble glucan synthesis were unable to colonize teeth as effectively as the parent strains, and caused fewer smooth surface caries lesions in an animal (rat) model. In contrast, soluble glucan formation was essential for colonization and caries-induction. The synthesis of intracellular storage compounds enables *S. mutans* to continue making acid even in the absence of dietary carbohydrates. Both chemically induced and defined mutants defective in intracellular polysaccharide (IPS) synthesis produced fewer caries lesions than parent strains when inoculated in pure cultures in gnotobiotic rodents. Mutants of *S. mutans* defective in either lactic dehydrogenase or FTF activity are also markedly less cariogenic in rat caries models while, in contrast, fructanase was shown not to be essential for virulence.

Three properties that are distinctive characteristics of cariogenic bacteria are:

(a) the ability to rapidly transport sugars, when in competition with other plaque bacteria;

(b) convert such sugars rapidly to acid; and

(c) the ability to maintain these activities even under extreme environmental conditions, such as at a low pH. Few oral bacteria are able to tolerate acidic conditions for prolonged periods, but mutans streptococci and lactobacilli are not only able to remain viable (survive) at a low pH, but are able to continue to metabolize and multiply, i.e. they are **acidogenic** (strongly acid producing) and **aciduric** (acid-loving).

These properties have also been studied using various mutants, although the results have not always been straightforward to interpret. Mutations that led directly or indirectly to inactivation of part of the PTS sugar transport system (e.g. an enzyme II for sucrose) or of the Msm transport system did not result in a decrease in the cariogenicity of strains (Table 6.7). These findings may not necessarily be that surprising, since mutans streptococci have multiple strategies to transport sugars, and systems such as the PTS are repressed under high sugar concentrations (*see* Chapter 4). Using similar reasoning, mutants lacking a specific adhesin (such as antigen I/II) are still able to colonize animals because species such as *S. mutans* attach to the acquired enamel pellicle via multiple adhesin-receptor interactions (*see* Chapter 5). Chemically induced mutants with reduced acid-tolerance have been shown to be less cariogenic, although the precise mechanisms behind this could not be determined. Microbial survival in acidic environments depends on the cell maintaining a favourable intracellular pH in spite of sharp fluctuations in external pH (*see* Chapter 4), and *S. mutans* achieves this by a number of specific mechanisms (*see* Chapter 4).

The importance that the combination of acidogenicity and acidurity confers on potentially cariogenic bacteria was shown in the laboratory using mixed culture competition studies. At a constant pH 7, *S. mutans* and *L. casei* were non-competitive and were only minor components (< 1%) of a microbial community, even when exposed to pulses of fermentable sugar (glucose). When the pH was allowed to fall after a glucose pulse, *S. mutans* and *L. casei* gradually increased in proportions until they eventually dominated (> 50%) the mixed culture at the expense of acid-sensitive species associated with enamel health (e.g. *S. gordonii, N. subflava*). As their proportions rose, so the rate and extent of the pH-fall increased.

Re-evaluation of the microbial aetiology of dental caries

A repeated feature of most of the clinical studies already described has been the occasional but consistent finding of carious sites from which no mutans streptococci can be isolated. This suggests that bacteria other than mutans streptococci can make a contribution to demineralization. Bacteria isolated from such plaque samples have been compared in their ability to lower the pH of laboratory media. While strains of *S. mutans* produced a final pH in the region of 3.95–4.10, a range of other streptococci achieved terminal values of pH 4.05–4.50. These strains are often numerically dominant, and belong to the *S. mitis*-group (especially *S. mitis, S. oralis* and *S. gordonii*), *S. salivarius*-group and *S. anginosus*-group; generally strains of *S. sanguis* are not acidogenic. Such findings reinforce the view that although mutans streptococci are clearly key causative organisms in enamel caries, other bacteria can contribute to, and modulate, the strength of the cariogenic challenge at a site.

The converse situation is also not uncommon, where mutans streptococci are found in high numbers but in the apparent absence of any demineralization of the underlying enamel. This may be due to the presence of lactate-consuming species (e.g. *Veillonella*), or to the production of alkali at low pH (e.g. ammonia production by urease or arginine deiminase activities of *S. salivarius* and *S. sanguis*, respectively). Other factors will also be significant, and these include the influence of the diet. In industrialized societies, a strong correlation between high sucrose intake and elevated levels of mutans streptococci has been found. A surprising observation in some developing countries in Africa has been the detection of high plaque proportions of mutans streptococci in the absence of a corresponding high level of caries. These mutans streptococci were found to have a similar potential to cause caries in controlled animal models as those strains from industrialized countries. The variation in disease outcome has been attributed to differences

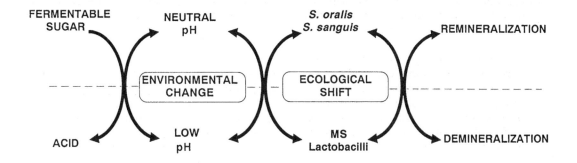

Figure 6.4 A schematic representation of the ecological plaque hypothesis in relation to the aetiology of dental caries. Frequent metabolism of fermentable sugars in dental plaque produces regular and prolonged conditions of low pH; this environmental change in plaque favours the growth of acid-tolerating bacteria (such as mutans streptococci (MS) and lactobacilli) at the expense of species associated with sound enamel. Such a change in the microflora predisposes a surface to demineralization. Disease could be prevented by not only targeting the putative pathogens, but also by interfering with the factors driving their selection. Reproduced with permission; Advances in Dental Research

in diet between industrialized and developing nations. The latter have lower levels of sucrose and increased amounts of starch in their diet; consumption of sucrose-containing snacks between meals is also uncommon. This may result in the development of plaque containing less glucan, with therefore an altered architecture, resulting in a low cariogenic challenge. Again, such observations serve to emphasize the multi-factorial nature of caries, which involves the interaction of an acidogenic/aciduric microflora on a susceptible surface in a conducive environment, and with frequent intakes of food containing retentive (i.e. sticky) and rapidly fermentable carbohydrates.

Collectively, these findings allow a model to be constructed to explain the changes in the ecology of dental plaque that lead to the development of a caries lesion. Cariogenic bacteria may be found naturally in dental plaque, but at neutral pH, these organisms are weakly competitive and are present only as a small proportion of the total plaque community. In this situation, with a conventional diet, the levels of such potentially cariogenic bacteria are clinically insignificant, and the processes of de- and remineralization are in equilibrium. If the frequency of fermentable carbohydrate intake increases, then plaque spends more time below the critical pH for enamel demineralization (approximately pH 5.5; *see* Figure 2.3).

The effect of this on the microbial ecology of plaque would be two-fold. Conditions of low pH favour the proliferation of mutans streptococci and lactobacilli, while tipping the balance towards demineralization. Greater numbers of mutans streptococci and lactobacilli in plaque would result in more acid being produced at even faster rates, thereby enhancing demineralization still further. Other bacteria could also make acid under similar conditions, but at a slower rate, but would be responsible for some of the initial stages of demineralization, or could cause lesions in the absence of other (more overt) cariogenic species in a susceptible host. If aciduric species were not present initially, then the repeated conditions of low pH coupled with the inhibition of competing organisms might increase the likelihood of colonization by mutans streptococci or lactobacilli. This sequence of events would account for the lack of total specificity in the microbial aetiology of caries and explain the pattern of bacterial succession observed in many clinical studies. This model forms the basis of the **'ecological plaque hypothesis'** (Figure 6.4). In this hypothesis, caries is a consequence of changes in the natural balance of the resident plaque microflora brought about by an alteration in local environmental conditions (e.g. repeated conditions of high sugar and low plaque pH). The hypothesis also acknowledges the dynamic relationship that exists between the microflora and the host, so that the impact of alterations in key host factors (such as saliva flow) on plaque composition is taken into account. This has a great significance for caries prevention, since implicit in the hypothesis is the concept that disease can be controlled not only by targeting directly the putative pathogens (e.g. mutans streptococci) but also by interfering with the factors that are driving the deleterious shifts in the balance of the microflora (e.g. lowering the acid challenge by reducing the frequency of sugar intake, or by using snacks containing sugar substitutes). These, and other caries-preventive strategies, are discussed in the next section.

Approaches for controlling dental caries

Mechanical removal of plaque by efficient oral hygiene procedures can almost completely prevent caries. Such measures are particularly effective when combined with a reduction in the amount and frequency of sugar intake. It is difficult, however, to alter established eating habits and to maintain a high degree of motivation for effective oral hygiene. Alternative preventive measures are under development which require little cooperation from the public.

Fissure sealants

Occlusal pits and fissures are the most caries-prone areas of the human dentition. Strongly adherent, self-polymerizing and UV-light polymerizing plastic sealant materials have been applied to fissures as a barrier against microbial attack. Problems surround the prolonged retention of these materials in the oral cavity and care must be taken to avoid sealing early caries lesions.

Fluoride

It has been known for over 40 years that the administration of fluoride systemically, via the water supply, can reduce the incidence of caries by at least 50%. The optimum concentration for maximal protection against caries is thought to be 1 part per million (1 ppm) but in many water supplies it naturally occurs at higher concentrations. Despite its proven value in

decreasing caries incidence, the addition of fluoride to the drinking water remains a controversial and emotive issue. Fluoride can also be added to table salt, milk and toothpastes. It is also used in a variety of mouthwashes and gels for topical use and in tablets for supplementation of the systemic effect, and has also been incorporated into thin films for coating teeth, topical varnishes and slow-release capsules. Fluoride is also available naturally in tea and the bones of fish (especially soft-boned sardines and salmon).

Ingested fluoride exerts its effect topically (if only transiently) and systemically after ingestion. Low levels of fluoride appear in oral fluids (saliva, GCF) and interact with the surface of the enamel of erupted teeth to form fluorapatite. Fluorapatite is thermodynamically more stable than apatite and resists acid dissolution to a greater extent than hydroxyapatite. Fluoride can also inhibit the metabolism of plaque bacterial populations (*see* Chapter 4; Figure 6.5) by:

1 reducing glycolysis by inhibition of enolase;
2 indirectly inhibiting sugar transport by blocking the production of PEP for the PTS system;
3 acidifying the interior of cells, and hence inactivating key metabolic enzymes;
4 interfering with bacterial membrane permeability to ionic transfer;
5 inhibiting the synthesis of intracellular storage (IPS) compounds, especially glycogen; and perhaps
6 by altering the structural integrity of plaque biofilms.

Dental plaque has been found to concentrate fluoride from ingested water. In areas where the concentration of fluoride in the water supply is less than 0.01 ppm, dental plaque has been found to contain 5–10 ppm. In water supplies supplemented with 1 ppm fluoride, concentrations of up to 190 ppm have been found in dental plaque. Much of this fluoride is bound to organic components in plaque, but there is also evidence that it can be released when the pH falls, and be bioavailable to interfere with acid production by plaque bacteria. The sensitivity of oral bacteria to fluoride increases as the pH falls, so that concentrations of fluoride that would be ineffective at resting pH values can be inhibitory at pH 5.0 or below. Mutans strepto-

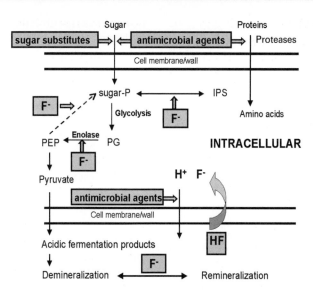

Figure 6.5 The site of action of some classes of inhibitors used in dentistry. F, fluoride; IPS, intracellular polysaccharide; PG, phosphoglycerate; PEP, phosphoenolpyruvate

cocci are particularly sensitive to low levels of fluoride at a moderately low environmental pH. Although surveys have failed to detect major changes in the qualitative and quantitative composition of plaque in humans residing in places with high or low natural levels of fluoride in the drinking water, fluoride is more likely to function prophylactically in these circumstances. Thus, mutans streptococci would be suppressed in plaque under conditions when they would otherwise be expected to flourish; the rate of change of pH in plaque would also be diminished. Laboratory evidence supports this hypothesis; using the previously described mixed culture system, *S. mutans* remained a minor component of plaque (<1% of the cultivable microflora) during glucose pulsing in the presence of 1 mmol/L sodium fluoride when, under similar circumstances, it had previously attained levels of 19% in the absence of fluoride. Other studies have shown that sufficient fluoride to affect the growth and metabolism of *S. mutans* can be released by acid attack from a fluoride-containing surface. Thus, fluoride can serve to stabilize the composition of the plaque microflora, a preventative mechanism which is consistent with the ecological plaque hypothesis.

Artificially high concentrations of fluoride, delivered to xerostomic patients by gels, did lead to the elimination of mutans streptococci from plaque of 10/33 patients after 5 years. Lactobacilli are innately highly resistant to fluoride, and were not affected by this gel therapy. In the laboratory, mutans streptococci can adapt to, and tolerate, even relatively high levels of fluoride. Concern has been expressed as to whether organisms might become resistant to fluoride due to the prolonged use of fluoride-containing toothpastes. Laboratory studies have shown that fluoride-resistance reduces the acidogenicity and cariogenicity of mutans streptococci, so that even if adaptation occurred, there would be no increase in caries risk.

There has been a dramatic fall in the prevalence of caries in many industrialized societies since the mid-1970s. This corresponds to the introduction of fluoride-containing toothpastes, and much of the benefit derived from fluoride is attributable to its delivery from this source. Although much of the anti-caries benefit of fluoride is due to topical and systemic effects on enamel, it is likely that there is also an antimicrobial effect. This antimicrobial effect can be enhanced by changing the counter-ion; thus, stannous fluoride is markedly more inhibitory to oral bacteria than sodium fluoride. Metal salts can be unstable in toothpaste formulations but, recently several products have been launched containing stannous fluoride. Other antimicrobial agents will be discussed in the next section.

Antimicrobial agents

The use of antimicrobial agents (not including antibiotics!) to control plaque has been advocated for a number of years. Some of these products are anti-plaque (and hence also anti-gingivitis), rather than just anti-caries, but a number of issues relevant to the control of caries will be discussed here.

Mouthrinses have proved to be a successful vehicle for the delivery of anti-plaque agents such as quaternary ammonium compounds, bisbiguanides, enzymes, metal salts, 'essential oils' and plant extracts; some examples are listed in Table 6.8. Because of the relatively short contact time between the inhibitor in the rinse and the mouth, the agents must bind effectively to oral surfaces (**substantivity**). Once adsorbed, such inhibitors are released slowly into the oral environment (especially saliva) and inhibit the growth or metabolism of microorganisms for prolonged periods even at sub-MIC concentrations (*see* Figure 6.5).

Table 6.8 Some classes and examples of inhibitors used as anti-plaque agents in mouthrinses and toothpastes

Class of inhibitor	Examples
Bisbiguanide	Chlorhexidine, alexidine
Enzymes	Mutanase, glucanase; amyloglucosidase-glucose oxidase
'Essential oils'	Thymol, eucalyptol
Metal ions	Copper, zinc, stannous
Plant extracts	Sanguinarine
Phenols	Triclosan
Quaternary ammonium compounds	Cetylpyridinium chloride
Surfactants	Sodium lauryl sulphate

The most effective antimicrobial agent for oral use has been chlorhexidine. This bisbiguanide has a broad spectrum of activity against yeasts, fungi and a wide range of Gram-positive and Gram-negative bacteria. Chlorhexidine can reduce plaque, caries and gingivitis in humans; it is not used for prolonged periods because of side-effects such as staining of teeth or mucosal irritation. At high concentrations, chlorhexidine is bactericidal and acts as a detergent by damaging the cell membrane. Chlorhexidine is substantive, and hence is bound to oral surfaces from where it is released gradually into saliva over many hours at bacteriostatic concentra-

tions. At these sub-lethal concentrations, chlorhexidine can:

1 abolish the activity of the PTS sugar transport system (*see* Chapter 4) and thereby markedly inhibit acid production in streptococci;
2 inhibit amino acid uptake and catabolism in *S. sanguis*;
3 inhibit a major protease (with arginine-x substrate specificity) of *P. gingivalis* (*see* Chapter 7); and
4 affect various membrane functions, including the ATP-synthase and the maintenance of ion gradients in streptococci.

Mutans streptococci are more sensitive to chlorhexidine than other oral streptococci, and this property has been exploited in those people at high risk of developing caries. Surveys in Scandinavia showed that subjects with salivary levels of mutans streptococci that were $> 10^6$ cfu/ml were at risk of developing caries. Levels of mutans streptococci could be reduced by professional oral hygiene, dietary counselling, topical fluoride and also by the use of chlorhexidine mouthrinses. While mutans streptococci were suppressed, other oral streptococci such as *S. sanguis* (associated more with enamel health) were relatively unaffected. This approach has also been applied successfully to expectant mothers. The suppression of mutans streptococci in mothers reduced the transmission of these potentially cariogenic organisms to the baby and delayed the onset of caries.

Chlorhexidine has proved to be of great clinical value in reducing plaque and caries in high-risk subjects (Table 6.9). Chlorhexidine can be delivered either by gel (e.g. as a 1% gel in a custom-fitted vinyl applicator), as a mouthrinse, or as a varnish. The varnish is able to slowly release chlorhexidine over a prolonged period. For example, mutans streptococci could not be detected in saliva during a mean period of 35 weeks in 21/33 volunteers treated with up to four weekly applications of a 20% chlorhexidine varnish. An extra layer of sealant or bonding resin has been applied over the chlorhexidine varnish to increase the retention of the antimicrobial for even longer. Combinations of chlorhexidine with other agents such as fluoride or thymol in varnishes has resulted in additive or synergistic benefits, e.g. in preventing caries in high risk patients such as those receiving radiation therapy for head and neck cancer. In these patients, the radiation therapy affects the salivary glands, and the reduced saliva flow is conducive to rampant caries. Daily fluoride mouthrinses and antimicrobial treatment with either 0.2% chlorhexidine mouthrinses or 1% chlorhexidine gel when the salivary levels of mutans streptococci exceeded $2x10^5$ cfu/ml were successful in preventing caries over a 12 month period.

Table 6.9 Effect of different methods of chlorhexidine treatment on mutans streptococci and dental caries

| Treatment | Reduction in | |
	mutans streptococci	Caries
Chlorhexidine:		
mouthrinse	+ / + +	None
gel	+ / + + +	Up to 81%
varnish	+ + + +	51%
Chlorhexidine + fluoride:		
mouthrinse	+ / + +	42%
gel	+ + +	89%
varnish	+ + + /+ + + +	Not tested
Chlorhexidine + thymol:		
varnish	+ + / + + +	Not tested

Toothpastes (dentifrices) are another vehicle for the unsupervised delivery of antimicrobial agents. Many proven antimicrobial and anti-plaque agents, such as chlorhexidine, are incompatible with components of toothpastes, and lose their bioactivity. A new phase of toothpaste development is under way based on the addition of compatible antimicrobial agents, either alone or in combination, to provide clinical benefit above that obtained just from fluoride and detergents. Some toothpastes contain Triclosan, which has a broad spectrum of antimicrobial activity against yeasts and Gram-positive and Gram-negative bacteria. Like chlorhexidine, it is also substantive and multi-functional in its mode of action. At sub-MIC concentrations, it can inhibit acid production by streptococci and protease activity by *P. gingivalis*. The anti-plaque activity of Triclosan has been enhanced by combining it with either a copolymer to boost its oral retention, or with zinc citrate. Zinc ions are also substantive and can inhibit sugar transport, acid production and protease activity. Combinations of agents (e.g. zinc citrate and Triclosan) can give additive clinical benefit. Enzymes have also been included in toothpastes. Examples include dextranases and glucanases (from fungi) to modify the plaque matrix and reduce plaque formation, and glucose oxidase and amyloglucosidase to boost the activity of the salivary peroxidase (sialoperoxidase) system (*see* Chapter 2). Plant extracts, such as sanguinarine, and tannins have anti-plaque activity and can inhibit glycolysis and glucosyltransferase activity, respectively. A number of products are formulated to reduce calculus formation (*see* Chapter 5); inhibitors of mineralization include polyphosphonates, zinc salts and pyrophosphates. Surface active agents, such as Delmopinol, are not antimicrobial, but they can prevent or reduce bacterial colonization of teeth, and are, therefore, useful compounds for the control of plaque-mediated diseases.

The regular, unsupervised use of antimicrobial agents from toothpastes and mouthrinses could lead to the disruption of the ecology of the oral microflora by either (a) perturbing the balance among the resident organisms, which might lead to the overgrowth by potentially more pathogenic species; or (b) the development of resistance. Guidelines are now laid down to ensure that manufacturers perform long-term clinical trials to confirm that these eventualities do not occur.

Sugar substitutes

Most humans enjoy and prefer to eat sweet substances. Unfortunately, many sweet foods are composed of mono- or disaccharides which are easily metabolized by plaque bacteria and predispose enamel to dental caries. To satisfy the human preference for sweet substances without causing caries the use of inert (non-metabolizable) dietary sweeteners has been proposed. These sugar substitutes function by stimulating saliva flow in the absence of a significant acid challenge to enamel (*see* Figure 6.6); indeed, the use of these agents can lead to the remineralization of enamel.

Artificial sweeteners are of two types: the intense type, many times sweeter than sucrose, and the bulk agents, which are usually not as sweet. The intense sweeteners include cyclamate, aspartame and saccharin. These agents are extremely sweet and their use has been proposed for drinks. These sweeteners have some weak antimicrobial effects, with aspartame and saccharin being capable of inhibiting

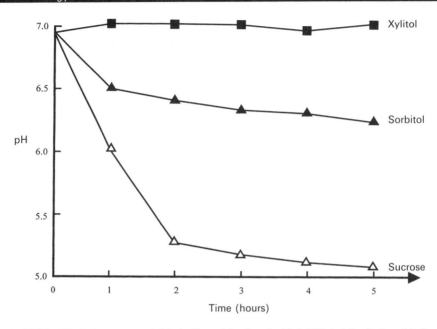

Figure 6.6 Typical fall in pH of plaque suspended in buffer and incubated with 0.75% (w/v) xylitol, sorbitol or sucrose

bacterial growth. The bulk agents, e.g. mannitol and sorbitol, are not as sweet as sucrose and are used, therefore, in the confectionery industry. The use of the bulk agents mannitol and sorbitol is based on the premise that they cannot be metabolized by the majority of plaque bacteria. Some oral bacteria, e.g. mutans streptococci, can metabolize these two sugar alcohols to acid, albeit slowly (Figure 6.6). The frequent use of sorbitol-containing products can also lead to increases in the numbers of sorbitol-fermenting bacteria in general, and in mutans streptococci in particular. Xylitol is another bulk sweetener, but it is not metabolized by plaque bacteria (Figure 6.6). In human trials, xylitol can reduce significantly the incidence of caries, both by reducing the frequency of acid attack on the enamel (*see* Figure 2.3) and by stimulating saliva flow, thereby encouraging remineralization. Xylitol is also transported into cells of mutans streptococci by the fructose-PTS where it enters a 'futile cycle' of phosphorylation, dephosphorylation and eventual expulsion. Xylitol also interferes with sugar metabolism of mutans streptococci by consuming PEP and NAD+ during the 'futile cycle' and competitively inhibiting glycolysis at the phosphofructokinase level by either xylitol-5-phosphate or xylulose-5 phosphate. This futile cycle reduces the rate of growth and acid production (from

exogenous sugars such as glucose) of cells, and leads to reduced levels of both mutans streptococci and caries in habitual users of xylitol-containing confectionery. Lycasin, a hydrogenated corn-starch syrup, has also been incorporated into confectionery with some success. The use of sugar substitutes is consistent with the 'ecological plaque hypothesis', since the prevention of periods of low pH in plaque during between meal periods would remove opportunities for the preferential growth of aciduric bacteria.

Replacement therapy

The possibility that antagonistic organisms could be exploited to control pathogens and prevent disease has been proposed for over 100 years, and is termed 'replacement therapy'. A major potential benefit of this approach is that it could provide life-long protection with minimal cost or compliance on behalf of the recipient, once colonization by an 'effector' strain has been achieved. There are two main approaches: the first is pre-emptive colonization, where key ecological niches (functions) within plaque are filled by a harmless or beneficial organism before the undesirable strain has had a chance to colonize or become established. The initial colonizer becomes integrated into the ecosystem and subsequently excludes the pathogen. Low-virulence mutants of mutans streptococci have been produced that are deficient in GTF or IPS production, or which lack lactate dehydrogenase activity, and which are designed to prevent subsequent colonization by 'wild-type' mutans streptococci. Similarly, genes encoding for alkali production are being cloned into acidogenic bacteria in order to reduce the acid challenge to enamel.

An alternative approach is to derive a more competitive strain that would displace a pre-existing organism from plaque. This strategy has the advantage that it is not dependent on treatment with the 'effector' strain at or before colonization by the undesirable organism. Examples of strains that have been 'auditioned' for this role include *S. salivarius* (TOVE-R), which has been shown to displace *S. mutans* from the teeth of rats and to inhibit caries, and a strain of *S. mutans* that had enhanced bacteriocin production. At present, such strategies have not been used extensively in human trials; assurances over the safety of such 'effector' strains will be required by both the authorities and by the public.

Vaccination and passive immunization

The oral cavity is provided with all of the components necessary to mount an effective immune response against micro-organisms (*see* Chapter 2). While the microbial aetiology of dental caries is not totally specific, considerable evidence implicates mutans streptococci as the major group of causative bacteria. These facts have led to the concept of vaccinating against dental caries using mutans streptococci (whole cell vaccines), or molecules derived from these bacteria (sub-unit vaccines), as an immunogen (**active immunization**). Indeed, studies using a vaccine based on *S. mutans* were initiated in Great Britain over 20 years ago. The early studies used crude whole cell preparations of *S. mutans* to protect primates. Although protection against caries and a reduction in the levels of mutans streptococci was achieved, concern was expressed over possible immunologically mediated tissue damage in humans following exposure to streptococcal antigens (as occurs in, for example, rheumatic fever). Indeed, in some animals vaccinated with whole cells of *S. mutans*, antibodies were formed which reacted not only with the bacteria, but also with heart tissue. Subsequent work has been directed

towards characterizing the antigenic composition of mutans streptococci and selecting individual purified antigens that will confer protection but lack any potential for human tissue cross-reactivity.

An alternative animal model has been adopted in the USA to study anti-caries vaccines, based on the development of caries on smooth surfaces in rats by *S. sobrinus*. Rodents have the advantage that, unlike primates, they are cheap and easy to maintain so that large experimental groups can be compared. Major differences in the morphology of teeth and in the composition of saliva, however, make rodents a less appropriate model of human caries than primates. Also, the development of caries by *S. sobrinus* is more by sucrose-mediated mechanisms, so that sub-unit vaccines in this model are directed towards generating antibodies against glucosyltransferases (GTF). Immunization of rats or hamsters with GTF preparations led to reduced plaque accumulation and caries, particularly on smooth surfaces, but similar vaccines did not give a good protective effect in primates, raising doubts about their potential effectiveness in humans.

Purified proteins present on the cell surface of *S. mutans* (e.g. antigen I/II, GTFs etc.) have been developed from studies of the primate model as immunogens for human anti-caries sub-unit vaccines. Antigen I/II (*see* Chapter 4) is a high molecular weight (mol. wt 185 000) protein that has been shown to confer protection in primates. It is also found in other species of oral streptococci, and so could give wide-ranging protection. In order to avoid the possibility of tissue cross-reacting antibodies being raised, peptides have been generated from the native antigen that confer protection without side-effects. Indeed, a peptide of only 3.8 kDa has been found to confer greater protection when topically applied to the gingivae than the parent molecule. The antigen stimulated IgG antibodies in GCF and sIgA antibodies in saliva. The protective mode of action probably involves preventing the adherence of mutans streptococci to teeth. Protection rates in primates have varied with the immunogen, the route of immunization, and whether the animals have been exposed to fluoride. Reductions in caries have ranged from 50–90%, although in one study, complete protection was achieved over a 3-year period.

The optimum route by which any vaccine might be administered for use in human trials has yet to be resolved. The possibilities include systemic injection (to generate circulating antibodies, especially of the IgG class, which would enter the mouth via GCF), oral vaccines, and local immunization (which elicit mainly an sIgA response). The host response will be influenced by the frequency and level of dosage needed, the age of the subject, and perhaps their prior experience of exposure to *S. mutans* antigens. Although potential vaccines against *S. mutans* have been manufactured to standards that satisfy the legislative authorities, there have been no major field trials to assess their efficacy in humans. This is because the incidence of caries has fallen dramatically in most industrialized societies during the time of the development of these vaccines, probably as a result of fluoride, while the public acceptance of new mass-vaccination programmes can be poor, even for serious medical infections. A major question facing health organizations is whether a vaccine is justified against a non-life threatening disease? It may be that vaccination could be considered of benefit to particular high-risk groups in the population. An interesting development to arise from the studies on vaccination is the concept of using pre-existing antibodies (**passive immunization**) to control putative pathogens. When the natural levels of mutans streptococci in the mouth were suppressed by chlorhexidine, the topical application to teeth of monoclonal antibodies directed against antigen I/II could prevent subsequent re-colonization by mutans streptococci in humans for up to 100 days, and protect against caries in primates. Similarly, bovine anti-mutans streptococci antibodies fed to gnotobiotic rats significantly reduced colonization by *S. mutans* and *S. sobrinus*, as well as caries on buccal, sulcal and approximal surfaces; specific monoclonal antibodies also reduced colonization of rats by *S. sobrinus*. Recently, it was demonstrated that transgenic plants could be genetically engineered to produce a monoclonal secretory antibody with specificity for antigen I/II of mutans streptococci. The dimeric nature of this antibody enabled it to persist intact for longer periods in the mouth than the parent antibody. Application to human volunteers from whom indigenous mutans streptococci had been cleared, resulted in prevention of recolonization by *S. mutans* for up to 4 months. This approach has many advantages that may enable it to form the basis of an alternative caries-preventive strategy for the future.

Summary

Numerous cross-sectional and longitudinal surveys have found a strong association between enamel caries and the levels of mutans streptococci in plaque. Early studies found an association between Actinomyces *spp. and root surface caries; subsequent work has reported stronger correlations with mutans streptococci and lactobacilli, while a recent study suggested a polymicrobial aetiology.*

The development of lesions on all surfaces appears to involve different waves of bacterial succession, reflecting changes in key ecological determinants over time. Mutans streptococci are implicated more with caries initiation, while lactobacilli and possibly A. odontolyticus *appear to be related to progression of enamel lesions. The association of mutans streptococci with dental caries is not unique; they can persist on surfaces without evidence of demineralization, while, in a small number of cases, caries can develop in their apparent absence, and other species (e.g. acidogenic, non-mutans streptococci) play a significant role. The progression of lesions can result in the invasion of dentine and pulp. The microflora is diverse from these infected sites, and a range of acidogenic and proteolytic Gram-positive and Gram-negative bacteria can be isolated.*

The properties of cariogenic bacteria that correlate with their pathogenicity include the ability to rapidly metabolize sugars to acid, especially at low pH, and to survive and grow under the acidic conditions so generated (i.e. acidogenicity and aciduricity). Additional properties include the ability to synthesize intracellular and extracellular polysaccharides. Strategies to control or prevent dental caries are based on (a) reducing levels of plaque in general, or specific cariogenic bacteria in particular, for example, by anti-plaque or antimicrobial agents; (b) using fluoride to encourage remineralization and to strengthen the resistance of enamel to acid attack; and (c) reduce bacterial acid production by avoiding the frequent intake of fermentable carbohydrates in the diet, by replacing such carbohydrates with sugar substitutes, or by interfering with bacterial metabolism with fluoride or antimicrobial agents. Other potential strategies include (a) enhancing the colonization resistance property of plaque by replacement therapy, whereby harmless strains may exclude or suppress cariogenic species, and (b) vaccination or passive immunization against mutans streptococci using sub-unit vaccines or specific antibodies, respectively.

Bibliography

Baehni, P.C. and Guggenheim, B. (1996) Potential of diagnostic microbiology for treatment and prognosis of dental caries and periodontal diseases. *Crit. Rev. Oral Biol. Med.,* **7**, 259–277.

Bowden, G.H.W. (1990) Microbiology of root surface caries in humans. *J. Dent. Res.,* **69**, 1205–1210.

Burne, R.A. (1998) Oral streptococci ... products of their environment. *J. Dent. Res.,* **77**, 445–452.

Dawes, C. and ten Cate, J.M. (eds) (1990) Fluorides: mechanisms of action and recommendations for use. *J. Dent. Res.,* **69**, 505–835.

Emilson, C.G. (1994) Potential efficacy of chlorhexidine against mutans streptococci and human dental caries. *J. Dent. Res.,* **73**, 682–691.

Gomes, B.P.F.A., Lilley, J.D. and Drucker, D.B. (1996) Clinical significance of dental root canal microflora. *J. Dent.,* **24**, 47–55.

Johnson, N.W. (ed.) (1991) *Risk Markers for Oral Disease,* Volume 1: *Dental Caries,* Cambridge University Press, Cambridge.

Kuramitsu, H.K. (1993) Virulence factors of mutans streptococci: role of molecular genetics. *Crit. Rev. Oral Biol. Med.,* **4**, 159–176.

Lang, N.P., Hotz, P.R., Gusberti, F.A. and Joss, A. (1987) Longitudinal clinical and microbiological study on the relationship between infection with *Streptococcus mutans* and the development of caries in humans. *Oral Microbiol. Immunol.,* **2**, 39–47.

Liljemark, W.F. and Bloomquist, C. (1996) Human oral microbial ecology and dental caries and periodontal diseases. *Crit. Rev. Oral Biol. Med.,* **7**, 180–198.

Loesche, W.J. (1986) Role of *Streptococcus mutans* in human dental decay. *Microbiol. Revs,* **50**, 353–380.

Loesche, W.J. and Straffon, L.H. (1979) Longitudinal investigations of the role of *Streptococcus mutans* in human fissure decay. *Infect. Immun.,* **26**, 498–507.

Marsh, P.D. (1994) Microbial ecology of dental plaque and its significance in health and disease. *Adv. Dent. Res.,* **8**, 263–271.

Russell, R.R.B. (1994) The application of molecular genetics to the microbiology of dental caries. *Caries Res.,* **28**, 69–82.

Sato, T., Hoshino, E., Uematsu, H. and Noda, T. (1993) Predominant obligate anaerobes in necrotic pulps of human deciduous teeth. *Microb. Ecol. Health Dis.,* **6**, 269–275.

Scheie, A.A. (1989) Modes of action of currently known chemical anti-plaque agents other than chlorhexidine. *J. Dent. Res.,* **68**, 1609–1616.

Schüpbach, P., Osterwalder, V. and Guggenheim, B. (1995) Human root caries: microbiota in plaque covering sound, carious and arrested carious root surfaces. *Caries Res.,* **29**, 382–395.

Tenovuo, J. (1991) The microbiology and immunology of dental caries. *Rev. Med. Microbiol.,* **2**, 76–82.

van Houte, J. (1994) Role of micro-organisms in caries etiology. *J. Dent. Res.,* **73**, 672–681.

Van Palenstein Helderman, W.H., Matee, M.I.N., van der Hoeven, J.S. and Mikx, F.H.M. (1996) Cariogenicity depends more on diet than the prevailing mutans streptococcal species. *J. Dent. Res.,* **75**, 535–545.

7

Periodontal diseases

The term 'periodontal diseases' embraces a number of conditions in which the supporting tissues of the teeth are attacked. The terminology that will be used in this chapter to classify periodontal diseases will relate to clinical descriptors such as the age group of the person affected (e.g. pre-pubertal, juvenile, adult), the rate of progress of the disease (rapid, acute, chronic), the distribution of lesions (localized or generalized), or whether there are any particular debilitating or predisposing factors (e.g. pregnancy, diabetes, HIV-infection) (Table 7.1).

Table 7.1 Different types of periodontal diseases

Common	Rare
Chronic marginal gingivitis	HIV-gingivitis and HIV-periodontitis
Chronic adult periodontitis	Pregnancy gingivitis
	Acute streptococcal gingivitis
	Viral gingivitis
	Acute necrotizing ulcerative gingivitis
	Juvenile periodontitis
	Pre-pubertal periodontitis
	Rapidly progressing periodontitis

Periodontal diseases are common; for example, in a national survey in the UK, 79% of dentate adults had bleeding gums, 88% had calculus and 69% had periodontal pockets, including 10% with deep pockets. Periodontal diseases are also expensive to treat; in 1995–96, the costs to the NHS in the UK for simple one-visit periodontal treatment was £104 million, with two- and three-visit treatments costing another £30 million.

In periodontal diseases, the junctional epithelial tissue at the base of the gingival crevice migrates down the root of the tooth to form a periodontal pocket (*see* Figure 2.1). This is as a result of direct action by the micro-organisms themselves, and as a result of the indirect, but potentially damaging, side-effects of the inflammatory response mounted by the host in response to plaque accumulation.

Ecology of the periodontal pocket: implications for plaque sampling

As discussed in Chapters 2, 4 and 5, the ecology of the gingival crevice is different to that of other sites in the mouth; it is more anaerobic and the site is bathed in gingival crevicular fluid (GCF). In disease, the crevice becomes a pocket, and the Eh falls to low levels (i.e. highly anaerobic), while the flow of GCF is increased. GCF delivers humoral and cellular defence factors, and also provides complex proteins and glycoproteins that serve as novel substrates for bacterial metabolism, e.g. iron and haeme-containing molecules. Unlike dental caries, many of the bacteria associated with periodontal diseases are asaccharolytic but proteolytic. A consequence of proteolysis is that the pH in the pocket during disease becomes slightly alkaline (pH 7.4–7.8) compared to almost neutral values in health (ca. pH 6.9). The growth and enzyme activity of some periodontopathogens, such as *P. gingivalis,* is enhanced by alkaline growth conditions. Likewise, the temperature of the periodontal pocket can increase slightly during inflammation, and this can affect gene expression by periodontal pathogens such as *P. gingivalis*, and alter the balance of some of the predominant organisms.

The flow of GCF can remove micro-organisms not attached firmly to a surface. The cementum surface of the tooth is colonized by Gram-positive bacteria belonging mainly to the genera *Streptococcus* and *Actinomyces*. Many putative periodontopathogens (*Prevotella, Porphyromonas, Fusobacterium* spp.) can attach to this layer of cells by co-aggregation (*see* Chapter 5). Likewise, black-pigmented anaerobes and *Peptostreptococcus micros* may persist in the pocket due to their ability to adhere to crevicular epithelial cells. Indeed, their attachment to these cells is markedly enhanced when the epithelium has been treated with proteases of bacterial or host origin.

When attempting to determine the microflora of a periodontal pocket, care has to be taken to preserve the viability of the obligately anaerobic species during the taking, dispersing, diluting and cultivation of the sample. Many of the critical issues were discussed in Chapter 4. Ideally, the sample should be taken only from the base of the pocket, near the advancing front of the lesion in order to avoid removing organisms that are not associated with tissue destruction, and which might obscure any association between specific bacteria and disease activity. The use of rigorous recovery approaches, together with the application of molecular techniques (e.g. amplification of 16S rRNA sequences by PCR) has led to the discovery of organisms never before described.

Evidence for microbial involvement in periodontal diseases

Evidence that bacteria are implicated in periodontal diseases has come from gnotobiotic animal studies. Germ-free animals rarely suffer from periodontal disease, although, on occasions, food can be impacted in the gingival crevice producing inflammation. Inflammation, however, is much more common and severe when specific bacteria, particularly some of those isolated from human periodontal pockets, are used in pure culture to infect the animals. These bacteria include streptococci and *Actinomyces* spp. but are more commonly Gram-negative, for example, *Actinobacillus, Prevotella, Porphyromonas, Capnocytophaga, Eikenella, Fusobacterium* and *Selenomonas* spp.. Furthermore, periodontal disease is arrested when an antibiotic active against the particular microbe is administered to the infected animal. In humans, evidence for the role of micro-organisms has also come from plaque control and antibiotic treatment studies. These latter types of studies, however, can give no information as to whether disease results from the activity of (a) a single, or only a limited number of species (the '**specific plaque hypothesis**'); or (b) any combination of a wider range of plaque bacteria (the '**non-specific plaque hypothesis**') (*see also* Chapter 6).

In order to test these 'hypotheses', a large number of cross-sectional epidemiological studies have been performed on patients with particular forms of periodontal disease. As with dental caries, a disadvantage of this type of study is that true 'cause-and-effect' relationships can never be determined. Micro-organisms that appear to predominate at diseased sites might be present as a result of the disease, rather than having actually initiated it. With the exception of gingivitis, longitudinal studies (which do not suffer from this drawback) are not usually possible because of the lengthy natural history of most forms of periodontal disease and the difficulties in predicting subjects and sites likely to become affected. Recently, as with dental caries, the '**ecological plaque hypothesis**' has been applied to explain the aetiology of periodontal disease. This hypothesis proposes that changes in local environmental conditions in the sub-gingival region (e.g. the increased flow of GCF that occurs during inflammation) favour the growth of the proteolytic and obligately anaerobic (and often Gram-negative) species at the expense of those seen in health. This results in a shift in the overall balance of the sub-gingival microflora, thereby predisposing a site to disease; this hypothesis will be described in more detail later in this chapter.

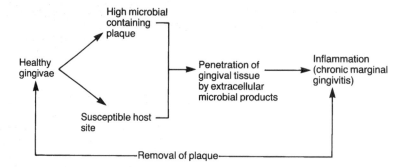

Figure 7.1 Schematic diagram of the aetiology of chronic gingivitis

Microbiology of periodontal diseases

Chronic marginal gingivitis

Chronic marginal gingivitis is a non-specific, inflammatory response to dental plaque involving the gingival margins. If good oral hygiene is restored, gingivitis is usually eradicated and the tissues becomes clinically normal again (Figure 7.1). Estimates of the incidence of gingivitis are difficult to determine but probably the whole dentate population is affected by this condition at some stage. Generally, gingivitis is regarded as resulting from a non-specific proliferation of the normal gingival crevice microflora due to poor oral hygiene.

The observation in the 1960s that gingivitis develops in a predictable and reproducible manner in volunteers who refrain from oral hygiene allowed the design of longitudinal studies to determine the bacteriological events that lead to disease.

The microflora associated with gingivitis is more diverse and differs in overall composition from that found in health. There is an increase (10–20-fold) in plaque mass, and there is a shift from the streptococci-dominated plaque of gingival health (Chapter 5) to one in which *Actinomyces* spp. predominate. The proportions of capnophilic (especially *Capnocytophaga* spp.) and obligately anaerobic Gram-negative bacteria also increase. An early study of 25 subjects suggested that specific relationships might exist between certain bacteria and particular stages in the development of gingivitis. When the gingivitis score was plotted as a function of the amount of plaque (plaque

score), the gingivitis score increased in two large increments. Proportions of *A. israelii* increased significantly from 13 to 26%, and *A. naeslundii* rose from 7 to 14% of the total cultivable microflora with the onset of a non-bleeding gingivitis. When the gingivitis progressed to a bleeding stage, black-pigmented anaerobes increased from 0.01 to 0.2% of the total microflora. The possible effect that bleeding might have had on the sub-gingival microflora is significant because black-pigmented anaerobes require haemin for growth and this can be derived from the degradation of proteins and glycoproteins present in GCF.

The potential diversity of the sub-gingival microflora, and the difficulties associated with data analysis, can be gauged from the results from two of the most comprehensive microbiological studies carried out so far. Around 160 different bacterial groups (taxa) were cultivated from four young adults participating in an experimental gingivitis study, while more than 100 non-spirochaetal taxa were isolated from 21 children and adults with naturally occurring gingivitis. In the former study, of the 166 taxa isolated, 73 showed a positive correlation with gingivitis, 29 were negatively correlated while the remainder either showed no correlation or were regarded as being present as a result of gingivitis. This last conclusion emphasizes the value of longitudinal studies. Despite the variability in the composition of the microflora between subjects, certain trends have emerged. The microflora becomes more diverse with time as gingivitis develops, although none of the taxa from either study were uniquely associated with gingivitis. However, some organisms are found more commonly in gingivitis and are rare in health. Some of the most likely aetiological agents in the experimental gingivitis study in young adults are shown in Table 7.2.

Table 7.2 Predominant bacteria of experimental gingivitis in young adult humans

Gram-positive bacteria	Gram-negative bacteria
Actinomyces israelii	*Prevotella oris*
Actinomyces naeslundii	*Prevotella intermedia*
Actinomyces odontolyticus	*Campylobacter* spp.
Propionibacterium acnes	*Wolinella* spp.
Lactobacillus spp.	*Veillonella parvula*
Streptococcus anginosus	*Fusobacterium nucleatum*
Streptococcus mitis	*Treponema* spp.
Peptostreptococcus micros	
Eubacterium spp.	

It is still not clear whether gingivitis is a necessary stage for the development of more serious forms of periodontal disease, or whether these can arise independently. Certainly some species that predominate in periodontitis, but which are not detectable in the healthy gingiva, have been found as a small percentage of the microflora in gingivitis. This suggests that environmental conditions which develop during gingivitis (e.g. bleeding, increased flow of GCF) may favour the growth of species implicated in periodontitis.

Chronic adult periodontitis

This is the most common form of advanced periodontal disease affecting the general population, and is a major cause of tooth loss after the age of 25 years. It differs from chronic marginal gingivitis in that in addition to the gingivae being involved, there is loss of attachment between the root surface, the gingivae and the alveolar bone, and bone loss itself may occur (Figure 7.2), giving an increased depth on probing (Figure 7.3), and bleeding. Factors that enhance plaque retention or impede plaque removal, such as sub-gingival calculus, overhanging restorations or crowded teeth, can predispose towards chronic periodontitis.

The inflammatory response to plaque is a basic host defence mechanism against microbial infections. Unfortunately, this host response also contributes to the destruction of tissues due to, for example, the release of lysosomal

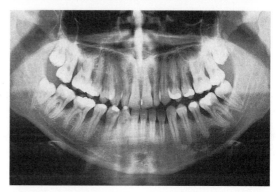

Figure 7.2 Radiograph of adult periodontitis showing extensive bone loss

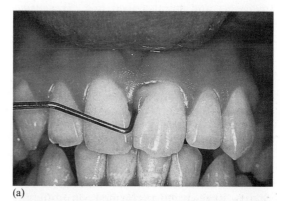

(a)

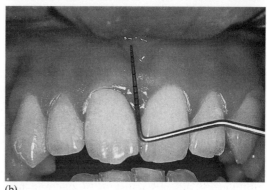

(b)

Figure 7.3 Use of a periodontal probe to determine the depth of a pocket: (*a*) the probe *in situ;* (*b*) the probe removed and overlaid on the tissues to show the extent of the loss of attachment

enzymes during phagocytosis, or to the production of cytokines that stimulate resident connective tissue cells to release metalloproteinases. Also, prostaglandins and cytokines generated during the inflammatory response can stimulate bone resorption (*see below*). The effectiveness of the inflammatory response can be gauged by the overall slow rate of progression of a lesion in normal individuals (with the result that tooth loss may take several decades to occur), compared to the rapidity and severity of periodontal diseases in subjects with impaired host defences. During pocket formation, there will be spells of disease activity followed by quiescent times, accompanied by healing.

Early studies of plaque associated with chronic periodontitis relied on microscopically observed, qualitative morphological descriptions of the micro-organisms present. Dark-field microscopy showed that many of the bacteria in plaque from patients with deep pockets were motile (probably *C. rectus* and *S. sputigena)* and spiral-shaped (e.g. *Treponema* spp.). Attempts have been made to use the presence of these morphotypes as the basis of a cheap and rapid test for use in the clinic to monitor the status of a pocket or effectiveness of treatment. Difficulties have arisen because many putative pathogens cannot be recognized on the basis of their cell morphology alone. Immunological probes, specific for targeted pathogens, can be used to detect selected bacteria directly in plaque samples without the need for lengthy cultural procedures.

Numerous cross-sectional microbiological studies have been performed on different patient groups with pockets of varying depths from a variety of geographical areas. All studies agree that the microflora is diverse and is composed of large numbers of obligately anaerobic Gram-negative rod and filament-shaped bacteria, many of which are asaccharolytic but proteolytic. These bacteria are often difficult to recover and identify in the laboratory and there is often conflicting evidence as to which organisms are the primary pathogens. Such studies have implicated certain clusters or combinations of bacteria with disease. Significantly, very different clusters of bacteria appeared to be able to produce an apparently similar pathological response. Thus, unlike some of the acute forms of periodontal disease, chronic periodontitis appears to result from the activity of mixtures of interacting bacteria.

In order to allow for the complexity of this microflora, some research teams screen routinely for the presence of almost 150 different microbial taxa in samples; for example, in one particularly comprehensive study, 136 distinct taxa were isolated from 38 sub-gingival samples from 22 adults. Few laboratories have the resources to monitor such a range of micro-organisms and so the majority of studies either restrict their screening to certain, pre-selected presumptive periodontal pathogens, or do not discriminate many of the ill-defined or more fastidious groups of micro-organisms. There is agreement that there is a progressive change in the composition of the microflora from health and gingivitis to periodontitis. This change involves not only the emergence of apparently previously undetected species, but also modifications to the numbers, or proportions, of a variety of species already present. Moreover, the changes in the microflora proceed in a manner which appears to be potentially highly variable both between individuals, and also at different sites in the same person.

Two theories have been proposed to explain the emergence of previously undetected species. It may be due to the selective growth (enrichment) of a micro-organism that is present in health in only very low numbers, due to a change in the environment during disease. Alternatively, it might be due to the exogenous acquisition of periodontopathic bacteria from other diseased sites or subjects. Some of the organisms that are considered to be potentially significant aetiological agents are listed in Table 7.3 (*see* opposite). There is a desire that a degree of specificity should exist in the microbial aetiology of periodontal diseases. As with many infections, it has been hoped that this specificity should be reflected in solitary or a very limited number of pathogenic species being implicated in periodontitis. Hopes that this indeed might be the case rose when it was observed that chronic periodontitis progressed not at a continuous slow rate, as was previously believed, but by distinct periods of disease activity over relatively short periods of time, followed by phases of quiescence or even repair. Thus, studies in which 'active lesions' had not been identified might have led to the inclusion of periodontal pockets which, at the time of sampling, were in remission and, therefore, possibly harbouring a 'non-active' microflora. This might have obscured significant associations of bacteria with those sites undergoing tissue destruction. Consequently, most recent studies have attempted to diagnose sites that are 'active' by comparing (a) changes in probing depth over short time periods, (b) detecting key enzymes, either of bacterial (e.g. arginine-specific) or host (e.g. elastase, cathepsin B)

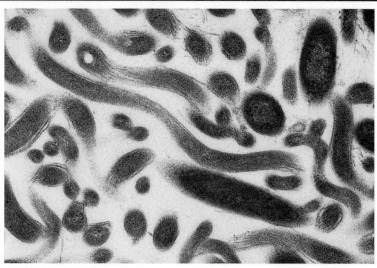

Figure 7.4 Electron micrograph of a sample from acute necrotizing ulcerative gingivitis (ANUG) showing spirochaetal cells

origin, or (c) inflammatory mediators (e.g. prostaglandin) and tissue breakdown products (e.g. glycosaminoglycans) in GCF.

The recognition by cultural studies of micro-organisms that are more commonly found in periodontal diseases than in health has enabled oligonucleotide probes to be constructed that are specific for these target species. These probes do not require the cultivation of slow-growing or nutritionally fastidious bacteria, and so hypotheses relating to the association of specific bacteria with different disease states can now be tested more rapidly and with more limited resources. Such studies have also tended to show that many of these putative pathogens can be found in health, but in extremely low numbers; their prevalence and concentration increase with the severity of disease at a site.

Table 7.3 Some bacterial species that have been commonly implicated in chronic periodontitis in adult humans

Gram-positive	Gram-negative
E. brachy	'B. forsythus'
E. nodatum	'B. pneumosintes'
E. timidium	F. nucleatum
P. anaerobius	P. gingivalis
P. micros	P. intermedia
	P. loescheii
	P. oralis
	C. rectus
	Treponema spp.

Studies have occasionally reported associations between streptococci and actinomyces with chronic periodontitis.

Acute necrotizing ulcerative gingivitis (ANUG)

Vincent's infection, or ANUG, is a painful, acute condition of the gingivae. It is characterized clinically by the formation of a grey pseudomembrane on the gingivae which easily sloughs off revealing a bleeding area beneath it. ANUG can usually be diagnosed by the characteristic halitosis (bad breath) it produces. Patients suffering from ANUG may be debilitated by another illness, or under acute emotional stress.

ANUG is a true infection and, unlike chronic marginal gingivitis, micro-organisms can be seen invading the host gingival tissues. In smears of the affected tissues the invading microbes resemble spirochaetes and fusiform bacteria (Figure 7.4). Early electron microscopic investigations showed that the invading micro-organisms consisted primarily of large and intermediate-sized spirochaetes which were present in the lesions in high numbers and in advance of other micro-organisms. A heterogeneous collection of micro-organisms have been isolated from ulcerated sites. Various spirochaetes (*Treponema* spp.) were found in high numbers (approximately 40% of the total cell count), but in view of the fuso-spirochaetal pattern characteristically observed by microscopy, the most unusual finding was the relatively low numbers of *Fusobacterium* spp. and the high proportions of *P. intermedia*, which averaged 3 and 24% of the total cultivable microflora, respectively. Metronidazole was effective in eliminating the fuso-spirochaetal complex from infected sites and this was associated with rapid clinical improvement. This study also concluded that disease was a result of an overgrowth of the resident microflora by obligately anaerobic species, probably as a result of selection through the availability of host-derived nutrients in individuals who had undergone stress or systemic disease.

Juvenile periodontitis

Juvenile periodontitis is a rare condition (affecting only around 0.1% of the susceptible age group) which usually occurs in adolescents. The disease appears to start around puberty, seems to be more common in girls, cases often cluster in families, and loss of attachment is rapid. Juvenile periodontitis also shows some racial predispositions, being slightly more common in people of West African and Asian origin.

Two forms of the disease have been described. In localized juvenile periodontitis (LJP) there is a distinct pattern of alveolar bone loss which is characteristically localized, for as yet unknown reasons, to the first permanent molars and the incisor teeth (Figure 7.5). In contrast, a generalized form has been described in which many teeth are affected. The aetiology of this particularly aggressive form of periodontal disease involves host and bacterial factors. The majority of patients with juvenile periodontitis have peripheral blood polymorphs (PMNs) with an impaired ability to react to chemotactic stimuli. This deficiency is coupled with, or is a direct cause of, the presence of relatively high numbers of *A. actinomycetemcomitans*. The microflora of plaque from patients with juvenile periodontitis is relatively sparse; considering the severity and rapidity of the tissue destruction and bone loss. There are relatively few micro-organisms present (approximately 10^6 cfu/pocket), belonging to only a limited number of species, and the majority of these are capnophilic Gram-negative rods. In some studies, *A. actinomycetemcomitans* could be recovered from 97% of affected sites and comprised up to 70% of the cultivable microflora. It has also been reported, however, that *A. actinomycetemcomitans* can be found quite commonly at healthy sites in some communities. For example, its prevalence was 13% in

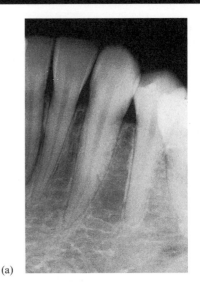

(a)

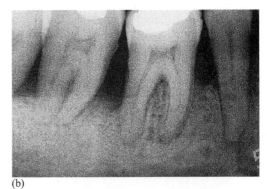

(b)

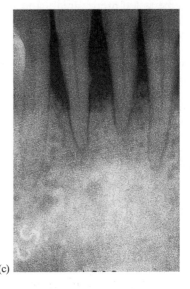

(c)

Figure 7.5 Radiograph of (*a*) normal periodontium, and (*b* and *c*) localized juvenile periodontitis. The level of bone is nearer the apex of the tooth in LJP

Finland and 20–25% in urban USA, perhaps again emphasizing the key role of the need for a susceptible host, while *A. actinomycetemcomitans* could not be recovered from some sites with the disease. Nevertheless, affected individuals tend to have elevated serum antibody titres to this micro-organism, while a reduction or elimination of this micro-organism results in a resolution of disease activity; recurrence of the disease is usually related to the re-appearance of *A. actinomycetemcomitans*. These findings have important implications in treatment design because tetracycline has been shown in clinical studies to be effective in eliminating *A. actinomycetemcomitans* from infected pockets, and resolving the clinical condition. This is in contrast to other forms of chronic inflammatory periodontal disease when metronidazole might be chosen because of its specific action against obligately anaerobic bacteria. Tetracycline does not always lead to complete elimination of *A. actinomycetemcomitans* from the pocket, and the combination of metronidazole and amoxycillin has been found to be particularly effective in these situations, particularly when combined with scaling and root planing.

Five serotypes of *A. actinomycetemcomitans* have been described (serotypes *a–e*), and more than one serotype can be found in the mouth of an individual. In general, serotype *b* strains are found more commonly in LJP patients than the other serotypes. Intra-family transmission of strains may occur, and molecular studies have provided evidence for the existence of virulent clones (*see below*).

Strains of *A. actinomycetemcomitans* produce a range of relevant virulence factors. These include a powerful leukotoxin (i.e. a protein toxic for polymorphs), LPS (endotoxin, which can stimulate bone resorption), and cell surface associated material, which induces resorption of bone. In addition, *A. actinomycetemcomitans* produces enzymes with the ability to degrade collagen, as well as other, less well-defined factors, that modulate the activity of the host defences. Histological studies have shown that *A. actinomycetemcomitans* can invade gingival connective tissues.

In contrast to most other forms of periodontal disease, therefore, LJP appears to result from the activity of a relatively specific microflora dominated by a single species. Some studies have found LJP sites in which *A. actinomycetemcomitans* is not necessarily the predominant micro-organism, which is analogous to the situation described in Chapter 6 with respect to dental caries and the presence of mutans streptococci. In these pockets, small spirochaetes, *E. corrodens*, *Wolinella* spp. and *F. nucleatum* are often numerous. Even when the presence of *A. actinomycetemcomitans* did correlate with LJP, its proportions ranged from 10 to 99% of the total pocket microflora in only 17% of 137 affected sites. In addition, 20% of sites contained from 1 to 10% *A. actinomycetemcomitans*, while 64% of sites harboured less than 1% *A. actinomycetemcomitans*. Some sites with active breakdown have no recoverable *A. actinomycetemcomitans* implying that, in a minority of cases, the same pathological condition can be caused by other micro-organisms.

In one of the few microbiological studies of generalized juvenile periodontitis, *Treponema* spp. were closely associated with disease (including morphotypes that could not be cultured but which could be distinguished by microscopy), as were *F. nucleatum*, lactobacilli, several species of *Eubacterium*, *Peptostreptococcus* spp., *P. intermedia* and *Selenomonas* spp.. The role, and therefore the significance, of most of these bacteria in disease has yet to be determined.

Other periodontal diseases

Acute, or exaggerated, forms of gingivitis can arise due to a variety of predisposing factors or circumstances. They are most commonly associated with HIV infection, diabetes, pregnancy, puberty, menstruation, stress, or the use of oral contraceptives. The microbiological findings from some of these forms of gingivitis and other periodontal diseases will be considered below.

HIV-gingivitis and HIV-periodontitis
HIV-positive patients can present with an atypical gingivitis which is characterized by a band-like marginal erythema, usually accompanied by diffuse redness, which extends into the vestibular mucosa. It may bleed easily, and not respond to treatment. The microflora has been determined using conventional cultural and indirect immunofluorescence techniques. HIV-gingivitis sites were commonly colonized by *C. albicans* and by a range of putative periodontopathogens including *A. actinomycetemcomitans*, *F. nucleatum* and *P. gingivalis*

Table 7.4 Percentage isolation frequency of some micro-organisms from the gingival crevice of healthy subjects, and from HIV-positive subjects with gingivitis or periodontitis

Micro-organism	HIV-negative patients (health and gingivitis)	HIV-positive patients with	
		Gingivitis	Periodontitis
A. naeslundii	NR	86	70
A. actinomycetemcomitans	2	65	74
E. corrodens	4	43	30
Capnocytophaga spp.	6	29	30
F. nucleatum	31	78	66
P. gingivalis	2	86	100
P. intermedia	31	100	90
C. rectus	15	43	60
C. albicans	3	49	74

NR, Not reported in this study, but commonly found in health

(Table 7.4), some of which are less common in chronic gingivitis.

HIV-positive patients can also suffer from an unusually severe and rapid form of periodontitis. The disease is generalized and is associated with blunted or cratered gingival papillae, loss of periodontal attachment, soft tissue ulceration and necrosis, as well as the more usual indicators of periodontitis (bone loss and bleeding). Indeed, there is a tendency towards spontaneous bleeding, and the condition is sometimes extremely painful. Preliminary studies suggest that the isolation frequency of a number of putative periodontopathogens such as *P. gingivalis*, *P. intermedia*, *F. nucleatum* and *A. actinomycetemcomitans*, as well as *C. albicans* was higher than at control sites. The predominant micro-organisms, however, were streptococci (mean proportion = 56% of the total cultivable microflora) especially *S. sanguis* and *S. mitis*, and anaerobic Gram-negative rods (24% of the total cultivable microflora). Black-pigmented anaerobes comprised over 12% of the microflora, and *P. intermedia* was the most prevalent species. The microflora of the HIV-gingivitis and HIV-periodontitis lesions are not markedly distinct, although the pathological consequences are quite different. This may be due to variations in the immune status of the respective groups.

Care must be taken in the treatment of these patients, as all procedures will result in bleeding, and the risk of cross-infection will be high (*see* Chapter 14). Patients are normally treated by conventional therapy, e.g. plaque control, scaling and root planing. This may be supplemented by chlorhexidine mouthwashes or local irrigation. Ulceration may respond to antibiotics such as metronidazole and amoxycillin.

Pregnancy gingivitis
The factors responsible for an exaggerated gingivitis in pregnancy have been linked to an increase in the proportions of the black-pigmented anaerobe *P. intermedia* during the second trimester, possibly due to the appearance of steroid hormones in GCF.

Acute streptococcal gingivitis
Acute streptococcal gingivitis is a condition affecting the gingivae which can result in severe illness. The gingivae become red, swollen and full of fluid (oedematous), the temperature is raised and the regional lymph nodes are also enlarged. If cultures are taken from the affected gingivae, a Lancefield group A streptococcus is usually isolated. Although a number of streptococci have been implicated in the aetiology of the disease, *Streptococcus pyogenes* is usually the pathogen responsible.

This disease is usually preceded by a sore throat and hence it is possible that there is a direct spread of *S. pyogenes* from throat to gingivae. One curious factor is that the disease persists for 6–15 days irrespective of penicillin treatment (the antibiotic of choice). It has been suggested that this persistence after therapy represents a secondary opportunistic viral infection, although as yet this is unproven.

Acute herpetic gingivitis
The majority of infectious cases of gingivitis are

bacterial in origin but occasionally viral gingivitis is seen, predominantly in young people. The commonest form of viral gingivitis is acute herpetic gingivitis, the causative agent of which is Herpes simplex type 1 (HSV-1). Acute herpetic gingivitis is seen usually in children and appears as ulcerated swellings of the gingivae which are acutely painful. The symptoms may persist for 7–21 days and herpetic lesions may concomitantly be present on lips or any area of the oral mucosa. The diagnosis is usually made on clinical criteria although cytological smears and cytopathic effects following culture have been used for confirmation; direct immunofluorescence is also used for diagnosis. Some antiviral agents (e.g. acyclovir and penciclovir) have been found to be effective treatments.

Pre-pubertal periodontitis

Destructive periodontal disease in the primary dentition can occur in a localized and generalized form. Localized pre-pubertal periodontitis usually has its onset before the age of 5 years. The gingival tissues have only minor clinical inflammation, dental plaque may be minimal, and the disease can usually be arrested by antibiotic treatment and mechanical periodontal therapy. Generalized pre-pubertal periodontitis occurs at the time of tooth eruption and severe gingival inflammation can be common. The disease can be refractory to most treatments, and may be associated with recurrent infections, and abnormalities of peripheral neutrophils and monocytes. Pre-pubertal periodontitis is rare, although in one recent study of over 2000 children in the USA, around 1% had radiographic evidence of bone loss. A higher prevalence of putative periodontopathogens such as *A. actinomycetemcomitans*, *P. intermedia*, *Capnocytophaga* spp. and *E. corrodens* have been found at diseased sites.

Rapidly progressing periodontitis

This is a poorly defined clinical condition, and it is not always clear whether such individuals could also be diagnosed as having generalized juvenile periodontitis. The amount of plaque is usually low at affected sites, which is surprising considering the rate of loss of attachment. In severe lesions, *P. gingivalis*, '*B. forsythus*', *F. nucleatum*, *A. actinomycetemcomitans* and *Campylobacter* spp. were found to predominate the microflora. This finding may again point to

major abnormalities in the functioning of the host defences in these individuals.

Cancrum oris (noma)

This is a highly tissue-destructive disease found mainly in Africa, and is associated with malnourished individuals. The disease process may involve three stages: (a) a staging period, where infection, e.g. measles, results in a lowered host resistance, and the appearance of oral lesions; (b) an infection period, where some trigger activates a polymicrobial infection, and (c) a tissue invasion and destruction phase, during which an acute ulcerative condition progresses to oro-facial gangrene, which is life-threatening. *Fusobacterium necrophorum* acquired from domesticated animals might be the trigger organism for the development of Cancrum oris.

Diabetes-associated periodontal disease

In general, patients with diabetes have more severe episodes of periodontal disease, especially in younger subjects whose condition is poorly controlled, compared with healthy controls. Diseased sites have higher proportions of *Capnocytophaga*, and other periodontal pathogens. Sometimes, non-oral bacteria (e.g. staphylococci) have been isolated. These changes in microflora may reflect a compromised host defence.

Bacteria and disease progression

The microflora associated with bursts of disease activity have been analysed in both chronic and acute forms of periodontal disease. In patients with localized juvenile periodontitis, periods of apparent disease activity were reflected in a less diverse microflora in which the absolute counts and proportions of only *A. actinomycetemcomitans* and *E. corrodens* were significantly higher. Similarly, in subjects described as having 'destructive periodontal disease', the isolation frequency of *P. intermedia*, '*B. forsythus*', *A. actinomycetemcomitans* and *C. rectus* was significantly higher at active sites. An alternative approach has been to determine the prevalence of three putative periodontopathogens at sites with active or inactive disease. *A. actinomycetemcomitans*, *P. gingivalis* or *P. intermedia* were isolated from 99% of progressing pockets but from only 40% of inactive sites. It was hoped that this finding might lead to a predictive test to identify sites at risk of future disease progression. When all three species were absent from a site, the probability of the pocket undergoing future progression was only 1%, but in a prospective study, only 20% of sites suffered attachment loss when one or more of these micro-organisms were present. Thus, as with the situation with mutans streptococci and dental caries, there is more chance of ruling out the possibility of disease when key micro-organisms are absent than predicting future episodes of disease when they are present.

Re-evaluation of the microbial aetiology of periodontal diseases

The data presented above concerning the predominant microflora associated with periodontal diseases are derived from numerous studies which, inevitably, do not have similar clinical or microbiological designs, and so may not always be directly comparable. For example, some study designs detect only the predominant micro-organisms, while others identify all of the colony types, and make no assumptions about the putative pathogens. In contrast, other studies use selective media to search specifically for and isolate pre-determined key micro-organisms, even when they might comprise only a small proportion of the plaque microflora.

The research team from the Virginia Polytechnic Institute, USA, has carried out the most comprehensive bacteriological studies of human periodontal disease. In a range of studies of the gingival crevice in health and disease from 300 people, 51 000 bacteria were isolated, and 509 distinct taxa were recognized, a significant proportion of which (141/509) were detected only once. The data from these studies have recently been pooled and re-analysed. This has the advantage that similar methods were used to identify a wide range of bacteria; in addition, these micro-organisms represented the predominant microflora (i.e. representing 10–90% of the total cultivable bacteria). A feature of this analysis was the clear demonstration that the severe diseases were associated with a greater diversity of Gram-negative species, while the range of Gram-positive species decreased with increasing disease severity (Tables 7.5 and 7.6). In particular, various species of *Actinomyces* and *Streptococcus* were

more associated with gingival health (*see* Table 7.6).

Table 7.5 Bacteria whose proportions in plaque rise with increasing severity of periodontal disease

Gram-positive	Gram-negative
E. alactolyticum	*A. actinomycetemcomitans*
E. brachy	*'B. gracilis'*
E. nodatum	*C. concisus*
E. saphenum	*C. rectus*
E. timidum	*C. curvus*
Eubacterium spp.[a]	*F. alocis*
L. rimae	*F. nucleatum*
L. uli	*P. denticola*
P. anaerobius	*P. intermedia*
	P. nigrescens
	P. melaninogenica
	P. oris
	P. tannerae
	P. veroralis
	P. gingivalis
	S. flueggei
	S. infelix
	S. noxia
	S. sputigena

[a] At the time of the study, these isolates could not be ascribed to a species.

The most commonly isolated species from all of the samples analysed were *A. naeslundii* and *F. nucleatum*, although the relative concentration of *A. naeslundii* tended to decrease as the severity of the disease increased, while *F. nucleatum* was closely associated with diseased sites. There are several subspecies of *F. nucleatum*; in disease, the most common subspecies was *F. nucleatum* subspecies *vincentii*, followed by subspecies *nucleatum* and subspecies *polymorphum* (ratio 7:3:2, respectively). *F. nucleatum* maintained its proportion as gingivitis progressed and as periodontitis developed; however, because of the corresponding increase in depth and volume of the periodontal pocket in disease, this represented an increase in cell mass of 10 000-fold.

The diversity of the microflora increased as the severity of periodontal disease rose (Tables 7.5, 7.7 and 7.8); this was assumed to be due to a stimulation of the growth of many species by the elevated flow of GCF. Many of the putative periodontal pathogens did not increase in

Table 7.6 Bacteria whose proportions in plaque decrease with the severity of periodontal disease

Gram-positive	Gram-negative
A. meyeri	*C. gingivalis*
A. naeslundii	*H. aphrophilus*
A. odontolyticus	*H. segnis*
Actinomyces spp.[a]	*Leptotrichia* spp.
E. sabbureum	*N. elongata*
R. dentocariosa	*N. mucosa*
S. gordonii	*V. parvula*
S. intermedius	
S. oralis	
S. salivarius	
S. sanguis	

[a]These strains could not be ascribed to a particular species.

prevalence until after the initial stages of inflammation (Table 7.7). Although spirochaetes can be detected at healthy sites, the isolation frequency of many species rose as gingivitis and periodontitis progressed (Table 7.8); this was particularly apparent for *T. denticola* and a 'large treponeme' that could be seen by microscopy, but as yet cannot be cultured. *Mycoplasma* spp. also increase in prevalence with disease severity (Table 7.8), but there is little information available as to their classification or disease potential.

None of the species listed in Tables 7.7 and 7.8 are present in high numbers at all sites or in all forms of periodontal disease. Periodontal diseases are a result, therefore, of the interaction and combined activities of a range of species; such diseases probably represent an example of 'pathogenic synergy', discussed later in this chapter).

The habitat and source of periodontopathic bacteria: implications for the aetiology of disease

The predominant bacteria found in the various types of periodontal disease are different from those that are prevalent in the healthy gingival crevice. One of the most intriguing questions in periodontology, therefore, concerns the reservoir and source of these potential periodontopathogens. Some periodontopathic bacteria can attach to mucosal surfaces, and a range of putative periodontal pathogens (including black-pigmented anaerobes, *Capnocytophaga* spp., spirochaetes and *Fusobacterium* spp.) were isolated from the dorsum of the tongue and from tonsils. Thus, the dorsum of the tongue may act as a reservoir for certain periodontopathic bacteria.

Usually the above putative periodontal pathogens are detected by culture only occasionally, and in low numbers, in the healthy gingival crevice. Studies using more sensitive immunological and molecular techniques, however, have found that putative periodontal pathogens, including *A. actinomycetemcomitans*, '*B. forsythus*', *C. rectus*, *P. gingivalis* and *T. denticola*, are more widespread than previously thought, but in numbers below those capable of detection by conventional cultural techniques.

In general, the putative periodontal pathogens are non-competitive with other members of the resident microflora at healthy sites, and remain at low levels; such levels would not be clinically significant. If plaque is allowed to

Table 7.7 Percentage of sites in which some putative periodontal pathogens were detected among the predominant microflora from a range of periodontal diseases

Bacterium	Periodontal disease							
	Health	GI1	GI2	MP	AP	GEOP	LJP	EOP
A. actinomycetemcomitans	0	0	9	4	6	0	6	5
'*B. gracilis*'	21	22	27	25	38	17	16	33
C. rectus	21	22	45	48	17	22	34	15
E. timidium	14	0	27	46	26	69	56	58
F. nucleatum	71	67	91	77	84	83	66	78
P. gingivalis	0	0	0	12	11	5	6	27
S. sputigena	7	0	18	19	31	28	19	42

GI1 and GI2, gingivitis; MP, moderate periodontitis; AP, adult periodontitis; GEOP, generalized early onset periodontitis; LJP, localized juvenile periodontitis; EOP, early onset periodontitis.

Table 7.8 Percentage isolation frequency of spirochaetes and mycoplasma from different forms of periodontal disease

Bacterium	Periodontal disease					
	Health	GI1	GI2	AP	GEOP	LJP
T. denticola	5	7	18	18	30	20
T. pectinovorum	8	6	21	20	17	23
T. socranskii subsp. *buccale*	13	10	25	20	20	13
subsp. *paredis*	3	5	9	8	3	—
subsp. *socranskii*	21	20	35	39	10	20
T. vincentii	16	13	21	15	3	3
Large treponeme	—	1	7	5	63	53
Mycoplasma	—	13	23	16	50	43

GI1 and GI2, gingivitis; AP, adult periodontitis; GEOP, generalized early onset periodontitis; LJP, localized juvenile periodontitis.

accumulate beyond levels that are compatible with health, then the host mounts an inflammatory response. The flow of GCF is increased, and this introduces into the crevice not only components of the host defences but also complex host molecules that can be catabolized by the proteolytic Gram-negative anaerobes. This change in the local environment will favour the growth of these putative pathogens at the expense of the species associated with gingival health. This can lead to a shift in the proportions of the resident sub-gingival microflora. This is analogous to the increases in mutans streptococci and *Lactobacillus* spp. seen prior to caries development following the repeated ingestion of dietary carbohydrates. Evidence for these shifts has come from laboratory studies. The growth of sub-gingival plaque on human serum (used to mimic GCF) led to the selection of species associated with periodontal destruction, such as black-pigmented anaerobes, peptostreptococci, *Fusobacterium* spp. and spirochaetes; most of these species could not be detected in the original samples. Likewise, a rise in pH from 7.0 to 7.5 (as can occur during inflammation) can allow *P. gingivalis* to rise from <1% to >99% of a microbial community of black-pigmented anaerobes. If similar events occur in a pocket, then periodontal diseases could be regarded as endogenous or opportunistic infections, caused by an imbalance in the composition of the resident microflora at a site, due to an alteration in the ecology of the local habitat. This view is formulated in the 'ecological plaque hypothesis' (*see also* Chapter 6), which describes the dynamic relationship between the resident microflora and the host in health and disease in ecological terms (Figure 7.6). A consequence of this hypothesis is that disease can be prevented not only by targeting the putative pathogens, but also by interfering with the environmental factors that drive the changes in the balance in the microflora, e.g. such as by reducing the inflammatory response, or by altering the redox potential of the pocket to prevent the growth of the obligate anaerobes. Other relevant changes in the local environment that could affect the host–microbe interaction could come from trauma, an alteration in the immune status of the host (e.g. during systemic disease or after drug therapy), or from smoking.

Periodontal diseases could also be regarded as exogenous infections because some of the causative bacteria, such as *P. gingivalis*, are not widely distributed in the healthy mouth and are not, therefore, regarded by some as members of the resident microflora. The use of molecular techniques to develop DNA fingerprints has shown that transmission of *P. gingivalis* and *A. actinomycetemcomitans* can occur among family members, with parents and children sharing strains with identical patterns. Likewise, some married couples have been shown to have the same clonal types of *P. gingivalis* and *A. actinomycetemcomitans*, indicating that these species can be transmitted between spouses on occasions. Intriguingly, there has been a report of a child with Papillon–Lefevre syndrome who was consistently re-infected with *A. actinomy-*

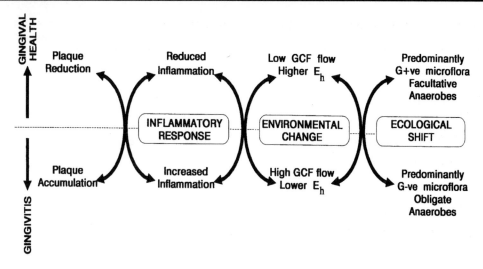

Figure 7.6 A schematic representation of the 'ecological plaque hypothesis' in relation to periodontal disease. Plaque accumulation produces an inflammatory host response; this causes changes in the local environmental conditions which favour the growth of proteolytic and anaerobic Gram-negative bacteria. Disease could be prevented by not only targeting the putative pathogens but also by interfering with the factors driving their selection. Reproduced with permission; Advances in Dental Research

cetemcomitans; the child apparently had acquired its biotype of *A. actinomycetemcomitans* from the family pet dog. Further studies will be necessary to determine whether other episodes of *Actinobacillus*-associated periodontal destruction in children also represent a zoonosis. If so, treatment might also involve elimination or suppression of putative periodontopathogens from their primary oral reservoirs. Even if a pathogen is acquired from another individual, it will be present initially at only low cell levels. As described earlier, a major ecological disturbance will have to occur at a site if these putative pathogens are going to be able to outcompete the other members of the plaque microflora, and achieve numerical significance.

Risk factors for periodontal diseases

An essential requirement for oral diseases, in addition to the presence of a pathogenic microflora, is the need for a susceptible host. As discussed above, ecological changes can occur within an individual pocket that result in the initiation of disease. There are also systemic factors that predispose a site or subject to disease. Large scale epidemiological surveys using multi-factorial statistical analyses to correct or compensate for confounding parameters such as gender, age etc. have identified (a) non-insulin-dependent diabetes mellitus (type II), especially in individuals in whom metabolic control is poor, and (b) tobacco smoking, as major risk factors. Smoking tobacco increases the risk of periodontal disease by two- to seven-fold, depending on the level of smoking. The sub-gingival microflora is different in smokers, and there are statistically higher proportions in plaque of '*B. forsythus*' and *P. micros*. There is evidence that chemical derivatives of nicotine present in GCF can augment the potency of some metabolites of periodontal pathogens and be toxic to host cells involved in wound healing. In addition, smoking can lead to a reduction in serum levels of IgG_2 and to impaired function of polymorphs.

Other risk factors for periodontal diseases include conditions associated with reduced neutrophil numbers or activity, or with neutrophil dysfunction such as that associated with LJP. Improvements in assessing accurately various human behaviours have enabled stress, distress and coping disorders to also be identified as important risk factors for periodontal disease.

Treatment and prevention of periodontal diseases

Plaque control

Plaque control is fundamental to (a) the prevention of gingivitis, (b) treatment of established disease (gingivitis or periodontitis) and (c) in the maintenance of health following effective treatment. Plaque control can be achieved by conventional oral hygiene measures such as toothbrushing and flossing, which can be augmented by professional prophylaxis during routine visits to the dentist.

As discussed in Chapter 6, a number of antimicrobial agents have been incorporated into toothpastes and mouthwashes, in order to provide anti-plaque and anti-gingivitis benefits. These agents include metal salts (e.g. zinc citrate), enzymes (e.g. glucose oxidase/amyloglucosidase), plant extracts (e.g. sanguinarine), bisbiguanides (e.g. chlorhexidine) and phenols (e.g. Triclosan). These antimicrobial agents can not only inhibit the growth of relevant sub-gingival bacteria, but can interfere with the expression of virulence determinants (e.g. protease activity) when present at sub-MIC levels. Their efficacy in preventing gingivitis has been demonstrated using an experimental gingivitis model in human volunteers. Mouthwashes containing chlorhexidine are also effective against established gingivitis; it is yet to be determined how effective antimicrobial agents delivered from toothpastes are in resolving pre-existing disease.

In more advanced forms of periodontal disease, treatment requires professional plaque control which in some circumstances may require surgery so that clear access to the root surface is achieved. In extreme cases, not only is there a need to remove plaque and/or calculus, but also the outer surface layers of cementum (root planing), because of the possible penetration into cementum of cytotoxic or inflammatory products of sub-gingival bacteria, especially endotoxin (lipopolysaccharide, LPS). Even after thorough root planing to remove obvious deposits of plaque and calculus, residual bacteria may still be present, and sites can be re-populated rapidly leading to further loss of attachment in some pockets. Consequently, post-surgical control of microorganisms is sometimes necessary. This again can involve meticulous supra-gingival plaque control (to reduce the likelihood of sub-gingival colonization) or the use of antimicrobial agents, such as chlorhexidine, or even systemic antibiotics, such as tetracycline, amoxycillin or metronidazole. Antibiotics should only be used in special circumstances, such as localized juvenile periodontitis or in refractory periodontal disease, because of the problems of antibiotic resistance. A preferred approach is to apply antimicrobial agents locally. This can be by hollow fibres impregnated with the drug of choice, by direct irrigation of the pocket, by inserting slow release materials such as acrylic or ethyl cellulose polymers, or by antibiotic-impregnated gels. Chlorhexidine, metronidazole and tetracycline have been successfully delivered in this way.

A novel approach to controlling specific pathogens in plaque in the future may involve photodynamic therapy. Periodontal pathogens, including *P. gingivalis*, *A actinomycetemcomitans* and *F. nucleatum*, are susceptible to killing by low power laser light once cells have been treated with low concentrations of a photosensitizer dye such as toluidine blue. This therapy could also be applied to cariogenic bacteria.

Refractory periodontal disease

In a small minority of cases, pockets with destructive periodontal disease fail to respond to conventional treatment even when augmented with antibiotic therapy. Microbiological findings indicated that these pockets did not form a homogeneous group in terms of the predominant species that were recovered. Three major groupings of bacteria were found involving different combinations of '*B. forsythus*', *F. nucleatum*, *C. rectus*, *S. intermedius*, *P. gingivalis* and *P. micros*.

Other reasons for pockets to be refactory to treatment include (a) the development of antibiotic resistance among the members of the pocket microflora following previous use of the antibiotic and (b) the inactivation of a drug by neighbouring bacteria. In a study of 52 patients, β-lactamase activity was detected in the GCF of 36% of 200 sites with pocket depths $> 3 \, mm$ and in 13% of 206 shallower pockets. The levels of β-lactamase activity were considered sufficient in 60% of the positive sites to inactivate the likely clinical levels of penicillin in GCF. Pockets may also appear refractory

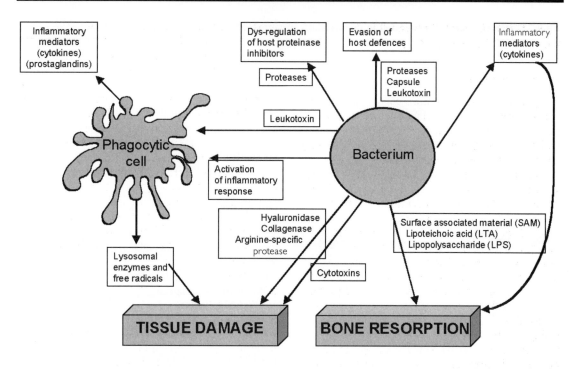

Figure 7.7 Diagram to illustrate the mechanisms by which plaque can cause damage to host tissues by direct and indirect routes of pathogenicity

due to an inappropriate drug being administered. In a large cross-sectional study of 500 patients with refractory sites, nearly one third of pockets were colonized by non-resident oral micro-organisms including yeasts (especially *C. albicans*), staphylococci, enterobacteria and *Pseudomonas aeruginosa*. When present, these micro-organisms could constitute between 20 and 40% of the microflora. All yeasts and the majority of enteric rods and pseudomonads were resistant to tetracycline, penicillin G and erythromycin. It may be necessary, therefore, to perform a microbiological screening in some refractory patients prior to treatment with antibiotics.

Pathogenic mechanisms in periodontal disease

The major forms of periodontal disease are characterized by the progressive destruction of the supporting tissues of teeth in the apparent absence (at least in the early stages) of significant tissue invasion. Tissue damage, therefore, must also be mediated by surface components and extracellular products of bacteria (Table 7.9). These bacterial products can cause destruction of gingival tissue by two mechanisms. In one, damage results from the *direct* action of bacterial enzymes and cytotoxic products of bacterial metabolism. In the other, bacterial components are only *indirectly* responsible, causing tissue destruction as the inevitable side-effect of the protective host inflammatory response to plaque antigens; this has been termed 'bystander damage' (Figure 7.7).

Indirect pathogenicity

Any sub-gingival plaque bacteria could be considered to be playing a role in tissue destruction via the indirect pathogenicity route if they contribute to an inflammatory host response. Bacterial antigens can penetrate the crevicular epithelium and stimulate either humoral or cell-mediated immunity. Humoral immunity results in the synthesis of immunoglobulins, which activate the complement cascade that leads to inflammation and the generation of prostaglandins. Prostaglandins

Table 7.9 Bacterial factors implicated in the aetiology of periodontal diseases

Stage of disease		Bacterial factor
Attachment to host tissues		Surface components, e.g. 'adhesins' Surface structures, e.g. fimbriae
Multiplication at a susceptible site		Protease production to obtain nutrients Development of food chains Inhibitor production, e.g. bacteriocins
Evasion of host defences		Capsules and slimes PMN-receptor blockers Leukotoxin Immunoglobin-specific proteases Complement-degrading proteases Suppressor T-cell induction

Tissue damage	(a) direct	**Enzymes**
		  'Arginine-specific' proteases
		  Collagenase
		  Hyaluronidase
		  Chondroitin sulphatase
		Bone resorbing factors
		  Lipoteichoic acid
		  Lipopolysaccharide (LPS)
		  Capsule
		  Surface-associated material
		Cytotoxins
		  Butyric and propionic acids
		  Indole
		  Amines
		  Ammonia
		  Volatile sulphur compounds

	(b) indirect	Inflammatory response to plaque antigens (*see text*)

are inflammatory mediators, and can stimulate bone resorption. Levels of prostaglandin in GCF correlate with periodontal status, and can act as molecular predictors of attachment loss. In contrast, cellular immunity leads to the release of cytokines from activated T-lymphocytes, and these modulate macrophage activity. Activated macrophages release cytokines that communicate with other host cells, and these interactions can lead to tissue damage. The cytokines include tissue necrosis factor (TNF-α), gamma-interferon (IFN-γ), and interleukin-1 (IL-1). Both IL-1 and TNF-α can induce the release of collagenase from a variety of connective tissue cells, including fibroblasts, and stimulate bone resorption.

Important host tissue cells in the gingival crevice include the pocket epithelium and the periodontal ligament. In addition to collagen, these cells are also made up of glycosaminoglycan (GAG) molecules linked to a protein core. The main proteoglycans of the gingivae and periodontal ligament are hyaluronic acid, heparin sulphate, dermatan sulphate and chondroitin sulphate 4. These proteoglycans can be degraded by elastase and cathepsin B which are present in the inflamed gingival crevice, and are probably derived from polymorphs, macrophages and fibroblasts. Mast cells can be found migrating through the junctional epithelium and into the pocket, and can release histamine and other vasoactive molecules, as well as a range of proteases.

Many of the host cells in the gingival crevice also contain proteinase inhibitors such as α-1-proteinase inhibitor and α-2-macroglobulin, which are responsible for inactivating proteases in the host tissues. These molecules enable the host to control the potentially destructive forces of the inflammatory response. As will be discussed in the next section, bacterial proteases can degrade these important control molecules, leading to further 'bystander damage' to tissues.

Direct pathogenicity

The putative pathogens produce a range of potential virulence factors that enable them to:

(a) colonize and multiply at sub-gingival sites;
(b) evade or inactivate the host defences;
(c) induce tissue damage; and on occasions,
(d) invade host tissues.

These virulence factors will be described in the following sections.

Colonization and multiplication

As discussed in Chapters 4 and 5, periodontal pathogens are able to colonize the sub-gingival environment by means of cell surface adhesins that interact with specific receptors. These may be located either on the root surface or on gingival epithelial cells, or the pathogens may co-aggregate with already attached Gram-positive bacteria such as streptococci and *Actinomyces* spp.. These putative pathogens produce a range of proteases and glycosidases in order to obtain nutrients from the catabolism of host molecules; often several species with complementary enzyme profiles combine to catabolize complex molecules. Bacteria such as *P. gingivalis* also possess haemagglutination and haemolytic activities, which may be a means of targeting appropriate substrates for the release of essential co-factors for growth, such as haemin, from host molecules. A lysine-x protease may degrade haemoglobin, and is essential for the growth of *P. gingivalis*.

Evasion and/or inactivation of the host defences

Phagocytic cells form the main defence strategy by the host against periodontal pathogens. As stated earlier, many strains of *A. actinomycetemcomitans* produce a powerful protein leukotoxin able to lyse human neutrophils, monocytes and a sub-population of lymphocytes, whilst other cell types (e.g. epithelial and endothelial cells, fibroblasts, erythrocytes, etc.) are resistant. The leukotoxin belongs to the RTX (repeats-in-toxin) family of bacterial pore-forming cytolysins; *C. rectus* also produces a leukotoxin.

In studies of strains of *A. actinomycetemco-mitans* isolated from several countries, especially those in northern Europe, a wide range of clonal types were recognized, suggesting that these were opportunistic pathogens (*see* Chapter 4). Strains of *A. actinomycetemcomitans* serotype *b*, however, have been recognized recently that over-produce their leukotoxin by up to 20 times that seen in other strains. These serotype *b* strains form a single clone, and are from individuals who can all be traced back to North West Africa, but who now live in various countries around the world. Several members of the families of these individuals have LJP. The same clone has not been isolated from Caucasians nor from healthy individuals, giving rise to the speculation that this might represent a specific, and highly infectious clone of a periodontopathogen.

Several periodontal pathogens produce ill-defined molecules that can inhibit the chemotaxis of polymorphonuclear leucocytes (PMNs), and interfere with their ability to kill bacteria or phagocytose cells. Several common sub-gingival species produce proteases that can degrade components of the immune response including immunoglobulins, complement and cytokines. Bacteria, including *A. actinomycetemcomitans* also exert an immunosuppressive effect, perhaps mediated by cell surface proteins, while *P. gingivalis* possesses a capsule, which protect cells against phagocytosis.

Induction of tissue damage

Members of the sub-gingival microflora can produce a range of enzymes that may play a direct role in the damage of host tissues in the periodontal pocket. For example, *P. gingivalis* has been shown to produce collagenases that can degrade type I and type IV collagen, although the majority of collagenase activity in GCF is host-derived. Once denatured, collagen may be broken down by bacterial proteases with a broader specificity. Other enzymes produced by sub-gingival bacteria that may damage tissues directly include hyaluronidase, chondroitin sulphatase and glycylprolyl peptidase. These enzymes can also be detected on outer membrane vesicles of Gram-negative bacteria; these vesicles can be shed from the cell surface during growth, enhancing the likelihood of tissue penetration by these enzymes (*see* Figures 3.3a and 4.3).

Once the integrity of the epithelium is

impaired, further damage might arise from the increased penetration of cytotoxic bacterial metabolites such as indole, amines, ammonia, volatile sulphur compounds (e.g. methyl mercaptans, H_2S), and butyric and propionic acids. *F. nucleatum* is the most commonly isolated species in periodontal pockets, and it produces large concentrations of butyrate and volatile sulphur compounds.

P. gingivalis has been shown to have the greatest proteolytic activity of the Gram-negative bacteria isolated in high numbers from sites affected by periodontal disease, and is the most virulent species when inoculated into animals in a simple pathogenicity test. The majority of this proteolytic activity has been characterized as an arginine-specific, cysteine protease, called gingipain. These proteases can degrade components of the host defences (immunoglobulins, complement, regulatory proteins), as well as host connective tissue proteins. These proteases may also play a key role in the indirect route to tissue damage by degrading inhibitors produced by the host to regulate host proteases involved in inflammation. Similarly, by destroying regulatory proteins the *P. gingivalis* proteases can activate the kallikrein–kinin pathway that increases vascular permeability, ensuring an increased supply of nutrients into the gingival crevice. The protease can also activate the complement system to provide C5a, a potent chemoattractant for neutrophils. These neutrophils release high concentrations of enzymes that can degrade constituents of connective tissue. These host proteinases attack other host regulatory proteins, thus producing a dysregulated and damaging host response. Other periodontal pathogens, including '*B. forsythus*' and *T. denticola,* also produce proteases with arginine-x specificity.

P. gingivalis produces other proteases. A thiol-proteinase has been proposed to contribute to the degradation of the collagenous periodontal ligament that connects teeth to alveolar bone (*see* Figure 2.1). Epithelial cells that surround the teeth produce matrix metalloproteinases that are usually secreted as inactive zymogens (inactive precursors). The thiol protease of *P. gingivalis* is able to activate some of these host degradative enzymes, which would promote accelerated tissue destruction *in vivo*. The production of some of these pathogenic determinants are up-regulated by environmental changes that occur during the transition from a normal gingival crevice to a periodontal pocket (e.g. increases in local pH, temperature and haemin concentrations).

A feature of advanced forms of periodontal disease is bone loss (*see* Figures 7.2 and 7.5). Molecules from periodontal pathogens (e.g. LPS, lipoteichoic acid and surface-associated proteins) have been shown in laboratory studies to cause bone resorption.

Invasion

Microbial invasion of the host tissues occurs in acute necrotizing ulcerative gingivitis (ANUG), where there is a consistent (but superficial) invasion of the gingival connective tissues by spirochaetes. Invasion also occurs in other acute forms of periodontal disease, e.g. localized juvenile periodontitis, in the later stages of severe chronic periodontitis, and in HIV-associated periodontal disease.

The invasion of gingival tissue by *A. actinomycetemcomitans* has been studied in detail. The mechanisms show some similarities with other intracellular pathogens, such as *Shigella flexneri* and *Listeria monocytogenes*, but there are also unique features, especially with respect to cell-to-cell spread. Contact between *A. actinomycetemcomitans* and a host cell triggers effacement of the microvilli, formation of 'craters' on the host cell surface, and rearrangement of host cell actin at the site of entry. Bacteria appear to enter the cell through ruffled apertures on the host cell surface, and entry occurs in a host-derived, membrane-bound vacuole. The host-derived vacuolar membrane that initially surrounds the internalized bacterial cells soon disappears and cells of *A. actinomycetemcomitans* grow rapidly intracellularly, and spread to neighbouring cells by using host cell microtubules. These protrusions contain cells of *A. actinomycetemcomitans*, and interconnect with other host cells, enabling cell-to-cell spread of the bacteria to occur.

Pathogenic synergism and periodontal disease

One of the most consistent and controversial features of the microbiology of periodontal diseases is the isolation of complex mixtures of bacteria from diseased sites. In particular, in chronic periodontitis, the composition of these

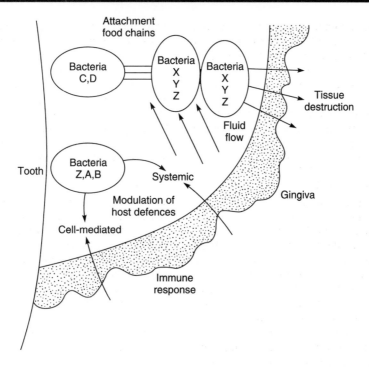

Figure 7.8 Pathogenic synergy in the aetiology of periodontal diseases. Bacteria capable of causing tissue damage directly (e.g. species X, Y and Z) may be dependent on the presence of other cells (e.g. organisms C and D) for essential nutrients or attachment sites so that they can grow and resist the removal forces provided by the increased flow of GCF. Similarly, both of these groups of bacteria may be reliant for their survival on other organisms (e.g. Z, A and B) to modulate the host defences. Individual bacteria may have more than one role (e.g. organism Z) in the aetiology of disease

mixtures can differ considerably both between and within studies of patients presenting with apparently similar clinical features. These variations might be explained by:

(a) differences in sampling and plaque-processing methods;
(b) difficulties in accurately diagnosing the clinical condition;
(c) plaque being sampled during both 'active' and 'inactive' phases of the disease; or
(d) the existence of clones of varying virulence.

For the establishment of disease, however, an organism must gain access to and adhere at a susceptible site, multiply, overcome or evade the host defences, and then produce or induce tissue damage (*see above*). A large number of virulence traits are needed, therefore, for each stage in the disease process (*see* Table 7.9), and it is unlikely that any single micro-organism will produce all of these factors optimally or in every situation.

An alternative explanation for some of the observed variations in microflora associated with periodontal disease could be that tissue destruction is a result of consortia of interacting bacteria. In this way, periodontal diseases are a particularly striking example of a **synergistic infection,** whereby micro-organisms that are individually unable to satisfy all of the requirements necessary to cause disease combine forces to do so. Thus, although only a few species (e.g. *P. gingivalis, P. intermedia, Treponema* spp.) produce enzymes that cause tissue damage directly, the persistence of these 'primary pathogens' in the pocket may be dependent on other organisms to provide means of attachment (e.g. receptors for co-aggregation on *Streptococcus* and *Actinomyces* spp.), or essential nutrients for growth (e.g. vitamin K, protohaeme, succinate; *see* Table 5.10). Similarly, the bacteria that support the growth of the 'primary pathogens' may also require other organisms to suppress or inactivate the host defences, or to inhibit competing organisms (e.g. by bacteriocin production) to ensure their survival. Bacteria could also have more than one function in the aetiology of periodontal disease and a schematic diagram illustrating this **pathogenic synergism** is shown in Figure 7.8. Our ability to interpret results from future microbiological studies of periodontal disease would be greatly enhanced if we knew more about the role (or niche, *see* Chapter 1) of particular species in the disease process. A micro-organism could still be highly significant in disease without necessarily having the potential to cause tissue destruction directly, while in other pockets, different bacteria could fill identical roles.

Predictors of disease activity

The study of the complex interactions that exist between host cells and the sub-gingival microflora has raised the possibility that markers or predictors of disease activity might exist that are more sensitive than existing crude indices, such as changes in probing depth, etc. Some of these have been discussed in various sections throughout this chapter, and include the following.

1. Sensitive and rapid tests (e.g. using immunological and oligonucleotide probes) for detecting putative pathogens.
2. Detection of selected enzymes in subgingival plaque or in GCF, e.g. a synthetic substrate (BAPNA: benzoyl arginine naphthylamine) that is hydrolysed by the arginine-specific proteases produced by *P. gingivalis*, '*B. forsythus*' and *T. denticola* to produce a coloured product has been incorporated into a rapid diagnostic kit. This test has been shown to be highly sensitive and specific at detecting enzyme activity, and in clinical studies, the test was capable of predicting sites at risk of attachment loss.
3. Detection of inflammatory mediators or tissue breakdown products in GCF. Paper strips can collect GCF from control and inflamed sites, and host enzymes can be measured (e.g. metallo-proteinases such as collagenase, cysteine proteinases such as cathepsin, and serine proteinases including elastase); levels of aspartate aminotransferase were found to correlate with gingival inflammation. Commercial chair-side tests have been developed that measure some of these enzymes.
4. Measurement of tissue degradation products, including glycosaminoglycans and their breakdown products, in GCF.
5. Detection of inflammatory markers, such as prostaglandins and cytokines such as IL-1 and IL-6. Levels of prostaglandins in GCF have shown a strong correlation with attachment loss, and values above a clear threshold were considered to be predictive of future disease activity.

Such tests could help with the diagnosis of a site, the monitoring of treatment, or possibly predict those at risk of future breakdown. Their use requires an understanding of the biological basis of the test, and the data obtained needs careful interpretation. This area is likely to be of increasing importance for the future.

Periodontal health and general health

Evidence now suggests that an association exists between periodontal disease and the general health of an individual, particularly with respect to cardiovascular disease, diabetes mellitus and a risk of pre-term labour and low birthweight infants. The hypothesis to explain this association is as follows. Periodontal diseases represent an inflammatory response by the host to the build up of dental plaque; these sub-gingival biofilms contain mainly Gram-negative species which possess LPS, and shed toxic metabolites and other molecules which induce prostaglandins and pro-inflammatory cytokines. The periodontium has a large surface area for contact between the host and the sub-gingival microflora, and, because it is so vascular, there is the opportunity that this site could act as potential systemic source of inflammatory mediators which could affect distant sites in the body.

In a carefully controlled study of 124 mothers, extensive periodontal disease was found to significantly increase the chance of pre-term, low birthweight babies. Based on their data, the authors concluded that 18% of the approximate 250 000 pre-term babies in the

USA could be attributed to periodontal disease. This finding has some experimental support since experimental periodontitis in the hamster can retard foetal growth, while infection of pregnant hamsters with *P. gingivalis* reduced foetal development by up to 25%. Correlations have also been found between the severity of periodontal disease and the risk of coronary heart disease and strokes. Again the hypothesis is that periodontal diseases provide a biological burden of LPS and pro-inflammatory cytokines (including IL-1, TNF-α, and prostaglandins) which serve to promote atherogenesis and thrombo-embolic events in the heart. These findings, if confirmed in subsequent studies, provide new opportunities for intervention strategies to reduce the incidence of these important medical conditions.

Summary

Periodontal diseases are a group of disorders that affect the supporting tissues of the teeth. The predominant microflora found in disease differs from that in health, but there is no single or unique pathogen. Most of the bacteria associated with disease are Gram-negative and obligately anaerobic, except for localized juvenile periodontitis, where the microflora is mainly capnophilic. Although the microflora in disease is diverse, certain species are found commonly at sites undergoing tissue breakdown; these include P. gingivalis, P. intermedia, A. actinomycetemcomitans, 'B. forsythus', C. rectus, F. nucleatum, Eubacterium spp. and spirochaetes. Many of these species are highly proteolytic and can degrade host tissues and/or components of the host defences including key regulatory proteins of the inflammatory response. Bacterial invasion of tissues is rare except in some acute conditions such as ANUG and localized juvenile periodontitis, and in more advanced stages of disease. Acute forms of periodontal disease may also be due to abnormalities in the functioning of the host defences; other risk factors include diabetes mellitus and smoking. Tissue destruction is generally mediated by bacterial cell surface proteases and extracellular cytotoxic compounds. Organisms can evade or subvert the host defences by the action of specific proteases and leukotoxin production, or by the presence of a capsule. Periodontal diseases involve the destruction of tissues directly by bacterial enzymes and indirectly as a consequence of the host inflammatory response ('bystander effect'). Periodontal diseases may also act as risk factors for more serious medical conditions, including pre-term, low birthweight babies and cardiovascular disease. Treatment and prevention of periodontal disease involves good oral hygiene, which may be augmented by the use of antimicrobial agents.

Bibliography

Addy, M. (1990) Chemical plaque control. In *Periodontics. A Practical Approach* (ed. B. Kieser), Wright, Oxford, pp. 527–534.

Baehni, P.C. and Guggenheim, B. (1996) Potential of diagnostic microbiology for treatment and prognosis of dental caries and periodontal diseases. *Crit. Rev. Oral Biol. Med.*, 7, 259–277.

Cutler, C.W., Kalmar, J.R. and Genco, C.A. (1995) Pathogenic strategies of the oral anaerobe, *Porphyromonas gingivalis*. *Trends Microbiol.*, 3, 45–51.

Darveau, R.P., Tanner, A. and Page, R.C. (1997) The microbial challenge in periodontitis. *Periodontol. 2000*, 14, 12–32.

Genco, R.J. (1996) Current view of risk factors for periodontal diseases. *J. Periodontol.*, 67, 1041–1049.

Genco, R., Hamada, S., Lehner, T., McGhee, J. and Mergenhagen, S. (eds) (1994) *Molecular Pathogenesis of Periodontal Disease*, American Society for Microbiology, Washington, DC.

Haffajee, A.D. and Socransky, S.S. (1994) Microbial etiological agents of destructive periodontal diseases. *Periodontol. 2000*, 5, 78–111.

Holt, S.C. and Bramanti, T.E. (1991) Factors in virulence expression and their role in periodontal disease pathogenesis. *Crit. Revs Oral Biol. Med.*, 2, 177–281.

Johnson, N.W. (ed.) (1991) *Risk Markers for Oral Diseases*. Volume 3, *Periodontal Diseases: Markers and Disease Susceptibility and Activity*, Cambridge University Press, Cambridge.

Lamont, R.J. and Jenkison, H.F. (1998) Life below the gum line: pathogenic mechanisms of *Porphyromonas gingivalis*. *Microbiol. Molec. Biol. Revs.*, 62, 1244–1263.

Manson, J.D. and Eley, B.M. (1995) *Outlines of Periodontics*, 3rd edn, Wright, Oxford.

Meyer, D.H. and Fives-Taylor, P.M. (1997) The role of *Actinobacillus actinomycetemcomitans* in the pathogenesis of periodontal diseases. *Trends Microbiol.*, 5, 224–228.

Moore, W.E.C. and Moore, L.V.H. (1994) The bacteria of periodontal diseases. *Periodontol. 2000*, 5, 66–77.

Newman, H.N. (1990) Plaque and chronic inflammatory periodontal disease. A question of ecology. *J. Clin. Periodontol.*, 17, 533–541.

Offenbacher, S., Katz, V., Fertik, G. *et al.* (1996) Periodontal infection as a possible risk factor for preterm low birth weight. *J. Periodontol.*, 67, 1103–1113.

Slots, J., Rams, T.E. and Listgarten, M.A. (1988) Yeasts, enteric rods and pseudomonads in the sub-gingival flora of severe adult periodontitis. *Oral Microbiol. Immunol.*, **3**, 47–52.

Travis, J., Potempa, J. and Maeda, H. (1995) Are bacterial proteases pathogenic factors? *Trends Microbiol.*, **3**, 405–407.

Wilson, M. and Henderson, B. (1995) Virulence factors of *Actinobacillus actinomycetemcomitans* relevant to the pathogenesis of inflammatory periodontal diseases. *FEMS Microbiol. Revs*, **17**, 365–379.

Zambon, J.J. (1997) Principles of evaluation of the diagnostic value of sub-gingival bacteria. *Ann. Periodontol.*, **2**, 138–148.

8

Acute bacterial infections

There are a number of acute bacterial infections that affect the oral cavity and most of these are opportunistic, i.e. arising from members of the host's own microflora. Oral infections caused by true pathogens (e.g. *Mycobacterium tuberculosis*) are comparatively rare, and more often affect medically compromised patients (*see* Chapters 12 and 13).

Opportunistic pathogens

Opportunistic pathogens are the most common type of infections in the oral cavity.

These infections arise from overgrowth of bacteria, or yeast species from within the oral microflora, due to a change in local environmental conditions. Oral infections may not be localized as bacteria can get into the bloodstream and colonize other tissues (*see* Chapter 1). Opportunistic infections occur when the numbers of micro-organisms within the microflora exceed a critical number. This number is called the **minimum infective dose** and can be measured in experimental animals. The minimum infective dose varies among microbes and can also vary between individuals as they often have different susceptibilities to microbial challenge. The minimum infective dose is also influenced by other predisposing factors which may affect the patient and some of these are shown in Table 8.1. Often these predisposing factors are temporary (e.g. short-term antibiotic therapy) and the infection can be resolved when the predisposing factor is removed. Unfortunately, if the predisposing factor is permanent

(e.g. loss of salivary gland function), then the opportunistic infection may be impossible to cure without recourse to antimicrobial therapy. Thus, the first principle in the treatment of opportunistic infections is to try and remove the predisposing cause.

Many oral opportunistic infections have unusual clinical features. In Chapters 6 and 7, the aetiology of dental caries and periodontal disease was described; these represent examples of opportunistic infections affecting structures unique to the mouth, i.e. the teeth and periodontal tissues. In this chapter other types of opportunistic infections will be described that are more acute in nature.

Opportunistic infections can be caused by a single micro-organism but this is unusual; more often, two or more microbial species are involved. In some acute infections, described later in this chapter, several micro-organisms may be isolated from the affected site and present a challenge to the diagnostic microbiologist as to the precise role of the constituent species in the disease process. The species of micro-organism causing opportunistic infection may also change as the infection progresses, reflecting ecological changes in the affected site. Examples of such changes include alterations in the type of nutrients available, shifts in pH, and the impact of host's defences. As explained earlier in this book, there is a direct relationship between the habitat and the microflora at a site. The characteristics of the habitat will determine both the types of micro-organisms able to grow, and the phenotype of those organisms. The action of the micro-organisms that grow in an

Table 8.1 Predisposing factors which result in oral infections

Predisposing factors	Possible effect on defence mechanisms	Oral infection
Physiological		
Old age and infancy	Diminution in salivary flow and immunoglobulin secretion	Candidosis, root caries
Pregnancy	Unknown	Gingivitis
Trauma		
Local	Loss of tissue integrity	Various opportunistic infections
General	General debilitation	Candidosis
Malnutrition	Deficiencies of trace elements, including iron and folate	Candidosis
Chronic long-term infection	General debilitation, xerostomia	Candidosis
AIDS	Reduction in T4 helper cell activity	Candida, geotrichium and other fungal infections, periodontal disease
Antibiotic therapy	Loss of colonization resistance, selection of resistant microflora	Candidosis, various opportunistic infections
Chemotherapy and irradiation	Xerostomia, local mucosal effects	Candidosis, caries
Oral malignancies	Xerostomia, loss or impairment of function of affected area	Caries, candidosis, Gram-negative bacterial colonization

infected site will also directly alter the habitat. Even infections caused by one species may have one or two other distinct subspecies present. An example of the diversity of subtypes present in oral infections are lesions caused by *Candida albicans*. One study has demonstrated three distinct subtypes of *C. albicans* present in chronic erythematous candidosis associated with the wearing of dentures. The effect of this multiplicity of causes of oral infections makes diagnostic microbiology of this area both complex and challenging. As indicated in the previous chapters on caries and periodontal diseases, a great deal of detailed knowledge has been obtained over the past two decades on the types of bacteria present at infected sites, and the virulence factors they produce, together with how these bacteria obtain their nutrients for growth, interact with microbial communities and evade host defences. It will become clear that we are only just beginning to understand how members of the resident oral flora can exploit their habitat and become opportunistic pathogens.

The microbiological diagnosis of acute oral infections

The diagnosis of acute oral infection is made by a combination of the patient's history, the presenting signs and symptoms and the results of special tests, which usually include microbiology. Often microbiological tests may be used for confirmation purposes as the treatment may have already started. Repeated microbiological sampling of a lesion may also allow monitoring of the efficacy of treatment (e.g. *Candida* infections) and help in the decision to continue, or discontinue, therapy. **Empirical therapy** is when antimicrobial therapy is prescribed without the benefit of microbiological investigations, which is common with many acute oral infections. The fact that numerous similar lesions have been sampled before allows the clinician to make a reasonable prediction as to the nature of the infecting pathogen, and to prescribe appropriate antimicrobial therapy. The pathogens causing lesions do show phenotypic change, and it is only by repeated sampling of the lesions that the clinician can obtain the information on which to base empirical therapy. Acute infective lesions do need careful sampling if the microbiological investigation is to be accurate. An aspirate is the appropriate sample if pus is present in large quantities. Studies have shown that microorganisms survive best in their own milieu, so pus aspirates are to be preferred for diagnostic purposes. If the lesion cannot be aspirated then a swab sample usually is taken. Plain dry cotton wool swabs are not very good at preserving the viability of oral micro-organisms, particularly obligate anaerobes; swabs in reduced transport fluid are to be preferred. The quality of the microbiological investigation is dependent on the speed of transfer to the laboratory, as oral anaerobes eventually become non-viable even on reduced transport fluid swabs and minor components become numerically dominant if allowed to exploit such conditions of storage. Ideally, microbiological specimens need to be transported to the laboratory during normal working hours and the clinician must provide all the relevant clinical information (e.g. antibiotics prescribed or already taken by the patient).

Conventionally, on arrival at the laboratory the samples will be first Gram stained and examined by light microscopy. This simple test gives a great deal of information as to the relative numbers of particular micro-organisms in the lesion, and the number of inflammatory cells (which is a measure of the severity of the inflammation). From the appearance of the micro-organisms on the Gram film it is often possible to make presumptive deductions as to what might be present in the lesion. The results of the examination of the Gram film may be useful in helping the clinician prescribe anti-microbial therapy. The sample will also be plated onto selective and non-selective agar-based media. The non-selective medium used is usually blood-based, the plates are grown anaerobically, and also aerobically in the presence of carbon dioxide to encourage the growth of capnophilic bacteria. The plates are usually grown at 37 °C and examined after incubation for 18–24 hours. Primary growth on the plates can usually be seen after 18 hours but some micro-organisms (e.g. the *Actinomycetes*) may take several days to grow. The primary plates are examined for the predominant microbial colonies and presumptive identifications can then be made. Identification of predominant colony types at a species level is made by establishing the nutritional requirements of the isolated bacteria (e.g. fermentation tests) and their constituent enzymes (e.g. using commercial kits), or by directly using nucleic acid or immunological probes (*see* Chapters 3 and 4). Representative colonies of the predominant micro-organisms are then plated onto fresh media and their sensitivity to antimicrobial agents tested. Oral microbiological investigations require personnel trained in this specialty who understand the significance of the type of micro-organisms causing these infections. Primary plates from oral lesions are often read by 'medical' microbiologists who are less experienced in these types of investigations; often the growth on these plates may be dismissed as merely 'Normal oral flora'.

It is accepted that the conventional culture approaches result in an underestimate of the full diversity of the micro-organisms present at a diseased site. This was discussed in Chapters 3 and 4, and in Chapter 7 in relation to the aetiology of periodontal diseases. Recent developments in molecular ecology have enabled the composition of complex microbial communities to be determined, without the bias of culture, from diverse habitats ranging from land-fill sites, geo-thermal vents and dento-alveolar abscesses. Studies have been made of pus from abscesses, in which the DNA is extracted from all of the microbial cells present. The 16S rDNA present is amplified by PCR using universal primers, and sequences compared to those in databases of known oral microflora. These comparisons have shown that unculturable and novel species are found in every sample, and can comprise over 25% of the microflora of each sample.

In Chapter 6, the concept of Koch's postulates was discussed in relation to oral disease and it was emphasized that both dental caries and periodontal diseases represent examples of polymicrobial infections. As such, Koch's postulates have to be modified to accommodate the fact that oral infections are often poly-microbial. The same concept applies to acute oral infections, they seldom have one agent responsible for the infection. Oral infections usually arise from the activity of at least two or more infective agents that are present as a result of the ecological pressures of the developing lesion. As a result, acute oral infections may present with a range of micro-organisms that reflect microbial selection as the lesion developed. As yet, the exact details of these selection processes are not fully understood.

The progression and principles of treatment of acute oral bacterial infections

When the predisposing factors allow, bacteria can multiply and cause acute infections. Acute infections usually result in **abscess** formation. An abscess is the localized collection of bacteria and their products, together with inflammatory cells, tissue breakdown products, proteins from serum and other organic material. Abscesses cause local tissue destruction directly from the pressure they exert, or by the action of the extracellular enzymes present within them. Most of the enzymes with tissue-damaging potential are derived from the bacteria but some will be from the host. Abscesses are also hypertonic with respect to their environment and exert pressure on the immediate environment. If the surrounding tissue is bone then osteoclastic factors may be induced and bone will be removed. In general, this effect of pressure causes bone to be removed in the path of least resistance and, in most cases, this is medullary bone. In places where the cortical plate of bone is thin, for example in the central incisor area, the abscess can break into the soft tissue and cause further inflammation. The presence of inflammation in the soft tissues is called **cellulitis**. Once the infection has penetrated soft tissue, it tracks along sheets of connective tissue, or fascia, causing local destruction. A further effect of this accumulation of pus and inflammation in the soft tissues is to limit the action of the oral musculature; this limitation is called trismus.

The effects of the inflammation and pus from the abscesses are not only local but can also exert a systemic effect (Figure 8.1). Bacterial metabolites, exotoxins and endotoxins, and altered host products enter the bloodstream and affect the temperature regulatory centre in the hypothalamus. The general body temperature is raised and the person is described as pyrexial. If the abscess is not treated then bacteria may enter the bloodstream and start to reproduce; this is called **septicaemia**. This condition is very dangerous as the bacteria may infect a vital organ such as the brain, kidney or liver and lead to failure of function; which can be fatal. Patients with septicaemia are clinically pyrexial and are often confused, transiently losing consciousness, or comatose. It has been estimated in the UK that 12 fatalities from dental abscesses still occur every year, usually as a result of gross dental neglect, dental phobia or medical compromise.

The deleterious effects of acute bacterial infections arise from the presence of pus. This provides a reservoir of material to enter the bloodstream, or for local destruction. The most effective way to deal with this problem is to get rid of the pus by draining it. The draining of

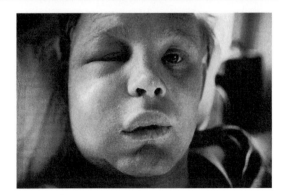

Figure 8.1 A patient with a large periapical abscess on the upper first permanent molar. Note the extensive swelling (cellulitis) and loss of normal facial contour

pus not only gets rid of most of the infecting micro-organisms but it also reduces them to numbers that can be dealt with by the normal host defences. Antibiotics (*see* Chapter 13) will not resolve pus unless the cause is dealt with and pus is drained. The use of antibiotics in acute abscesses is to limit the spread locally and to prevent metastasis to other organs. Antibiotics will not usually act in the centre of an abscess as the pH and the hypertonic conditions will not allow the antimicrobial to interact with the bacteria. Antibiotics are also destroyed by some bacterial enzymes (e.g. penicillins can be inactivated by beta lactamase production; several oral bacteria produce this enzyme). Abscesses are polymicrobial and the production of antibiotic-neutralizing enzymes by one species may cause significant cross-protection of other potentially sensitive organisms. Thus, the definitive treatment for an abscess is drainage and the use of an antibiotic is an adjunct to prevent gross local and systemic spread. In addition to drainage and antibiotic therapy, rehydration of the patient is necessary. Patients with acute oral bacterial infections are often dehydrated because they do not eat and drink. Dehydration alone can cause the patient to feel unwell and this problem can be easily resolved by requesting the patient to drink fluids or if in hospital by giving an intravenous drip to replenish the fluids.

Abscesses can drain by breaking down the oral mucosa and releasing the pus into the oral cavity. This can result in an acute abscess becoming chronic. Often chronic abscesses are long-standing and their oral aperture, called the sinus, may become epithelialized. Such chronic

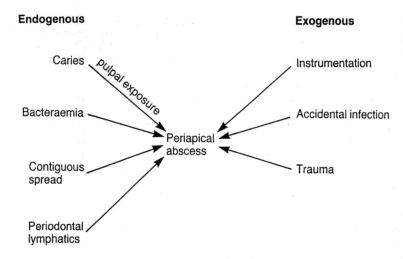

Endogenous   **Exogenous**

Caries

Bacteraemia

Contiguous
spread

Periodontal
lymphatics

pulpal exposure

Periapical
abscess

Instrumentation

Accidental infection

Trauma

Figure 8.2 Scheme for the routes of infection resulting in a periapical abscess

abscesses do not heal as the pathology that caused their formation is still present; if the sinus becomes blocked then they may become acute again. The **primary** treatment of an abscess is drainage but the **secondary** treatment is to remove the cause.

Dento-alveolar abscesses

The dento-alveolar abscess (synonyms: the periapical abscess, dental abscess) is a collection of pus in the pulp, or around the root of the tooth. Dento-alveolar abscesses can result from death (necrosis) of the pulp, usually from the progression of dental caries. There are other causes of dento-alveolar abscesses and these are shown in Figure 8.2. The micro-organisms involved in the progression of a dento-alveolar abscess are difficult to study as once sampled the lesion is destroyed and no further information can be obtained. A diverse range of facultative and obligate anaerobes are found in dento-alveolar abscesses (Table 8.2); the species that are present reflect the ecological conditions prevailing at that site. Detailed microbiological studies of dento-alveolar abscesses do not help define the pathogenesis of these lesions, but only identify the organisms present at that time. The majority of dento-alveolar abscesses are usually infected with endogenous bacteria. Exogenous bacteria such as *Staphylococcus* spp. may be found in oral abscesses, but only if the patient is medically

compromised (*see* Chapter 9), or if cross-infection has occurred during operative procedures.

Table 8.2 Bacteria commonly isolated from dento-alveolar abscesses

Facultative bacteria	Obligate anaerobes
S.angionosus	Anaerobic cocci
S.oralis group	*Prevotella oralis*
mutans streptococci	*Peptostreptococcus* spp.
Lactobacillus spp.	*Porphyromonas* spp.
Actinomyces spp.	*Porphyromonas endodontalis*
Haemophillus spp.	*Veillonella* spp.
	Prevotella spp.

Adapted from Lewis *et al.*, 1990

In order to survive in an abscess bacteria have to gain nutrients and to overcome the host defences. Abscess size and spread has been shown in some studies to be related to the number of viable bacterial species present. Abscesses with up to three different bacterial species present tend to be small, not to spread and to be less painful. In contrast, abscesses from which six or more bacterial species can be cultured tend to spread and be more painful. The reason for this critical number of bacterial species is not precisely known but is probably related to bacterial synergism (*see* Chapter 5) and pathogenic synergism (*see* Chapter 7). The bacteria in abscesses with six or more species present form what has been called a consortium or microbial community, which can be viewed as a kind of partnership for mutual benefit. In a consortium, bacteria usually express different additional phenotypic characteristics from those exhibited by any of the bacteria when in pure culture. In experiments where multiple bacterial species from dento-alveolar abscesses have been isolated, proteolytic activity may be enhanced several-fold compared to that expected from the sum of the activity of each species when grown in pure culture. The change and enhancement of phenotypic expression that helps bacterial growth in the tissues is a property of a consortium. The nutrient source in infected tissues is predominantly serum-derived proteins and there may be some tissue components degraded by bacterial action. As discussed in Chapters 4 and 5, the degradation of these complex host molecules (many of which are glycoproteins), requires the concerted action of several species with complementary patterns of glycosidase and protease activities. The micro-organisms that appear to have a key role in degrading serum proteins and in the establishment of a bacterial consortium are *P. oralis*, *P. intermedia*, *P. endodontalis* and *P. gingivalis*. These micro-organisms not only degrade serum proteins but can also cleave IgG and other immunoglobulins and negate this important part of the host's defences. Other molecules involved in the host defences can also be degraded by some of the broad-spectrum bacterial proteases. These micro-organisms can also obtain iron and haemin (necessary for their growth) from iron-containing molecules such as albumin, haptoglobin, haemopexin and transferrin. It is possible that some of the *Prevotella* and *Porphyromonas* species as well as *A. meyeri,* degrade proteins into suitably sized peptides that can be used by peptide-requiring organisms such as *E. lentum*, *F. nucleatum*, *P. micros* and *S. intermedius*. Other species, such as *Streptococcus* spp., may be involved in removing sulphate and carbohydrates from the side chains of the host glycoproteins. Metabolic bacterial products such as hydrogen sulphide, indoles and amines also have deleterious effects on host defences by inactivating polymorpho-nuclear leucocytes and preventing complement action; in addition, some of the acidic products of metabolism are also cytotoxic. Thus, the bacteria in a consortium have properties that enhance their infectivity in a manner similar to that described in Chapter 7 with respect to pathogenic synergism in periodontal diseases.

The detailed microbiology of dento-alveolar abscesses is still not fully resolved. Many micro-organisms do not appear to grow well *in vitro* even though they can be seen by microscopy. Some micro-organisms such as *B forsythus*, *F. nucleatum* and *Eubacterium* spp. can be difficult to culture from dento-alveolar abscesses, even though they can be detected in large numbers using other techniques. Methods based on amplification of 16S rRNA have shown that not all taxa are cultured in the laboratory, whilst others are underestimated (*see* Chapter 3). An example of this is *P. endodontalis* which is frequently detected by molecular methods but rarely by culture. Other clones have been obtained that resemble a water-borne pathogen or a novel species that is directly related to the genus *Prevotella*. The use of molecular biological techniques should elucidate more about these bacteria which are either difficult to grow, or are not grown reproducibly by conventional culture techniques.

The principles of treatment of the dento-alveolar abscess have been discussed in the previous section. Drainage of the abscess is obtained by incising the tissue, removing the tooth, or by opening the pulp chamber and cleaning out the necrotic pulp. If the patient has a raised temperature or there is gross local spread then antibiotics can be used. These antibiotics prevent metastatic spread and reduce local spread; they are not a definitive cure for the abscess. There is a paucity of clinical evaluations of the efficacy of antimicrobials in dento-alveolar abscesses. Table 8.3 shows some of the antibiotics most commonly used for dento-alveolar abscesses. From the known microbiology of dento-alveolar abscesses, antibiotics that have an effect on oral facultative micro-organisms, particularly oral streptococci, and obligate anaerobes would be ideal. There is also a paucity of information as to the duration of antimicrobial therapy. What is known is that courses of antibiotics of longer than 5 days are not necessary if the patient is recovering. Recent studies have advocated the use of 2- or 3-day courses of antimicrobials, or the use of large bolus doses at the time of drainage and a similar dose 6 hours afterwards. Provided the patient is recovering, and the secondary treatment has been done, the antibiotics may then be safely discontinued.

Table 8.3 The antimicrobial agents used in the therapy of dento-alveolar abscesses and their action

Antibiotic	Effective against:	Comments
Amoxicillin	Oral streptococci, and some obligate anaerobes	Useful antibiotic, well absorbed, high serum concentrations
Ampicillin	Broad spectrum	Not always well absorbed, susceptible to penicillinases (β-lactamases)
Cephalexin	Oral streptococci, obligate anaerobes	Well absorbed
Cephradine	Oral streptococci, anaerobes	Well absorbed
Clindamycin	Oral streptococci, obligate anaerobes	Well absorbed, but can cause antibiotic-associated colitis
Erythromycin	Limited efficacy for oral bacteria	Not well absorbed, bacteriostatic agent only
Metronidazole	Obligate anaerobes	Well absorbed
Phenoxymethypenicillin	Oral streptococci, some obligate anaerobes	Poorly absorbed, susceptible to penicillinases (β-lactamases)

Ludwig's angina

Ludwig's angina is a cellulitis involving the submental, sublingual or submandibular spaces between connective tissues and muscles (fascial spaces). It is usually secondary to a dental abscess or follows tooth extraction. It can be associated with infection of the submandibular salivary glands and also trauma to the floor of the mouth. The infection distends the spaces in the neck which become tense and hard. The tongue may be displaced back into the oropharynx. This infection is serious as it can affect the parapharyngeal spaces and block the airway necessitating a tracheotomy (an incision into the trachea to re-establish the airway). Fatalities from this condition used to be common, as is reflected in the term 'angina', which means choking and suffocation.

The treatment of Ludwig's angina is high doses of antibiotics, surgical drainage, or both. These lesions are often very large, tense swellings in the neck, and yet when they are incised they often yield very little pus. The absence of pus from some cases of Ludwig's angina supports the conclusion that the bulk of some lesions is made up of inflammatory fluid. Prolonged courses of antibiotics are necessary for all cases of Ludwig's angina, usually administered by the intravenous route. Penicillin or amoxycillin, often supplemented with metronidazole, are effective. Ludwig's angina can sometimes be managed conservatively without surgery to the neck. This conservative management will only succeed if the odontogenic cause of the Ludwig's angina is removed.

The micro-organisms isolated from cases of Ludwig's angina are varied. The usual bacteria reported are *Prevotella*, *Porphyromonas*, *Fusobacterium* and *Streptococcus* spp., but coliforms have also been isolated. The diversity of the bacteria that can be isolated from Ludwig's angina makes it important to establish the identity of the organisms so that appropriate antibiotic therapy can be given. Fortunately, Ludwig's angina is rare in the modern antibiotic era.

Pericoronitis

Pericoronitis is inflammation of the soft tissues that surround the crown of a partially erupted tooth. It is most common between the ages of 17 and 25 years and is usually associated with wisdom teeth, although any tooth can be involved. The soft tissues around the tooth become inflamed and may impinge on the teeth in the opposite jaw. The inflammation can cause spasm in the adjacent muscles and restrict opening of the mouth (trismus). The treatment of pericoronitis is local debridement of the pocket around the tooth, usually by irrigation, and if necessary the use of antimicrobials; metronidazole is the drug of choice. If the responsible tooth is blocked from erupting (impaction), then the treatment is to extract it.

Microbiological studies of pericoronitis are limited; some studies have looked at the pus associated with acute infections while others have investigated more chronic conditions. There is general agreement that pericoronitis is a polymicrobial infection with obligate anaerobes predominating. *P. intemedia*, *Peptostrep-*

tococcus micros, *Fusobacterium* spp. and *S. mitis* are amongst the predominant bacteria found in acute pericoronitis. *P. gingivalis,* a bacterium found in advanced forms of periodontal disease, is usually not isolated. The lack of isolation of *P. gingivalis* has been interpreted as meaning that pericoronitis is not a modified form of periodontal disease.

Periodontal abscesses

Periodontal abscesses arise in pockets associated with diseases of the periodontium. This lesion is not uncommon yet its precise pathogenesis is still unknown. It is thought to arise by deep periodontal pockets becoming occluded, or blocked, with bacteria in them. Other explanations of the aetiology include trauma to the area and implantation of foreign material. The lesion is usually very painful, especially on biting, with swelling in the affected area. The treatment is drainage of the area either by extraction or by incision. If the tooth is retained then further periodontal treatment is essential and may involve surgery.

The bacteria causing lateral periodontal abscesses are usually anaerobes, especially Gram-negative rods. Occasional *Actinomyces* spp. are isolated. If antibiotic therapy is deemed necessary then metronidazole is the antimicrobial of choice, with or without amoxycillin.

Osteomyelitis

Infections of the bone – either acute or chronic – are called osteomyelitis. The incidence of osteomyelitis in industrial societies has decreased considerably in recent years, although the exact reason for this is not clear. Osteomyelitis affects predominately the medullary part of the bone, but the cortical plate and periosteum may also be affected. The signs of osteomyelitis are severe pain, enlarged lymph nodes and pyrexia. If the mandible is involved there may be paraesthesia (tingling) or altered sensory sensations. The soft tissues over the lesion may be distended and eventually burst to expose the bone. The bone may contain pus and there may be a sinus tract. It is now rare for osteomyelitis to follow a dental abscess, an event not unusual a quarter of a century ago. The other factor that can lead to osteomyelitis

is severe trauma caused by fracture of the jaws where there is exposed bone, but even this is not a common cause of this condition. Osteomyelitis can be acute or chronic, and affect either the maxilla or the mandible. The microbial cause of osteomyelitis was thought to be *Staphylococcus* spp.*,* particularly *S. aureus.* Recent studies have implicated obligate anaerobes in this infection, particularly Gram-negative rods including *Fusobacterium* spp.

There are chronic forms of osteomyelitis which affect the mandible and the maxilla. In these, the symptoms are less well pronounced and the lesions usually less extensive. In recent years another type of osteomyelitis has been recognized called osteoradionecrosis. This latter condition develops when the jaws are irradiated for neoplastic (cancerous) conditions. After irradiation the bone loses its blood supply, because the arteries shut down, and dies, leaving spicules of dead tissue (sequestrae).

The treatment of osteomyelitis is either surgical or with antibiotics. Surgery is used to remove any sequestrae and other dead tissue, and this allows healthy bone to regenerate. Such surgery is not without problems as there is a risk of further infection and the remaining bone may be weakened and vulnerable to fracture. Antibiotic therapy has to be prolonged to ensure that the infecting agent is killed, but often the osteomyelitis becomes chronic and surgery may be indicated. Loss of dead bone after surgery may necessitate further reconstruction operations and grafting.

The most difficult form of osteomyelitis to treat is when it occurs during irradiation of the bone. Surgery in an area where bone is being irradiated is seldom successful and is highly susceptible to secondary infection. Antibiotic therapy may also be unsuccessful due to the problems of penetration of the antimicrobial into the necrotic bone. Removal of teeth or oral surgery is best done before any irradiation is started, but unfortunately this is not always practicable.

Dry sockets

One localized form of osteomyelitis is the dry socket. This occurs after tooth extraction where the socket fails to heal. The clinical appearance of a dry socket, as its name implies, is of an empty socket with no organization or blood clot. It is usually very painful and tender to touch. The micro-organisms isolated from dry sockets are often sparse and usually obligately anaerobic. *Prevotella* spp. and *Fusobacterium* spp. have been isolated, but so also have *S. aureus* and *Actinomyces* spp. There is still some debate as to whether dry sockets are caused by trauma to the bone, or infection, or both. Some patients have a history of dry sockets following extractions. The use of prophylactic metronidazole appears to prevent the development of the condition, suggesting that dry sockets may in many instances be due to anaerobic infection. The preoperative use of chlorhexidine, placed subgingivally prior to extraction, prevents dry sockets; this again suggests an infective aetiology. There is however, undoubtedly a traumatic element to dry sockets with the local bone sustaining damage during the extraction.

The treatment of dry sockets is by local debridement and the placement of obtundent and antiseptic dressings. As has already been mentioned, the use of metronidazole in addition to local treatment is often helpful if there is systemic involvement and evidence of infection.

Infections associated with osseointegrated implants

The placement of implants into the maxilla or mandible is now becoming common. These implants, usually of metal or ceramometallic complexes, are placed in prepared cavities in the bone. The preparation of the bony cavity is critical, as if the temperature of the bone exceeds 4 °C during the drilling, then it will be irreparably damaged. Damaged bone will not regenerate or form a physical bond with the implant and, in addition, it is susceptible to infection. After the implant has been allowed to integrate with the bone, usually for months, it is re-exposed surgically. The fabricated superstructure, usually a denture or some other form of tooth replacement, is put into place.

The junction between the implant and the oral tissue has been the subject of extensive study, and appears in some respects to mimic the junction between teeth and gingivae. This area can become colonized with oral micro-organisms and usually the microflora is diverse, with obligate anaerobes predominating as this type of plaque biofilm matures. There is some

evidence that exudates derived principally from blood, do seep through the oral/implant junction and this will affect the ecology of the area in a similar way to that described earlier for gingival crevicular fluid.

Infections of implants tend to occur either almost immediately after placement or some months later. Those that occur at placement usually are as a result of poor surgical and aseptic technique and they can be due to oral micro-organisms such as the streptococci, or exogenous bacteria (e.g. *S. aureus*). There is little evidence that prophylactic antibiotics help to prevent these early infections and the usual result is abscess formation and the removal of the implant. Infections that occur some time after placement of the implants may still be due to poor placement technique that has caused necrotic bone. In order to keep free from infection, meticulous oral hygiene maintenance of the implant site is essential.

The composition of the microflora from both the stable and failing implants (sometimes termed peri-implantitis) has been determined. In edentulous patients, the organisms that establish on successfully integrating titanium implants were similar to the mucosal microflora on the adjacent alveolar ridge. Over 80% of the microflora were Gram-positive, facultatively anaerobic cocci, while black-pigmenting anaerobes and *Fusobacterium* spp. were isolated only occasionally; spirochaetes were never detected. In contrast, failing sites were colonized by higher proportions of motile bacteria, and spirochaetes could be detected; around 40% of the cultivated bacteria were Gram-negative obligately anaerobic rods. Other studies have detected periodontopathogens such as *P. micros*, *C. rectus*, *P. intermedia* and *P. gingivalis* at infected implant sites. In addition, non-oral bacteria have so been recovered from sites with failing implants. Thus it is always important to do a comprehensive microbiological investigation of failing sites so that appropriate antibiotics can be used to reduce the microbial load.

Infections associated with endodontic treatment

Infections associated with the pulp of the tooth (the root canal) are difficult because of the site being sampled. The pulp of the tooth is sited in a small tapering tube (the root canal), in which different bacteria may colonize at various levels. Approaches to sampling have been varied, employing simple paper points, or barbed broaches (tapering instruments) covered in cotton wool. Clinical treatment of infected root canals used to involve taking paper point samples to ensure that the area was sterile. In practice, this procedure was very difficult to do without introducing exogenous contamination from the mouth, and it is no longer recommended.

Microbiological studies of root canals have shown that the infection is polymicrobial with up to 20 different bacteria being involved (*see* Chapter 6). Obligate anaerobes account for over 60% of the flora cultivated from infected root canals, and the principal isolates from root canals have been found to be *Peptostreptococcus micros*, *P. melaninogenica*, *Prevotella oralis*, *Eubacterium* spp. and *Fusobacterium* spp.. The data presented so far suggest that there are definite associations of bacteria present which depend on the clinical state of the root canal. Painful teeth and infected root canals associated with swelling, have been found to be infected with combinations of *Peptostreptococcus micros* and *Prevotella* spp. When the root canal is 'wet' and discharging the principal isolates were *Prevotella* spp. and *Eubacterium* spp. and drainage to create aerobic conditions is essential.

Summary

A number of acute oral infections can affect the oral cavity and they are usually polymicrobial and opportunistic in nature (e.g. dental abscesses and osteomyelitis). The bacteria present usually form consortia and can derive their nutrients from proteolytic activity on serum-derived proteins. As with all infections with pus formation, treatment is by drainage, removing the cause and adjunctive antibiotics. Antibiotic therapy is usually empirical, the clinician basing the choice of antibiotics on the most likely aetiology of the infection based on previous studies.

Dento-alveolar abscesses can contain a diverse collection of bacteria, some of which cannot as yet be cultivated in the laboratory. The microflora of dento-alveolar abscesses appear to act synergistically and form consortia. The formation of a consortium may offer an advantage in protecting the infecting micro-organisms against host defences. A range of Gram-negative anaerobes are also cultured from pericoronitis and from infected osseointegrated implants. The aetiology of Ludwig's angina and dry sockets is not clearly understood. Studies are necessary utilizing the modern classifications to determine which bacterial species are present in acute oral infections.

Bibliography

Book, I., Frazier, E.H. and Gher, M.E. (1996) Microbiology of periapical abscesses and associated maxillary sinusitis. *J. Periodontol.*, **67**, 608–610.

Dymock, D. (1996) Molecular analysis of the microflora associated with dento-alveolar abscesses. *J. Clin. Microbiol.*, **34**, 537–542.

Gomes, B-P., Lilley, J.D. and Drucker, D.B. (1996) Association of endodontic signs and symptoms with particular combinations of specific bacteria. *Int. Endont. J.*, **29**, 69–75.

Jansen, H-J., van der Hoeven, J.S., Goertz, D. and Bakkereren, J.A.J.M. (1994) Breakdown of various serum proteins by periodontal bacteria. *Microb. Ecol. Health Dis.*, **7**, 299–305.

Lewis, M.A.O., MacFarlane, T.W. and McGowan, D.A. (1990) A microbiological and clinical review of the acute dentoalveolar abscess. *Br. J. Oral Maxillofac. Surg.*, **28**, 359–366.

Mombelli, A. (1993) Microbiology of the dental implant. *Adv. Dent. Res.*, **7**, 202–206.

Mombelli, A., Buser, D., Lang, N.P. and Berthold, H.O. (1989) Suspected peridontopathogens in erupting third molar sites of periodontally healthy individuals. *J. Clin. Periodontol.*, **17**, 48–54.

Wade, W.G., Gray, A.R., Absi, E.G. and Barker, G.R. (1991) Predominant cultivable flora in pericoronitis. *Oral Microbiol. Immunol.*, **6**, 310–312.

9

Chronic oral infections (including infections in medically compromised patients)

In the previous chapters the importance of a homeostatic oral microflora for the maintenance of health has been stressed. When the natural balance of the oral commensal flora is disrupted, for example following antibiotic therapy, then opportunistic infections can occur. These opportunistic infections arise from overgrowth of individual microbial species that are usually only minor components of the oral microflora: such overgrowth can often result in chronic lesions. The progress and treatment of these chronic oral lesions is affected by the patient's underlying medical condition. A good example of the effect of a medical condition affecting the oral microflora is seen in patients irradiated for the treatment of cancer. Irradiated patients have profound changes to their oral microflora and may develop unusual infections, which can be difficult to resolve. Any therapeutic regime that affects the quality and flow of saliva, or the integrity of the oral mucosa directly, can cause profound changes to the oral microflora; these changes will be discussed later in this chapter.

The oral cavity is affected by a number of chronic infections that produce slowly enlarging swellings (e.g. tuberculosis) which patients can mistake for cancerous growths. As a consequence of fear of cancer, these swellings can often attain quite a considerable size before the patients seek help. Some chronic lesions develop from acute infections; a good example of this is the chronic apical abscess. As with all oral lesions, chronic infections need both clinical and microbiological investigations to ensure that treatment is adequate and appropriate.

Chronic periapical abscess

The chronic periapical or dental abscess usually develops from an acute apical abscess (*see* Chapter 8). The lesion can become chronic when the pus from an acute periapical abscess drains. This drainage can be as a consequence of surgery, or by the pus tracking to the surface of the oral mucosa and penetrating it. If the chronic infection is not treated then a sinus may form, which is a passage from an abscess to an external surface lined with epithelium. A schema for the interaction of chronic and acute periapical abscesses and their sequelae is shown in Figure 9.1. Chronic dental abscesses can often be present for long periods and the sinus will periodically leak pus. The development of the chronic abscess from an existing acute lesion can often be deduced from the patient's history. Patient's will often report an initial history of severe throbbing pain, characteristic of an acute abscess, which progresses into chronic, dull, intermittent discomfort. What has happened in this situation is that the abscess has been acute and painful whilst the pus is confined; the discomfort lessens once the pus is released by sinus formation and drainage. The patient usually reports that the affected tooth is tender to percussion and there is a bad taste, which is due to the pus. Often when the patient is examined there is sinus formation which may yield pus on gentle massage.

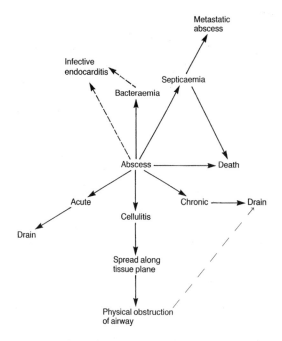

Figure 9.1 The possible sequelae from an abscess in the oral cavity

There is a real paucity of definitive published reports on the microbiology of chronic dental abscesses. Information tends to be limited to atypical anecdotal case reports involving unusual staphylococcal or streptococcal species. Clinical experience from diagnostic laboratory investigations shows the microflora cultured from chronic abscesses tends to be similar to that found in acute lesions, but sparser in cell numbers. The microflora of pus from chronic abscesses is polymicrobial, containing a diversity of obligate and facultatively anaerobic species. Chronic abscesses with sinuses are subject to secondary infection from exogenous sources. Patients may touch them, or apply medicaments, introducing bacteria such as *S. aureus* to the area. The introduction of virulent exogenous micro-organisms such as staphylococci may precipitate acute exacerbations.

The treatment for chronic periapical abscesses is either by extraction of the affected tooth, root canal therapy (endodontics), or by surgically excising the infected tissue and the tip of the tooth root (apicectomy). If the abscess has been present for a long time then the chronic infection may cause excessive granulation (fibrous) tissue to form, which is an attempt by the body to wall off the area, and to limit spread. The granulation tissue can eventually replace the abscess cavity and a periapical granuloma may form; these usually resolve after the tooth is treated. The presence of chronic infection, and bacterial toxins, in the periapical area can stimulate growth of the epithelial remains of tooth-forming tissue and a cyst will form. A cyst is an epithelial-lined cavity, and this can continue to grow after the tooth is removed. Cysts may need further surgery to remove them, and they can also become infected and painful. Usually antibiotics are not required for the treatment of chronic periapical abscesses, granulomas, or cysts as operative intervention suffices.

Actinomycosis

Actinomycotic infections are usually chronic, long-standing infections of the head and neck that follow mild trauma (e.g. tooth extraction, or a blow to the jaw). The usual clinical appearance of actinomycotic lesions is a chronic, slowly enlarging lesion at the angle of the jaw, with multiple external sinuses and induration of the skin (Figure 9.2). In actinomycotic lesions thick yellow fluid pus is expressed from the sinuses which contains yellow, granular particles, often referred to as 'sulphur granules'. These granules are yellowish-coloured aggregates of actinomyces filaments, and may inhibit the penetration of antibiotics into the lesion (Figure 9.3). Actinomycosis rarely penetrates bone and usually only affects the lower jaw. The lesion is slow-growing and produces a granulomatous reaction which tries to 'wall off' the chronic actinomycotic infection; this results in the formation of fibrous pus-filled cavities or locules. The granulomatous nature of the lesion is important for its eradication, as these fibrous locules must be surgically broken down to get rid of the pus and resolve the lesion. The slow, insidious nature of the growth of actinomycotic lesions may cause patients to delay seeking treatment due to fear of a cancerous growth.

There have been a number of reports that the microbiology of some actinomycotic lesions may be varied. *Actinomyces* spp. have been isolated in high numbers from acute dental abscesses. The *Actinomyces* counts in these lesions suggest strongly that the micro-organism is involved with an acute disease process, but their role is unclear. It is probable, there-

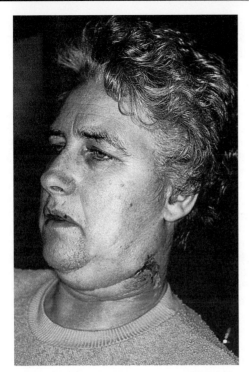

Figure 9.2 The clinical appearance of cervicofacial actinomycosis

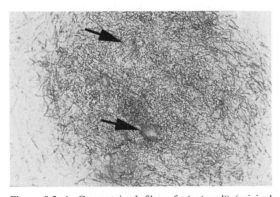

Figure 9.3 A Gram-stained film of *A. israelii* (original magnification ×100). Note the filamentous branching filaments and the tendency to form granular masses (arrows)

fore, that some actinomycotic lesions arise from acute infectious which eventually become chronic.

The majority of all actinomycotic lesions (90%) occur in the cervicofacial region (neck and face), and most of these are at the angle of the lower jaw. The remaining 10% of lesions are predominantly abdominal and, rarely the

infection can be disseminated throughout the body. Disseminated infections can occur in medically or immunologically compromised patients and can be fatal when they affect a vital organ (e.g. the brain). The usual isolate from disseminated lesions is a pure growth of *A. israelii*. Actinomycotic lesions have been increasingly reported in association with intrauterine devices, principally the birth control coil, and investigations of these infections have given information about the growth conditions of *Actinomyces* spp. *in vivo*. Actinomycosis probably occurs in this area as the strongly reducing effect of the metals in coils reduces the redox potential in the area, which is ideal for the growth of *Actinomyces* spp. Many of these coils contain copper, which has been shown to encourage the growth of *Actinomyces in vitro*. Almost invariably the isolate from infected coils is *A. israelii* together with scanty growths of streptococci, lactobacilli and a wide variety of obligate anaerobes. Infections associated with coils can lead to abscess formation in the fallopian tubes or ovaries, and this may result in sterility.

Actinomycosis is a true opportunistic infection. The major sites from which *Actinomyces* spp. can be isolated from the mouth are approximal plaque, the gingival crevice and tonsillar crypts. *A. israelii* is still the most frequent isolate, being recovered from over 90% of lesions. The actinomycetes have recently been reclassified (*see* Chapter 3), and no microbiological studies from clinical specimens have been reported using the new schema for identification. In addition, to the *Actinomyces* spp. other bacteria associated with actinomycosis include *A. actinomycetemcomitans*, haemophili, propionibacteria, *Prevotella* and *Porphyromonas*. The role of the other microorganisms found in actinomycotic lesions is not known. The proportion of other bacterial isolates present in actinomycosis varies from none to about 25% of the viable count.

The diagnosis of actinomycosis, in its chronic form, is usually made on the basis of the clinical presentation and history. Sometimes the lesion is biopsied and the chronic granulomatous nature of the lesion can be confused with other connective tissue disorders. Misdiagnosis of actinomycosis occurs particularly if the bacteria have been 'washed out' in the preparation of the histological slide from a biopsy. A cultured aspirate sample often gives definitive growth of the actinomycete, but care needs to be taken to get the specimen to the laboratory quickly to keep the organisms viable. Gram-stained films of samples from the lesion often reveal the characteristic 'sulphur granules,' and this may be enough to make a presumptive diagnosis of actinomycosis (*see* Figure 9.3). Further evidence of the presence of an *Actinomyces* spp. can be obtained if the Gram stain is modified with an eosin counterstain. The eosin counterstain may adhere to peripheral filaments and produce a 'clubbing' effect which may help diagnosis. In most cases, a presumptive diagnosis can be made from the clinical presentation and the Gram film; treatment can be instigated reliably from this information. Growth of the *Actinomyces* spp. can take up to 10 days before the primary isolate appears; it is advisable therefore to anaerobically incubate the primary plates for at least 14 days. Antibiotic sensitivity testing of *Actinomyces* spp. is best done by measuring inhibition of the growth of colonies overlaid with antibiotic-containing agar. Disc diffusion plates are not reliable for sensitivity testing of *Actinomyces* spp., due to the slow growth of *A. israelii* which results in dissemination of the antibiotic.

The treatment of actinomycosis, in its chronic form, is by thorough surgery on the lesion to break down the fibrous locules, and instigation of prolonged high-dose antibiotic therapy. Penicillin used to be the antimicrobial of choice, but intramuscular injections were necessary to attain the serum concentrations required; this was both inconvenient and painful for the patient. Oral amoxycillin is now the preferred antimicrobial treatment, as many *Actinomyces* strains are not very susceptible to penicillin. Amoxycillin is usually given intravenously before, and during the operative period, and then orally for 4–6 weeks afterwards. Minocycline has been used successfully in patients who are allergic to penicillin. The acute lesions, where *Actinomyces* have been found in high numbers, usually resolve following surgery and often do not require any antibiotic therapy.

Tuberculosis

It is an astonishing fact that one-third of the world's population is infected by tuberculosis. The incidence of this disease in Western countries is increasing alarmingly every year.

There are 10 million new cases of tuberculosis (TB) every year, and the disease causes 3 million deaths every 12 months. Tuberculosis is caused mainly by *Mycobacterium tuberculosis* but *M. bovis*, *M. africaneum*, *M. avium-intracellulare*, *M. fortuitum*, *M. kansasii* and *M. scrofulaceum* also cause disease. *M. tuberculosis* is a slow-growing organism taking 3–6 weeks to grow on Lowenstein–Jensen medium. Improved detection techniques using radioactive labelling of metabolites can reduce the detection time to 10–15 days. PCR methods, which at present are not commercially available, may allow detection of TB within one day. TB is transmitted by droplet infection, usually by coughing, sneezing or talking, and can remain viable in the air for long periods of time; it is not spread by touching.

Primary infection is usually in the lungs with secondary infection spreading to other sites. Secondary infection usually occurs in patients who are medically or immunologically compromised. The AIDS epidemic has seen a concomitant rise in the incidence of TB, but malnutrition, poor living conditions, organ failure, or alcoholism are the main predisposing conditions.

Oral lesions of TB used to be rare but, with the advent of AIDS, they have become more common. The usual oral site to be affected is the tongue, which may be swollen or ulcerated and painful (Figure 9.4). TB lesions in the mouth are usually related to the distribution of lymphoid tissue, but they have been reported on the gingivae, the floor of mouth and the lips. Osteomyelitis of the maxilla and mandible have also been reported to be caused by tuberculosis, as has parotid infection.

One of the major problems in the treatment of TB is multiply resistant strains of *M. tuberculosis*; these strains are resistant to at least two anti-tuberculous drugs. Since *M. tuberculosis* takes so long to grow, and antimicrobial sensitivity testing takes a further protracted period of time, treatment is usually started long before the susceptibility of the strain is known. If multiply resistant strains are present then this initial treatment can often be inappropriate and need modification. The usual combination of drugs used to treat TB is isoniazid, rifampicin, ethambutol and pyrazinamide taken in combination for up to 9 months. The patient's complete compliance is absolutely essential if the TB is to be cured;

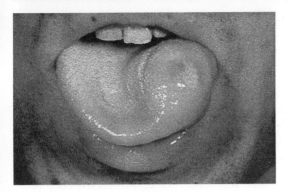

Figure 9.4 *M. tuberculosis* infection of the tongue. Note the unilateral swelling and the tendency to ulcerate

unfortunately this can often be a problem, and incomplete drug regimens encourage the emergence of resistant isolates.

Salivary gland infections

Salivary glands can be infected by bacteria, viruses and fungi. Bacterial infections of salivary glands usually do not occur if their output is normal, as any bacteria in the duct is flushed out, or inhibited by salivary antibacterial substances (*see* Chapter 2). When salivary gland function is impaired, bacteria can enter the duct and pass to the glands, where infection results. Figure 9.5 shows the predisposing factors for salivary gland infection. The most common salivary gland to be affected is the parotid. The submandibular gland is the second most affected and, as with the parotid, the infection can be due to bacteria or viruses, and rarely to fungi. The only fungi reported to infect salivary glands are *Candida* spp. and *Aspergillus*. Infection of the salivary glands usually causes enlargement of the gland and

often pain. If the duct becomes blocked, then the patient may suffer pain and swelling due to saliva retention, especially prior to meals, when saliva is generated.

Another consequence of salivary gland infection is xerostomia, or dry mouth. This can be very distressing for the patient, who will find it difficult to eat and speak. The oral mucosa will be dry and susceptible to infection by *Candida* spp. (*see* Chapter 11). Xerostomia is, however, a subjective term and often patients with quite adequately saliva-lubricated mouths may complain of dryness. It can be seen that xerostomia may be due to a number of causes which can predispose to salivary gland infection (Figure 9.5). Xerostomia can also cause significant changes in the oral commensal microflora. Studies on patients who have salivary gland impairment, for example due to Sjögren's syndrome, have shown that the numbers of micrococci, *S. salivarius* and *Veillonella* were reduced and there was a concomitant increase in staphylococci and candida.

Chronic bacterial infections of salivary glands are difficult to study because they are awkward to sample without contamination from the oral microflora. The usual method of sampling infected salivary glands is to pass a catheter into the duct and up into the gland. Any pus present in the gland can be directly sampled by aspiration. Usually the gland is massaged, pus is released and sampled at the gland aperture, where it is often contaminated by the resident oral microflora. The initial studies of bacterial salivary gland infections reported that the chief pathogens were staphylococci. These studies were done prior to the routine use of sterile gloves, so that these organisms may have been due to contamination by hand flora. Recent studies, using more appropriate sampling techniques which protect

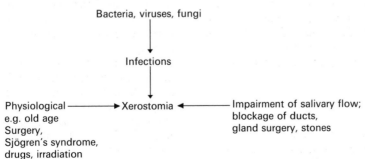

Figure 9.5 Predisposing factors to salivary gland infections

against hand flora contamination, have shown that staphylococci are not responsible for the majority of bacterial salivary gland infections. There appear to be two types of bacterial microflora associated with salivary gland infections: these are (a) mixtures of oral streptococci and aerobic Gram-negative bacilli, and (b) obligate anaerobes. Salivary gland infections with mixtures of facultative and aerobic Gram-negative bacteria appear to be associated with patients who are medically compromised and have these bacteria present in their oral microflora (*see below*). The micro-organisms found in these mixed infections are combinations of *E. coli, Pseudomonas, Serratia* and *Klebsiella* spp. No detailed investigations of the combinations or incidence of these Gram-negative facultative and aerobic species in salivary gland infections have been reported. The obligate anaerobic bacteria that infect salivary glands have been described as 'oral bacteroides spp.', but this group have been reclassified mainly into *Porphyromonas* and *Prevotella* spp. A detailed clinical investigation of salivary gland infections appears to be necessary to resolve some of the unanswered questions about the identity of the infecting anaerobic bacteria.

The treatment of bacterial salivary gland infections depends on the infecting microorganism. If pus is present in the gland, then drainage is essential, either through the duct, or by surgical intervention. The diagnostic microbiology laboratory is essential for the instigation of antimicrobial therapy, which is necessary in the majority of salivary gland infections. Metronidazole is the antimicrobial of choice for anaerobic infections, but for Gram-negative facultative and aerobic infections microbiological investigations are essential, as the antibiotic sensitivities of these microorganisms cannot be predicted with any certainty.

Acute suppurative salivary gland infection is usually due to bacteria gaining access to the salivary glands following blockage of ducts, or following xerostomia due to drugs with saliva-inhibiting (antisialagogic) properties. The usual gland to be affected is the parotid and there may be uni- or bilateral involvement. Acute pain and swelling in the gland area is often associated with limitation of mouth opening and a rise in temperature. The diagnosis of acute suppurative salivary gland infection is usually from the clinical appearance and from laboratory investigations. As described above, taking an uncontaminated sample from the duct orifice is often difficult, but usually possible. Direct extraoral sampling of the gland by aspiration with a wide bore needle may also be useful. The micro-organisms that cause acute suppurative salivary gland infections are usually bacteria and the most commonly reported taxa are *Staphylococcus aureus* and haemophili. One extensive study has implicated anaerobic bacteria in the aetiology of these infections. The study was done before the reclassification of anaerobes but it is likely that *Porphyromonas* and *Prevotella* spp. are implicated in these lesions. These acute suppurative infections require antimicrobial therapy and usually it is prescribed empirically. Penicillinase-resistant penicillin derivatives such as flucloxacillin are the antimicrobials of choice. If the infections are due to a blockage in the duct then surgery may be required, after the infection has resolved.

A number of viral infections affect the salivary glands, including mumps, cytomegalovirus, herpes, Coxsackie and parainfluenza viruses. Mumps is by far the most common viral infection of the salivary glands. Mumps is an RNA paramyxovirus that is about 200 nm in size, helical and enveloped. The incubation period of mumps is 18–21 days from inoculation. It is spread by droplet infections, or saliva transmission during kissing, and it is common in school age children, where mini-epidemics occur. The patient is infectious for up to 2 weeks after clinical symptoms develop. The usual symptom of mumps is swelling of the parotid glands and the submandibular is also swollen in 10% of cases. The swelling of the salivary glands is due to inflammation that does not produce pus. A prodromal period of nonspecific fever and a sore throat may also occur.

The diagnosis of mumps is usually made on the basis of the clinical presentation. Laboratory diagnosis can be made by complement fixation of the 'S' or soluble antigen, which is derived from the nucleoprotein core of the virus particle. S antigen is present in the acute phase of the illness and then declines. There is another antigen called 'V' which derives from the surface of the viral particle, the concentration of this antigen rises during active infection and then diminishes as the patient recovers. The disease is usually self-limiting, and most patients have a complete recovery with con-

Table 9.1 A classification of medically compromised patients

Disorder	Example	Oral complications
Endocrine disorders	Diabetes mellitus	Oral fungal infections
Cardiovascular problems	Mitral valve dysfunction	Infective endocarditis
Respiratory disorders	Asthma	Susceptibility to oral fungal infection
Neurological disorders	Epilepsy	Gingival hyperplasia and periodontal disease
Bleeding disorders	Haemophilia	Prolonged bleeding
Neoplastic disease	Oral carcinoma	Dental caries and irradiation mucositis following treatment
Chronic infection	Tuberculosis	Oral tuberculosis
Immunological disorders	AIDS	Oral fungal infections

comitant lifelong immunity. It is the antibody to the V antigen that gives lifelong immunity.

Gonorrhoea

Gonorrhoea is a sexually transmitted disease caused by the Gram-negative diplococcus *Neisseria gonorrhoea*. The usual site for infection is the genital organs and perianal area, but increasingly, this bacterium is affecting the mouth because of oral sexual practices. The usual initial symptoms are a burning or itching sensation in the mouth, which becomes very painful and is associated with a bad taste. The lymph nodes are enlarged and there may be a fever. Any part of the oral mucosa may be involved with inflammation, vesicle formation and, occasionally, pseudomembrane formation, but the tonsils and oropharynx are most commonly involved. The lesions can be so painful that eating and speaking can become difficult and there may be excessive salivation. This primary infection may lead to disseminated systemic infection.

The diagnosis of gonorrhoea may be difficult on clinical grounds, but the presence of Gram-negative diplococci, particularly intracellularly in polymorphonuclear leucocytes, may give a presumptive diagnosis. Culture of the bacteria on a semi-selective medium after incubation for 48 hours in the presence of 10% (v/v) carbon dioxide usually confirms the diagnosis. Treatment is dependent on the sensitivity of the bacteria after culture. The usual treatment of oral gonorrhoea is high doses of either amoxycillin or tetracycline but, unfortunately, some strains are now resistant to both of these antimicrobial agents and spectinomycin or 4-quinolone may be necessary to effect a cure.

Infections in medically compromised patients

The term 'medically compromised patient' is not precise and is often used arbitrarily. A good working definition of a medically compromised patient is one who, by virtue of his or her medical condition, or its treatment, is susceptible to infection, or to serious complications. Medically compromised patients can be classified in various ways and Table 9.1 shows one classification. The table is by no means exhaustive and for a fuller description of medically compromised patients the reader is referred to the textbooks of oral medicine in the reference list at the end of this chapter.

The oral cavity of medically compromised patients is altered by the changes that occur either in the mucosa itself, salivary flow, or in the constituents of saliva. Most of the infections that occur are opportunistic or, in the case of herpes, reactivated. Many of the infections that occur in medically compromised patients arise as a result of the treatment of the underlying medical problem. Table 9.2 shows some of the drugs that are used in medically compromised patients and the infections that can result from their use.

Some of the most difficult oral infections to treat are in patients who have neoplastic diseases and who undergo irradiation therapy, or receive cytotoxic drugs. Oral infections in patients with conditions such as malignant tumours, leukaemia and AIDS were little understood until recently, when intensive investigations have given insight into how they occur. In health, the oral mucosa is covered in a glycoprotein called fibronectin which favours the colonization of Gram-positive micro-organisms (*see* Chapter 4). The mucosa is not

Table 9.2 Infections following treatments used for medically compromised patients

Treatment	Condition	Pathology
Cytotoxic drugs	Oral neoplasia, AIDS	Candida, bacterial infection
Steroids	Asthma	Fungal infection
Epanutin	Epilepsy	Gingival overgrowth, periodontal disease
Irradiation	Oral neoplasia	Mucositis, ulceration
Immunosuppressive therapy	Rejection of transplants	Gingival overgrowth

Table 9.3 The 'abnormal' bacteria that have been isolated from the mouths of medically compromised patients

Condition and treatment	Bacteria and fungi isolated from the mouth
Irradiation for tumours of the head and neck	*E.coli*, pseudomonads, enterobacter, *Klebsiella*, *Staphylococcus* spp., *Candida* spp., *Acinetobacter* spp.
Cytotoxic treatment of leukaemias	*E.coli*, pseudomonads, enterobacter, *Klebsiella*, *Staphylococcus* spp. and oral streptococci, *Candida* spp.
Cytotoxic therapy for other tumours	*Proteus*, *E. coli*, pseudomonads, enterobacter, citrobacter, *Staphylococcus* spp.
Cerobrovascular accidents (strokes)	*Staphylococcus* spp., *Haemophili*, Enterobacteraceae and *Candida* spp.

colonized by aerobic Gram-negative bacilli because they are unable to attach permanently to the oral mucosa, probably due to their lack of appropriate specific adhesins. In addition, the salivary defence mechanisms (*see* Chapter 2) also prevent the attachment of Gram-negative bacilli, and in particular aerobes. When the oral mucosa is irradiated, or treated with cytotoxic agents, the surface fibronectin is altered by removal of the terminal sugar in the oligoside chain, probably by the action of an enzyme called elastase; the origin of this enzyme is probably from the tissue affected. The epithelium then becomes susceptible to colonization by Gram-negative bacilli, including aerobes such as *Pseudomonas* spp. The salivary flow is also diminished, its composition changed, and this favours the colonization of exogenous Gram-negative bacteria. There is also a concomitant overgrowth by yeasts such as *Candida albicans* and this may produce oral candidosis. Often an oral condition called mucositis appears, which starts as a reddened inflamed area and can ulcerate, or form pseudomembranes. Mucositis induced by cytotoxic agents, or irradiation can be very severe and can cause intense pain, difficulties in swallowing, or speech. In some cases it can lead to the suspension of treatment and intragastric feeding. Mucositis was thought to be due to oral candidosis, but aggressive treatment with oral or systemic antifungal agents does not eradicate the lesions, although it reduces the fungal counts. Sequential quantitative microbiological samples from irradiated patients of the oral mucosa and the saliva have shown that there is a progressive increase in the numbers of aerobic Gram-negative bacilli. The studies of medically compromised patients have shown that enterococci, pseudomonads and *Acinetobacter* spp. can be found in the oral cavity (*see* Table 9.3), in addition to occasional *Staphylococcus epidermidis* and *S. aureus*. There is now strong and compelling evidence that the abnormal colonization by Gram-negative bacteria is the cause of the mucositis, and an example of the breakdown of colonization resistance in the oral cavity.

The Gram-negative bacteria that colonize patients receiving treatment for neoplastic conditions shows diversity of species (Table 9.3) but the bacterial numbers usually increase with the progression of treatment. There are very few longitudinal studies of patients receiving anti-neoplastic treatment but all have shown an increase in abnormal Gram-negative bacteria as treatment progresses. Abnormal oral carriage is important because it can lead to serious threats to the longevity of the patient. Oral Gram-negative carriage can be associated with septicaemia and other serious febrile episodes, and these can be life-threatening. In patients with cerebrovascular accidents (strokes), oral Gram-negative carriage can lead to aspiration pneumonia, which is a serious potentially life-threatening complication. Patients with strokes may have no swallowing reflex to protect the lungs from being infected from saliva that descends down the trachea, and which can cause pneumonia.

Gram-negative oral bacterial colonization is therefore abnormal and indicative of profound and as yet not fully understood changes to the mouth and saliva. Since abnormal Gram-negative carriage can have so many deleterious effects it is important to prevent, or control it. The first attempts to control oral Gram-negative bacterial carriage were done on patients with oral mucositis and were successful. There have now been 46 controlled trials in the past 13 years of what has been called 'selective decontamination' in the prevention of mucositis, or abnormal colonization by Gram-negative bacteria. Selective decontamination is the use of prophylactic antibiotics to prevent the infection by endogenous, or exogenous micro-organisms. The agents used in the oral cavity are usually a combination of topical amphotericin, polymyxin E and tobramycin used as a paste. The amphotericin reduces the colonization by yeasts whilst polymyxin E and tobramycin act synergistically to kill, or reduce the counts, of Gram-negative bacteria. The use of selective decontamination reduces oral mucositis to simple erythema, and has been shown to decrease morbidity and mortality. Selective decontamination with the combinations of antibiotics described has also been shown to preserve the normal oral Gram-positive and anaerobic microflora. The use of selective decontamination is now widely used in the USA and in most parts of Europe, and has been shown to be of great benefit to compromised patients receiving potentially damaging treatments.

The acquisition of abnormal oral Gram-negative bacteria is now well recognized as a problem in medically compromised individuals, but it is the role staphylococci play in deleterious effects to these patients that is less well studied. The acquisition and carriage of, in particular, *S. aureus* and *S. epidermidis* in the oral microflora was first described over 20 years ago. There are considerable variations in the proportions of the oral microflora that is staphylococcal; some workers have suggested that it accounts for up to 50% of the total viable bacterial count. Septicaemia has been reported to be caused by *S. aureus* arising from oral sources, thus, the presence of these bacteria in the mouth is potentially serious. Further studies are needed to resolve how staphylococci are acquired by medically compromised patients and their exact role in disease.

Summary

Chronic periapical abscesses usually result from drainage of an acute dento-alveolar abscess. There is a paucity of information concerning the microflora associated with chronic abscesses and no detailed studies have been published since the reclassification of the obligate anaerobes. The microflora of chronic abscesses is thought to be similar in composition to acute abscesses, with a mixture of facultative and obligate anaerobic bacteria.

Cervicofacial actinomycosis is usually a slow-growing lesion that occurs at the angle of the mandible and is often secondary to trauma. The lesion classically contains filamentous forms of Actinomyces *spp. which aggregate into yellow-coloured 'sulphur' granules. Other bacteria such as* Actinobacillus actinomycetemcomitans *and* Haemophilus *spp. may also be present. The treatment of actinomycosis is usually drainage and long courses of antibiotics.*

Tuberculosis now affects a third of the world's population and is a major problem for healthcare workers. It can produce lesions in the oral cavity but this is not common. It is now often seen in patients with AIDS.

Once the homeostasis of the oral microflora is disturbed then the oral tissues are susceptible to opportunistic infections. Infections can also come from the acquisition of exogenous bacteria and in particular Gram-negative bacilli. Patients who are receiving treatment for neoplastic disease can acquire abnormal colonization of Gram-negative and positive bacteria, including E. coli, Pseudomonas, Acinetobacter *spp. and* Staphylococcus *spp. The abnormal colonization of the mouth can produce mucositis and lead to septicaemia and aspiration pneumonia. Attempts have been made to prevent abnormal colonization of the mouth by Gram-negative bacteria by the use of topical agents which are bacteriocidal for these micro-organisms; this therapy has been successful in preventing colonization in some conditions.*

Bibliography

Bagg, J. (1996) Tuberculosis: a re-emerging problem for health care workers. *Br. Dent. J.,* **180**, 376–381.

Baxby, B., van Saene, H.K.F., Stoutenbeek, C.P. and Zandstra, D.F. (1996) Selective decontamination of the digestive tract: 13 years on, what it is and what it is not. *Intens. Care Med.,* **22,** 699–706.

Lamey, P.J., Boyle, M.A., MacFarlane, T.W. and Samaranayake, L.P. (1987) Acute suppurative parotitis in outpatients; microbiological and post-treatment sialographic findings. *Oral Surg., Oral Med., Oral Pathol.,* **63**, 37–41.

MacFarlane, T.W. (1984) The oral ecology of patients with Sjögren's syndrome. *Microbios.,* **41**, 99–106.

Samuels, R.H.A. and Martin, M.V. (1988) A clinical and microbiological study of actinomycetes in oral and cervicofacial lesions. *Br. J. Oral Maxillofac. Surg.,* **20**, 458–463.

Scully, C. (1992) Infections in the immunocompromised patient. *Br. Dent. J.,* **172**, 401–407.

Scully, C., Flint, S.R. and Porter, S.R. (1996) *Oral Diseases,* 2nd edn, Martin Dunitz, London.

van Saene, H.K.F. and Martin, M.V. (1990) Do microorganisms play a role in irradiation mucositis? *Eur. J. Clin. Microbiol.,* **9**, 861–863.

Tyldesley, W.R. and Field, E.A. (1995) *Oral Medicine,* 4th edn, Oxford Medical Publications, Oxford.

Oral viral infections

Oral viral infections are common and it has been estimated that over 90% of the population are affected by them at some time. They produce a variety of pathological changes to the oral mucosa, some of which resolve and others can cause more permanent damage. The principal viruses that infect the oral cavity are herpes, Coxsackie group A, measles, mumps (*see* Chapter 9) and papilloma virus.

Table 10.1 Classification of herpes viruses

Numerical classifica-tion	Biological classifica-tion	Synonyms	Oral lesions
Type 1	alpha	Simplex type 1	Cold sores
Type 2	alpha	Simplex type 2	Ulceration
Type 3	alpha	Varicella-zoster	Chickenpox; herpes zoster
Type 4	gamma	Cytomegalovirus	Ulceration
Type 5	beta	Epstein–Barr	Glandular fever
Type 6	beta		Ulceration

Herpes virus infections

A total of eight herpes viruses have been described that infect humans, although little is known of two of them. The most common classification of these viruses uses a numbering system and this is shown in Table 10.1. Herpes viruses have also been classified on the basis of their biological properties into three subfamilies: Alphaherpesvirinae, Betaherpesvirinae and Gammaherpesvirinae. The Alphaherpesvirinae are rapidly growing, highly cytolytic viruses and most have the capacity to establish latent infections. Human herpes viruses in the Alphaherpesvirinae group are HSV type 1 (human herpes virus 1), HSV type 2 (human herpes type 2) and varicella-zoster virus (human herpes 3).

The Betaherpesvirinae have a long reproductive cycle usually in secretory, lymphoid kidney and other tissues and include human cytomegaloviruses (herpes virus type 5) and herpes type 6. The Gammaherpesvirinae cause latent infections in lymphoid tissue and Epstein–Barr virus (herpes type 4) is a member of this subfamily.

Herpes type 1

Almost 100% of the population have been infected with herpes type 1 by the time they are 15 years old. Most primary infections are symptomless but they can be reactivated and produce oral lesions. Herpes is a large DNA double-stranded virus which is very infectious relative to other oral viral infections (Figure 10.1). There is a common misconception that herpes is only transmitted whilst oral lesions are present. Recent studies have shown that herpes type 1 can be detected by PCR methods (*see* Chapter 2) from saliva even when oral herpetic lesions are absent; it may, therefore, be continually shed into saliva. The virus is transmitted usually during infancy by direct contact, often between mother and child. In AIDS patients significant and almost continual herpetic shedding can be detected. Saliva must therefore be considered as a vector of herpes type 1 infections at all times.

Primary herpetic infections are often symptomless. The virus attaches to the oral mucosa on heparin sulphate moieties of mucosal proteoglycan residues. Fusion of the viral envelope and the cell plasma membrane occurs and the viral capsid and DNA enter the cell and move into the nucleoplasm. The virus can remain dormant in this state until the replicative state occurs. When the virus is reactivated the viral DNA is replicated, cleaved and packaged into capsids in the nucleus. The virus acquires an envelope by budding through

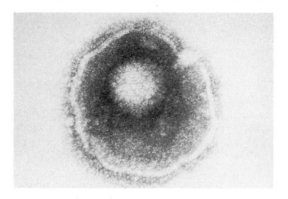

Figure 10.1 A photomicrograph of herpes type 1 virus (original magnification approx. ×100 000). Note the loose voluminous envelope and the capsid containing numerous capsomeres

modified areas of the nuclear membrane. Epithelial cells infected with herpes do not survive as host cell protein production is switched off and messenger RNA function is lost; the infected epithelial cell eventually lyses.

In addition to entering epithelial cells, some viral particles lose their envelope and are rapidly transported back along sensory nerves to the regional ganglia. The method of this transportation of the nucleocapsid to the regional ganglion is often described as being due to rapid retrograde axonal flow, but the precise details of this process are still to be elucidated. The passage from mucosa to ganglion is very rapid; experimental animal studies have shown that this takes less than 2 minutes from inoculation of the virus. Once entry has been gained into the ganglion the virus remains **latent** as a circular piece of extrachromosomal DNA called an episome.

The **primary** lesion of herpes is often symptomless but in some patients severe illness may be present. In the severe form the lymph nodes are enlarged and there may be pain in the mouth which may spread to the throat. Eventually small vesicles form usually on the gingivae, the tongue and the cheek mucosa. These vesicles are usually quite small and not in any particular formation, but are very painful (Figure 10.2). In infants the formation of the vesicles may be accompanied by excessive salivation, irritability and swollen lips. The vesicles rapidly break to leave small ulcers with red halos which heal without scarring. Rarely, herpes type 1 infection spreads to involve the whole of the gums, which are swollen and bleed

easily. The maximal period of viral replication is just before the vesicles form and this is called the **prodromal phase**. When the vesicles rupture large numbers of viruses are released into the saliva, and hence there is a high risk of transmission of the infection to anyone in contact with the affected person. The infections usually heal uneventfully within about 10 days. Primary infections generate antibody formation but this does not prevent recurrence of lesions probably because the virus is protected by its

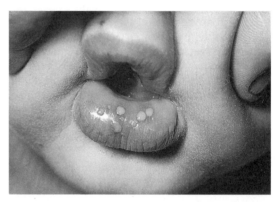

Figure 10.2 A primary herpes type 1 lesion in a one-year-old child. Note the characteristic 'cold sore' vesicles

site in the ganglion or in the epithelial cell.

Although almost all the population is known to be infected with herpes type 1, only about 20–30% suffer from **recurrent** lesions. These lesions arise through reactivation of latent viral DNA from the regional sensory ganglia. The stimulus for the formation of recurrent lesions can be sunlight, stress, minor trauma or menstruation. The exact mechanism of reactivation of herpes type 1 is still unknown and two theories have been postulated to explain what happens. The 'ganglion trigger' theory suggests that reactivation is due to a stimulus to the ganglion which causes the virus to be transported to the epithelium to cause infection. There is little experimental evidence to prove or disprove the 'ganglion trigger' theory, and it does not explain the fact that shedding of virus occurs in the absence of clinical disease. The most widely accepted theory of reactivation is the 'skin trigger' theory which postulates that the virus is being continually reactivated, travelling constantly from the ganglion to the skin and producing foci of potentially infected sites in the epithelium. Under normal circumstances the foci are eliminated by defence mechanisms, but if the conditions are favourable then clinical lesions can appear. This theory does not explain the reactivation of the virus in the ganglion and hence the two postulates are often combined into a 'ganglion and trigger' theory.

Clinical recurrent herpes type 1 lesions are preceded by a prodromal phase of variable length but usually no more than 2 days. The prodromal symptoms are altered sensations felt in the affected areas called hypoaesthesia. The commonest hypoaesthesia sensations are tingling, itching, or burning and it is at this time that maximal viral replication is occurring. After the prodromal phase, vesicles start to appear at the junction of the lip and the mouth; this area is called the vermilion border. The vesicles get bigger and coalesce to produce the typical 'cold sore'. When the cold sore bursts the area is very sore but heals without scarring within 7–10 days.

Oral herpes type 1 infections are usually confined to the mouth but in patients who are medically compromised (*see* Chapter 13) the virus may cause extensive infection of the mouth and spread to the skin. In patients with AIDS, or other conditions affecting the immune response, the virus can enter the bloodstream and travel to the brain, kidney or other vital organs and be fatal.

The diagnosis of herpes type 1 infection is usually made on the basis of the characteristic clinical signs and symptoms and there may be no necessity for any microbiological investigations. Atypical herpes type 1 or suspected type 2 infections require further laboratory investigations. Herpes type 1 can be grown in tissue culture and it produces a characteristic cytopathic effect, but this method of detection has been superseded by the use of fluorescent antisera. Monoclonal fluorescent-labelled antisera provide a quick, cheap method of detection of herpes virus and require no special equipment. The simplest and quickest method of herpes detection is by the use of monoclonal fluorescent antisera specific to either type 1 or 2. Samples of vesicle fluid are taken and spread onto a microscope slide and the monoclonal antiserum is applied, then washed and examined for residual fluorescence. Swabs or smears from cold sores can be used for diagnostic purposes but may give false-negative results.

PCR can also be used for detection of herpes especially where low concentrations of virus are present, but this is still predominantly a research tool.

The main treatment of herpes type 1 infection is with aciclovir or penciclovir which interfere with viral replication. Both aciclovir and penciclovir are nucleoside analogues, which interfere with replication of DNA by attachment to the developing chain and stopping it lengthening. Aciclovir can be used topically, orally or intravenously and has few side-effects. This antiviral agent is best applied in the prodromal phase of cold sore development when viral replication is maximal. Aciclovir has been in use for over a decade and resistant herpes type 1 viruses have been found, but these are less pathogenic and do not appear to present a significant clinical problem. Penciclovir is a newer topical agent that has been shown to shorten the length of the herpetic lesion, particularly if applied in the prodromal phase.

Herpes type 2

This virus was thought to only infect the genital area but it is now often isolated from the oral cavity. Type 2 produces similar lesions to type 1 and can cause primary and secondary lesions. It is difficult to distinguish between the two viral infections on clinical criteria and other laboratory tests are used (e.g. fluorescent antibody tests). Herpes type 2 is now becoming more common in the oral cavity probably as a result of altered sexual practices. It can cause serious infections in neonates, which can be oral, or more generalized, and associated with high temperatures. Herpes type 2 has been strongly associated with cancer of the cervix but there have been no reports of its being associated with oral neoplasia. The treatment of herpes type 2 infections is with aciclovir.

Herpes type 3

Herpes type 3 is also called varicella-zoster virus and is responsible for chickenpox in its primary infection, and shingles in its reactivated form.

Chickenpox
This is one of the most common childhood illnesses but it can also affect adults. It is spread by droplet infection, particularly from saliva

and nasal secretions, to the upper respiratory tract where it may gain entry to the bloodstream and spread to other parts of the body. The incubation period is 15–20 days, when the characteristic rash appears. In some patients oral ulcers 2–3 mm in diameter appear before the skin eruptions; these can be found anywhere in the mouth. The oral lesions are painful and consist of ulcers surrounded by a red annulus of inflammation. Often the ulcers go undetected as the classic vesicular eruptions, predominantly on the head and trunk, dominate the clinical presentation. The skin vesicles burst within a few hours and are extremely itchy; they eventually become dry and crusty, and heal without scarring. The patient is infectious during the development of the infection but not after the skin vesicles have healed. Antibodies to chickenpox develop and are protective for life, but do not prevent shingles.

The diagnosis of chickenpox is made from the characteristic clinical presentation of the disease and laboratory tests are therefore not usually necessary to make the diagnosis. The virus is slow-growing and can be difficult to grow in tissue culture; serological tests are used for its detection and these include complement fixation and a rise in antibody titre. Treatment of chickenpox is usually palliative but in medically compromised patients (*see* Chapter 13) aciclovir is used as there is a danger of systemic complications.

Zoster

Herpes zoster infection is due to reactivation of herpes type 3 from a sensory ganglion. The virus is latent in the ganglion from previous chickenpox infection and is reactivated, producing characteristic vesicular eruptions along the course of the sensory nerve (Figure 10.3). The commonest affected area is the thorax, but the branches of the trigeminal may also be affected in 10–15% of patients. The vesicles are closely grouped together along the distribution of the nerve and are often described as a 'belt of roses from hell'. The vesicles are extremely painful and eventually heal, but whilst they are present they may infect others. In about 15% of individuals there may be some residual damage to the sensory nerve varying from altered sensation to excruciating residual pain. In the oral cavity, post-shingles trigeminal neuralgia may occur especially in adults, but it is rare in children.

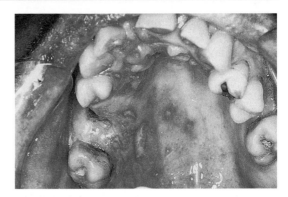

Figure 10.3 Oral herpes type 3 infection (Varicella zoster) often called shingles. Note the linear formation of the ulcers along the distribution of the palatal nerves

The diagnosis of shingles is made on clinical evidence but if laboratory confirmation is required then the methods described for chickenpox (*see above*) are used. Treatment of shingles with aciclovir is important in adults as it helps to prevent post-herpetic neuralgia.

Herpes type 4

Herpes type 4 is often called cytomegalovirus and is a rare cause of disease in the oral cavity. It can cause sore throats and occasionally atypical ulceration of the oral mucosa. It is diagnosed by direct immunofluorescence demonstration of the virus on smears from the lesions. Treatment is with ganciclovir and foscarnet.

Herpes type 5

Herpes type 5 is the Epstein–Barr virus, named after the two virologists who first observed it by using electron microscopy to examine cultures of lymphoblasts. This virus causes infectious mononucleosis, or glandular fever. The disease is caught from saliva during intimate contact with someone who has the disease, or is recuperating from it; kissing is often described as the act of transmission. The incubation period is long (from 4 to 7 weeks) and there is a low grade fever, tonsillitis, tiredness and generalized lymphadenopathy. In the early stages of the disease, in a minority of cases, the oral cavity is affected at the junction of hard and soft palates. Small clusters of fine petechial haemorrhages occur which may coalesce to form a white pseudomembrane.

The diagnosis of infectious mononucleosis is made on haematological grounds since atypical mononuclear cells are present in large numbers. Specific tests such as the detection of Epstein–Barr capsid antigen by immunofluorescence is also useful. This virus has strong links with Burkitt's lymphoma and nasopharyngeal carcinoma.

Herpes type 6

This virus is found to be latent in lymphoid tissue. It has been described as being associated with facial rashes in babies and oral ulceration has been associated with it. In addition, cervical lymphadenopathy has also been described. The incidence of infection and routine tests for the detection and identification of this virus are still to be described.

Herpes type 7 and 8

Little is known about these viruses except that they are associated with Kaposi's sarcoma and AIDS patients. They are herpes viruses from their appearance, serology and structure, but their precise incidence is unknown.

Coxsackie viruses

Coxsackie are enteroviruses that affect the gut and are named after the village in New York where these viruses were first isolated; they are classified into types A and B and the subspecies are numbered. Coxsackie virus types A4, A5, A9 and A16 cause hand, foot and mouth disease and herpangina is caused by A2, A4, A5 and A8 types.

Hand, foot and mouth disease

Hand, foot and mouth disease is a Coxsackie viral infection which usually occurs in episodic outbreaks and affects the body areas described in its name. Usually children are infected but adults, particularly in hospitals, may also contract the disease. The incubation period is usually from 5 to 7 days. In the incubation period the patient may have a headache and a sore throat. Eventually the mouth is affected with vivid red, painful ulcers being found in the oral cavity, particularly associated with the opening of the parotid duct. Lesions also appear on the hands and feet and are bright red spots that can be painful. The disease is self-limiting and heals usually without complication. The diagnosis is usually made on clinical grounds, since serology is difficult as many of the enteroviruses have antigenic groups which cross-react. No treatment is usually necessary for this condition as healing occurs spontaneously.

Herpangina

Herpangina is a relatively common condition in children which is often not diagnosed. It is spread by droplet infection and by the faeco-oral route. The incubation period is short, usually about 2 or 3 days, after which the posterior part of the mouth becomes inflamed. The oropharynx develops papular lesions which have small greyish centres and are surrounded by a halo of inflammation. The lesions are very painful and last for about 3 days before healing spontaneously without scarring. Herpangina can be accompanied by quite a severe fever and malaise. The diagnosis is usually made on clinical grounds.

Measles

Measles is a common disease of childhood that is spread by droplet infection from the upper respiratory tract and is highly infectious. The disease initially causes a high fever, but just before this, small lesions appear in the mouth called Koplik's spots. The spots in the mouth are tiny bluish grey, surrounded by purplish red area and are usually on the already erythematous mucosa. Koplik's spots are transitory and do not persist for more than 24 hours. The patient then develops a characteristic rash of measles associated with a high fever.

The laboratory diagnosis of measles is usually unnecessary as the clinical presentation is characteristic. Measles is usually not treated as most patients get better, but respiratory and systemic complications can occur.

Papilloma viruses

Papilloma virus infections are becoming increasingly common, particularly in patients with AIDS. The infections usually cause warts at the angles of the mouth or intraorally. There is some discussion as to which of the papilloma viruses cause oral warts but those with DNA types 6, 11 and 16 have been identified. The warts are often described as condylomata acumatum which are large accumulations of keratinized tissue. There is a strong association between DNA type 6, 11 and 16 and cancerous change and this may occur in oral warts. Excision and biopsy are necessary if oral warts start to get bigger or if they appear reddened and ulcerated.

Summary

A variety of viral infections affect the oral cavity, most of which are due to herpes virus. By far the most common viral infections are due to herpes type 1, which is responsible for cold sores. There are seven other herpes viruses which are found in the oral cavity and give rise to a variety of lesions. Other viruses affecting the oral cavity are measles, mumps, Coxsackie and papilloma viruses.

Bibliography

Alford, C.A. and Brit, W.J. (1990) Cytomegalovirus. In *Virology,* 2nd edn (B. Fields, R. Knipe, R. Channock, J. Hirsch, T. Melnick, T. Monath, and B. Roizman, eds), Raven Press, New York, pp. 1981–2010.

Chang, Y., Cesarman, E., Pessin, M.S. *et al.* (1994) Identification of herpes-like virus DNA sequences in AIDS associated Kaposi's sarcoma. *Science,* **266**, 1865–1869.

Epstein, M.A. and Achong, B.G. (1986) Introductory considerations. In *The Epstein–Barr Virus: Recent Advances* (M.A. Epstein and B.G. Achong, eds), Heinemann Medical, London, pp. 1–11.

Roizman, B. (1982) The family herpesviridae: general description, taxonomy and classification. In *The Herpes Viruses,* Volume 1 (B. Roizman, ed.), Plenum Press, New York, pp. 1–23.

Timbury, M.C. (1991) *Medical Virology,* 9th edn, Churchill Livingstone, London.

11

Oral fungal infections

In the past decade oral fungal infections have dramatically increased in incidence. Part of this increase has been due to the heightened awareness and diagnosis of oral fungal infections by clinicians, but another reason has been the AIDS pandemic (*see* Chapter 12). The acquired immunodeficiency syndrome is a good example of one essential feature of oral fungal infections in that they usually arise when the host is compromised. Oral fungal infections are usually 'diseases of the diseased' and some predisposition has to occur in the host for the host to be affected. This is important to understand as the cure of fungal infections must also necessitate removing, or alleviating the predisposing condition.

Fungi are divided into those that reproduce sexually, i.e. by the fusion of two gametes (perfect fungi), and those that are asexual (imperfect fungi). Oral fungal infections by perfect fungi are still rare, but increasing in incidence, particularly in immunocompromised individuals. Table 11.1 lists the principal fungi reported to infect the oral cavity.

The most common fungi to cause oral problems are the imperfect yeasts and of these Candida species account for the majority of the infections. *Candida albicans* is by far the most commonly isolated fungus from oral infections but other species may also be isolated. Table 11.1 shows some of the principal *Candida* species that have been isolated from oral infections. It has been recognized in the past decade that many oral infections due to *Candida* may have two, or three yeast species present. The exact role of these species of *Candida* is still unknown; they may contribute

to the pathogenic process or, may just be secondary colonizers of the infected area. Certainly some *Candida* species other than *C. albicans* are capable of causing infections on their own (*see* Table 11.1). Some imperfect yeast species (e.g. *C. krusei*) are becoming increasingly important clinically as they are often resistant to some of the azole agents that are used to treat these infections

Table 11.1 The principal fungi that may infect the oral cavity

Yeasts	Other fungi
Candida albicans	*Aspergillus* spp.
Candida tropicalis	*Mucor* spp.
Candida krusei	
Candida guilliermondii	
Candida parapsilosis	
Candida glabrata (syn *Torulopsis glabrata*)	
Geotrichium spp.	

Candida albicans

There has been a dramatic increase in the interest in this fungal pathogen and an understanding is now emerging about the pathogenic potential of this complex micro-organism. *C. albicans* is found in the oral cavity of approximately half the population, although estimates of its incidence do vary, according to the type of population sampled, the sampling method, the conditions of culture and the identification methods employed. The yeast has been found on all mucosal surfaces, but the main oral site

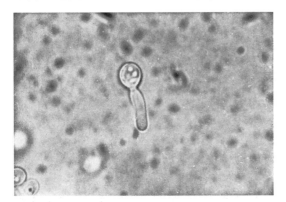

Figure 11.1 Growth of *C. albicans* for 2 hours at 37 °C in serum showing the formation of a hyphae (germ tube) from the blastospore (original magnification approx. ×100). This illustrates the dimorphic forms of *C. albicans*

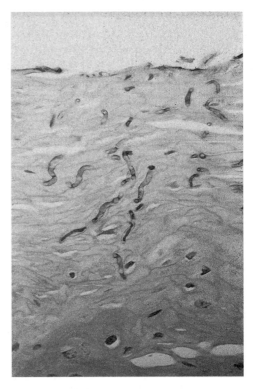

Figure 11.2 Hyphae of *C. albicans* invading oral epithelium (Periodic Acid Schiff's reagent; original magnification ×100). Notice the fungal hyphae at approximately 90° to the surface of the epithelium and only extending into the tissue as far as the granular layer

where it is most often found is the tongue, particularly in the posterior dorsum area in the region of the circumvallate papillae. The yeast can be a part of the resident microflora but when the ecosystem is changed (for example when broad spectrum antibiotics are administered), then overgrowth can occur and infection results.

C. albicans is often described as a dimorphic fungus in that it exists in blastospore and mycelial forms (Figure 11.1). It is in fact a trimorphic fungus because when it is put into certain specialized growth media (e.g. corn meal agar), small highly refractive spores called chlamydospores, are formed. The exact function of chlamydospores is still unknown and they are not found in oral candidosis, but they are useful for the laboratory identification of *C. albicans*. There is still considerable debate about the role of blastospore and mycelial forms of *C. albicans* and the transition between the two forms. It has been suggested consistently that the transition from the blastospore (yeast) to a mycelium, often called a Y to M transformation, is synonymous with a change from a commensal to a pathogenic state. There is no doubt that increased numbers of mycelia are found in oral *C. albicans* infections; however, they can also be seen in healthy mouths. Mycelia-deficient *C. albicans* have been isolated from infected oral sites and appear to cause infection in experimental animals. In general, the transformation from yeast to mycelia may be important, but is not always a prerequisite for infection to occur.

The mycelia can in some conditions penetrate the oral tissues, but curiously they only invade the keratin and granular layers of the epithelium, never the whole thickness (*see* Figure 11.2). When seen in biopsied tissues, the mycelia appear to invade roughly at right-angles to the surface of the epithelium. The mycelia also appear to penetrate straight through the epithelial cells, leaving an annulus of viable cell around the fungus. The reasons for this curious mode of invasion are not clear. It has been suggested that the mycelia penetrate the epithelium to obtain nutrients and to prevent displacement by desquamated oral epithelial cells. At present, both of these explanations are plausible and have scientific support.

Recent studies have shown that some *C. albicans* strains are capable of phenotypic changes. This was first noticed when selected strains were able to change their colonial morphology after subculture. Strains were able to change from smooth to rough colonial morphology. Comparison of the yeast DNA from the original and subcultured colonies has shown that the genotypic characteristics of both are identical. The conclusion is that the strains have undergone phenotypic change which has resulted in a change in colonial morphology. The ability of *C. albicans* strains to undergo phenotypic change can have more serious ramifications, particularly in relation to drug therapy. It has been found that AIDS patients with oral *C. albicans* infections, who have been treated with fluconazole, sometimes do not respond to the azole treatment. Laboratory investigation of sequential isolates from such infections has shown that the infecting strain is identical throughout, but that the sensitivity to the azole has changed and the MIC has increased; this is as a result of phenotypic change. The mechanism for this change in azole sensitivity has still to be elucidated, but it has now been described in *C. albicans* strains from non-AIDS patients.

The virulence factors of *C. albicans* have been and are still the subject of intensive investigation as their elucidation may provide insights into the pathogenesis of infection and ultimately lead to new and improved treatment modalities. What has been shown conclusively is that some strains of *C. albicans* are more virulent than others due to their different phenotypic characteristics. Crucial to establishment of differential virulence among *C. albicans* isolates has been the development of reliable methods for the recognition of different strains. Early attempts at distinguishing *C. albicans* strains relied on the inhibition of isolates to a variety of chemicals; a method called the resistogram technique. Resistograms are very inoculum-dependent and hence the slightest increase in yeast numbers could result in a change in the apparent resistance patterns obtained. This method has been superseded by 'genetic fingerprinting' of the DNA of *C. albicans*. In this method, the *C. albicans* DNA is extracted from the blastospore and 'cut' into fragments by restriction endonuclease enzymes (*see* Chapter 3). The DNA fragments are then separated by electrophoresis and this produces a characteristic set of bands which are unique to that strain. This technique called restriction fragment length polymorphism or RFLP. It is the starting point for evaluating different virulence factors of *C. albicans* strains.

The known virulence factors of *C. albicans* are listed in Table 11.2. It has been established that strains of *C. albicans* adhere specifically to oral epithelial cells and to polymethylmethacrylate which is used to make some types of dentures. The adhesion to epithelium is mediated by lectin-like components of *C. albicans* that interact with surface mono- or disaccharide components of the host (*see* Table 11.2). This adhesion is enhanced in the hyhal form of the fungus as more of these lectin-like components are present. When the hyphae penetrate the surface epithelium is disrupted by extracellular neutral and acidic proteases from *C. albicans* and more potential adhesion sites are exposed.

Table 11.2 Virulence factors of *Candida albicans*

Mechanism	Molecular factor
Adherence	Extracellular enzymes
	protease
	lipase
Dimorphism	Unknown
Interference with defence mechanisms	
phagocytosis	Toxins, metabolites
immune defences	Toxins, metabolites, acidic produts
complement	Nitrosamines
Synergism with other bacteria and yeasts	Unknown

In erythematous candidosis, *C. albicans* has been shown to adhere strongly to polymethylmethacrylate (acrylic). The adhesion to acrylic is probably mediated by a multi-functional adhesin protein, which has been identified on the surface of *C. albicans* hyphae; this adhesin has yet to be fully characterized. This specific adhesion to acrylic confers an ecological advantage to *C. albicans* in denture wearers in that the yeast can remain in the mouth independent of the oral mucosa.

Once *C. albicans* has adhered to a mucosal surface a commensal saprophytic existence can be established and the fungus competes for nutrients with other micro-organisms in the immediate vicinity. If the resident microflora is disrupted and the growth of the candida is unrestricted then infection occurs. Hyphae penetrate the epithelium with the help of the aspartyl proteinases and phospholipases, which have been shown to be associated with pathogenic strains. The penetration of the oral epithelium by the hyphae is resisted by a number of host defence mechanisms. Once the surface layer of the epithelium is crossed an intraepithelial inflammatory response develops and phagocytic macrophages and polymorphonuclear leucocytes (PMN) migrate to the area. PMNs are able to phagocytose *C. albicans,* usually after opsonization by immunoglobulins, or after exposure to complement. The granules in PMNs are highly efficient at lysing *Candida.* PMNs also produce lactoferrin and oxygen intermediates which have high anti-fungal activity. In addition, the lysis of PMNs releases a 30 kDa protein that is highly fungistatic. Macrophages adhere to *Candida* cells through a membrane-mannose receptor, or by attachment to vitronectin (a glycoprotein cell adhesion and spreading factor found in plasma and extracellular matrix). Macrophages can, in addition to their phagocytic function, produce nitrogen monoxide, which is highly fungicidal. *C. albicans* is not without its own defence mechanisms to these deleterious host defence effects. Phagocytosis of *C. albicans* by PMNs or macrophages can be resisted by the production of inhibitory acidic peptides and other extracellular glycoproteins and metabolites.

Very little is known about the virulence factors of other *Candida* spp., probably because they have not been so extensively studied as *C. albicans*, but *C. tropicalis* also produces extracellular proteolytic enzymes. *C. krusei* has also received some attention, mainly because azole-resistant strains have been isolated from patients with AIDS (*see* Chapter 12).

Candidosis: definition, laboratory diagnosis and clinical classification

Candidosis is the correct term for infections caused by *Candida* species as the suffix *-osis* describes fungal infections, and will be used throughout this text. The term candidiasis is sometimes used by clinicians to describe these infections, but technically this is incorrect, as the suffix *-iasis* is usually reserved to describe parasitic infections.

Oral candidosis is usually a secondary infection to some other local or systemic factor. The predisposing factors that lead to oral candidosis are numerous and virtually any perturbation of systemic health or well-being can cause overgrowth of *Candida*. The main predisposing factors that may lead to oral candidosis are shown in Table 11.3.

Table 11.3 Predisposing factors for oral candidosis

Local	Physiological
Trauma	Infancy
Occlusion	Old age
Maceration	
	Hormonal states
Saliva	Diabetes
Xerostomia	Hypothyroidism
Sjögren's syndrome	Hyperparathyroidism
Radiotherapy	Hypoadrenocortical activity
Cytotoxic therapy	
	Nutrition
Diet	Hypovitaminosis
High carbohydrate	Iron deficiency
	Malnutrition
Infection	
Any systemic long-standing infection	
Human immunodeficiency virus infection	

Laboratory diagnosis of oral candidosis

The diagnosis of oral candidosis is usually made on the basis of the medical history of the patient and the clinical presentation. Many of the types of oral candidosis described are so characteristic in their presentation that they often can be diagnosed without laboratory investigation. If microbiological tests are done these are usually swabs, imprint cultures, rinses, smears and incisional or, less commonly, excisional biopsies. Table 11.4 shows the types of oral candidosis and the samples that may be taken.

The samples generated must be used with care if a definitive diagnosis is to be made. Smears from the lesion are usually taken with a blunt instrument (e.g. a tongue depressor) from the surface of the affected area; the smears are placed between two microscope slides for transport to the laboratory. In the laboratory, they are stained with Periodic-Schiff's reagent which reacts with the mannans and other carbohydrates in the fungal walls of *Candida* species. The stained slide is then examined

Table 11.4 The laboratory samples that can be taken for the laboratory diagnosis of oral candidosis

Condition	Sampling method	Comments
Acute pseudomembraneous	Smear, swab, rinse, imprint culture	Smear shows the presence of hyphae and the pseudomembrane Swab, rinse imprint culture, allow definitive diagnosis
Acute erythematous	Smear, swab, imprint culture	Smear not always diagnostic. Other samples are preferable
Chronic plaque-like or nodular	Biopsy	Biopsy is mandatory to exclude neoplasia
Chronic erythematous	Smear, swab, rinse, imprint culture fitting surface	All may be diagnostic but swabs, smears and imprint culture should include the denture-
Chronic pseudomembraneous	Smears, swabs, imprint culture	Smear shows the presence of hyphae and the pseudomembrane. Swabs, rinses and imprint give definitive diagnosis
Candida-associated angular cheilitis	Swabs and smears	Smears may not be diagnostic. Swabs are to be preferred to elucidate the presence of bacteria
Chronic mucocutaneous candidosis	Biopsy	Biopsy is required for definitive diagnosis

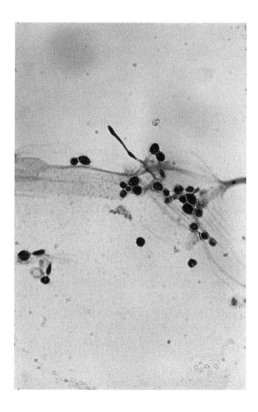

Figure 11.3 Smear from oral candidosis stained with periodic acid Schiff's reagent (original magnification approx. ×100). Note the hyphal and blastospores present in this smear

microscopically and blastospores and hyphae can then be seen (*see* Figure 11.3).

The presence of a large number of hyphae and blastospores is often interpreted as candidosis but this may not be always correct. Candidal hyphae may be found in the resident microflora and smear samples must therefore be interpreted with care. Swabs and rinses, in contrast, give a quantitative estimate of the number of yeasts present. A heavy or confluent growth from a rinse or swab after inoculation on Sabouraud's medium allows a more definitive estimate of the yeast population and distinguishes, on quantitative criteria, between the commensal and the pathogenic state. A light growth of yeasts (e.g. 10–20 colonies for a given area sampled), is taken as growth from a commensal site; greater than this is indicative of pathogenicity. The yeasts cultured can be identified from swab or rinse samples and their sensitivity to anti-fungal agents determined. The quantitative testing can be further refined by the use of imprint cultures. In this technique, a piece of foam soaked in a liquid growth medium is pressed on the mucosal surface and then transferred and inoculated on the surface of a Sabouraud's agar plate and cultured overnight. The number of colonies in each area sampled can then be calculated (Figure 11.4). Biopsies also can give information as to the presence, or absence, of hyphal invasion but

Table 11.5 Classification of primary oral candidosis

Current nomenclature	Synonym	Revised nomenclature
Acute atrophic candidosis	Thrush	Acute pseudomembraneous
Acute atrophic	Candida glossitis or antibiotic sore mouth	Acute erythematous
Chronic hyperplastic	Candida leukoplakia	Chronic plaque-like,
		Chronic nodular
Chronic atrophic	Denture-induced stomatitis or denture sore mouth	Chronic erythematous
		Chronic pseudomembraneous
Acute or chronic angular cheilitis	Perleche	Candida-associated angular cheilitis

Adapted from Samaranayake and MacFarlane (1990)

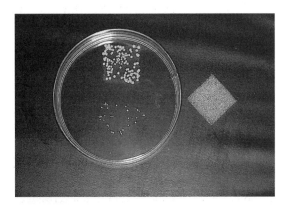

Figure 11.4 Quantitative assessment of *Candida* present on oral mucosa. The sparse growth was obtained after 24 hours incubation aerobically at 37 °C is an example of the commensal state. The confluent growth is from a case of oral candidosis

more importantly they can diagnose the effects of the yeasts on the tissues. Biopsies are mandatory where neoplastic change is suspected.

Clinical classification of oral candidosis

The classification of oral candidosis used to be based on the presence of acute and chronic inflammation. All the other forms of candidosis were classified as miscellaneous. This simple classification has proved unsatisfactory, particularly in the description of some presentations of oral candidosis associated with AIDS. A revised and more appropriate classification of oral candidosis is shown in Table 11.5. This classification will be used throughout this book.

Acute pseudomembraneous candidosis

Acute pseudomembraneous candidosis is a disease usually seen in newly born children, old and debilitated persons and medically compromised persons.

In newly born children the oral cavity is sterile and can become contaminated from the birth canal during parturition. The lack of a competitive oral microflora in the newborn allows any *Candida* present to flourish and to cause an infection. The infection in children can be quite acute, resulting in excessive salivation, a raised temperature and refusal of the child to eat. The cause of acute pseudomembraneous candidosis in the elderly is less well defined. It may be due to malnourishment, debilitation, xerostomia (or qualitative changes in saliva), or impairment or atrophy of host defence systems.

Acute pseudomembraneous candidosis is also seen in patients infected with the Human Immmunodeficiency Virus (*see* Chapter 12). The presence of acute psudomembraneous candidosis in such patients is usually indicative of a diminution in white cell counts and the progression to AIDS (*see* Chapter 12). This form of candidosis in HIV infected individuals may be progressive and lead to oesophageal or tracheal involvement. Oesophageal involvement may cause difficulty in swallowing and tracheal candidosis may lead to life-threatening *Candida* lung abscesses. The usual cause of this form of oral candidosis is *C. albicans* alone, but in some cases two or three of the other *Candida* species shown in Table 11.1 may also be present.

Acute pseudomembraneous candidosis presents

clinically as white or yellowish plaques; the plaques are variable in size and distribution. Histologically, the white plaques consist of mucosal cells and hyphal elements and when removed leave a raw bleeding area underneath. This form of oral candidosis is usually painful due to the acute inflammation but in some patients it may cause minimal discomfort despite extensive pseudomembrane formation.

Acute erythematous candidosis

Acute erythematous candidosis is characterized by an acute inflammatory reaction of the area affected. It can occur following suppression of the oral bacterial microflora following treatment with broad spectrum antibiotics and hence is often called antibiotic sore mouth. Typically, tetracycline usage is associated with acute erythematous candidosis but other antibiotics may also be implicated. Usually the tongue is involved and it becomes depapillated and sensitive to hot, cold, spicy or salty stimuli. The tongue becomes shiny in appearance due to the depapillation and histologically the epithelium is thinned and atrophic. This category of oral candidosis has been extended to include some of the mucosal changes seen in AIDS patients, where usually the palate is the area affected.

The condition is diagnosed by its classical clinical appearance and the supplementary laboratory tests (*see* Table 11.4). If the condition is caused by the use of broad spectrum antibiotics then stopping the agents may be enough to resolve the condition, together with some topical treatment. Stopping the antimicrobial is not always possible, however, so an anti-fungal agent may be used, not as a cure, but to provide some relief. Where the condition is associated with HIV infection, then a combination of topical and systemic antifungals is necessary for treatment as the condition is seldom contained by just one type of treatment.

Chronic plaque-like and nodular candidosis

These are two clinical variants of a hyperplastic epithelial change where the mucosa appears to develop a plaque-like or a nodular appearance. This condition is distinguished from pseudomembraneous candidosis in that the plaque or nodules cannot be dislodged by gentle rubbing with a blunt instrument to leave a raw bleeding area underneath. When chronic plaque-like or nodular candidosis is biopsied, or surgically removed, histological examination shows it to consist of a grossly thickened and hyperplastic epithelium penetrated by occasional hyphal elements of *C. albicans*. These two types of oral candidosis are clinically important, as 5–11% of the lesions may become cancerous. It is mandatory that these lesions are biopsied, preferably with excision, but this will depend on the size of the lesion. If the lesion is too big for removal, and the diagnosis is confirmed by biopsy as chronic plaque-like or nodular candidosis, then it can be treated with systemic fluconazole, when it will often regress. The lesion will need regular review and if any erythematous areas develop subsequently then it will need further biopsy. The presence of erythematous areas in a chronic plaque-like or nodular oral candidosis can be indicative of cancerous change. If the second biopsy shows any neoplastic change, then the lesion needs more radical treatment.

There has been a debate about whether plaque-like or nodular lesions are caused by *C. albicans*. The other argument to explain the presence of *C. albicans* is that it is a secondary fungal infection on a pre-existing hyperplastic epithelium. The fact that mucosal lesions of this kind can resolve following systemic anti-fungal treatment is supportive of *C. albicans* playing an important role in the development of these hyperplastic lesions and, most probably, their change to a neoplastic state. In addition, certain strains of *C. albicans* are capable of changing some as yet unidentified salivary components into nitrosamines, which are known carcinogens. In summary, all of the evidence supports *C. albicans* as having a pivotal role in the development of plaque-like and nodular forms of oral candidosis and their potential for neoplastic change.

Chronic erythematous candidosis

This is usually associated with the wearing of dentures. The mucosa is erythematous but not painful and may only be discovered during a routine examination. If the lesions are associated with a denture then the lesion will be delineated by the extent of the mucosal coverage of the denture. Chronic erythematous candidosis is usually associated with upper partial or full dentures, as these are in close apposition to the mucosa and tend to be more conducive to the accumulation of plaque on the fitting surface. Lower dentures tend to be less stable and it is unusual to see this condition below them. The pathogenesis of this condition is still the subject of some debate but is associated with both plastic and metal dentures.

The lesion is associated with poor oral hygiene and the formation of biofilms of mixtures of fungi and bacteria on the denture. The biofilm on the denture-fitting surface causes mucosal inflammation, which is usually of three types. The first type is a localized pinpoint hyperaemic type; the second a more extensive erythematous mucosal reaction; the third a granular or nodular type of reaction, principally involving the central palatal areas. The condition can usually be partially resolved by improving the denture hygiene and avoiding continuous wearing of the dentures. This evidence supports the contention that it is a mixture of tissue trauma and microbial factors causing the condition. Often there is a history of high fermentable carbohydrate intake in this condition, which could be associated with the production of carboxylic acids by yeast species; these acids are known to be an irritant to mucosal tissues.

Chronic erythematous candidosis is common and in one survey was found to affect almost 60% of elderly denture wearers. The principal yeast isolated from this condition is *C. albicans*, but others, including *C. tropicalis*, *C. stellatoidea*, *C. parapsilosis*, *C. guillermondii* and occasionally *Rhodotorula* spp. and *C. glabrata* may be found. The treatment is to improve the denture cleaning, apply topical anti-fungals and to avoid continuous denture wearing. Chronic erythematous candidosis may be seen in some patients with AIDS who do not wear dentures, particularly on the palate; it is usually indicative of falling white cell counts.

Chronic pseudomembraneous candidosis

This condition is clinically identical to the acute form except that it is chronic and always painless. The usual yeast isolate from this condition is *C. albicans*; other yeasts are seldom present. It is usually found in patients with AIDS and may be a poor prognostic indicator for longevity. It is also found occasionally associated with chronic erythematous candidosis in patients who wear poorly cleaned dentures continuously. It is treated with topical or systemic anti-fungals.

Angular cheilitis

Angular cheilitis is characterized by erythematous areas at the angles of the mouth. It can occur at any age but it is often associated with old worn-out dentures which fail to support the face and which create folds at the angles of the mouth; there is often a concomitant chronic erythematous candidosis beneath the denture. The folds at the angles of the mouth become sodden with saliva and infected with *C. albicans* and members of the skin microflora, principally *Staphylococcus aureus*. The infection can spread from the angles to infect the lips, which may bleed, ulcerate and be very painful.

The treatment of this condition is by renewing the dentures and ensuring the tissue folds at the angles are supported by a new prosthesis. The infection usually needs treatment with an agent active against both bacteria and fungi, since both are usually found in this lesion. Miconazole is usually the anti-fungal of choice because it is active against *Candida* spp. and some Gram-positive bacteria, including staphylococci. Occasionally, angular cheilitis does not resolve despite appropriate anti-fungal treatment and concomitant prosthetic treatment. This failure to resolve is usually due to a residual staphylococcal infection, and topical treatment with fucidic acid usually resolves the problem. *Candida*-associated angular cheilitis can also be seen in patients without dentures. It can be indicative of a folic acid deficiency and replacement therapy often results in complete resolution.

Other forms of secondary oral candidosis

Chronic mucocutaneous candidosis

This is not a single condition but a spectrum of problems that affect the mouth, skin and fingernails. The initial lesions in the oral cavity appear as chronic or acute pseudomembranes; eventually these change to become hard, keratinized areas, particularly involving the vestibular area of the lip. The skin lesions may be granulomatous, appearing on the face and scalp, and often there is concomitant chronic fingernail infection. Some forms of this condition have a familial link whilst others do not have a genetic basis. Chronic mucocutaneous candidosis can be associated with multiple endocrine problems or it can have a late age of onset, usually in males.

The condition can generally be managed with systemic anti-fungals and is fortunately rare. *C. albicans* is usually isolated from chronic mucocutaneous candidosis and it is usually treated with systemic azoles. Azole-resistant strains of *C. albicans* have been isolated from this condition and this is probably another example of phenotypic change in this fungus after prolonged use of static anti-fungals.

Cheilo-candidosis

This is a condition that principally affects the lips, which become heavily infected with *C. albicans*. The lesions can affect both lips, although the patient is otherwise healthy. The lips become swollen, crusted and painful and infected, usually, with *C. albicans*. The precise aetiology of this condition is still unknown, but it is thought to be associated with some epithelial abnormality, or a reaction to excessive exposure to the sun. Cheilo-candidosis usually responds to topical or systemic antifungal therapy.

Treatment of oral candidosis

Oral candidosis is usually a secondary infection superimposed on other medical problems. The infection will not usually resolve until the predisposing factor is removed. Often it is impossible, or difficult, to cure or correct the underlying predisposing condition (e.g. AIDS), and therefore the oral fungal infection has to be managed palliatively. Oral candidosis is most often undertreated and may recur. It is essential, if recrudescence is to be avoided, to get both a clinical and mycological cure (i.e. the yeasts must be eradicated). In clinical practice, the establishment of a mycological cure can be monitored by microbiological sampling throughout therapy until the yeasts are eradicated. If laboratory monitoring is not possible,

then treating the patient for a period of time which is roughly twice that required to eradicate the clinical symptoms usually suffices.

The principal anti-fungals available for the treatment of oral candidosis are the polyenes and the azoles. The polyenes, amphotericin and nystatin, have been used for over 30 years. They have almost perfect properties for topical agents, in that they are not absorbed through the gut and resistance to them is almost unknown. The polyenes are available for treatment in a variety of formulations, including suspensions, pastilles and lozenges. If the polyenes are to be effective they must be retained in the affected area for periods of hours to kill the yeasts present. It is important therefore to choose the oral formulation best able to remain on the lesion.

There have been a large number of azole compounds developed for the treatment of fungal infections, but most of these are not suitable for oral lesions. All of the azoles are fungistatic for *Candida* species. It is very important, therefore, to treat the underlying predisposing condition of the oral candidosis when using azoles if resolution is to be achieved. The azoles used for oral candidosis are miconazole, fluconazole, ketoconazole and itraconazole. Miconazole is a topical agent which is fungistatic and has some bacteriostatic action; it is therefore useful in the treatment of mixed bacterial and fungal infections (e.g. angular cheilitis). Fluconazole is a systemic agent which is active in saliva and has been used for most oral fungal infections; it can affect the liver in high doses. Ketoconazole is a systemic anti-fungal whose principal use is in the treatment of chronic mucocutaneous candidosis; again, high doses can have a hepatatoxic effect. Itraconazole is not very effective against oral candida infections.

Azole resistance has been described on the basis of both clinical and laboratory evidence. The measurement of azole resistance in the laboratory is not easy, as the exact minimum inhibitory concentration is often difficult to assess for these static agents. The problem with assessing azole resistance in the laboratory is determining the end point. Tests have now been devised which involve dilution assays that work reproducibly but need careful controls. Many of the descriptions of the emergence of resistance could be due to phenotypic change, particularly in *C. albicans* and *C. krusei* strains.

Summary

Oral candidosis is usually a secondary infection superimposed on another medical condition. A mixture of Candida *spp. can usually be isolated from oral candidosis, but* C. albicans *is the principal pathogen.* C. albicans *possesses a range of virulence factors that can be phenotypically expressed and enhance its pathogenic potential. These virulence factors in* C. albicans *include adhesins and the ability of hyphae to secrete aspartyl proteinases and phopholipases. The laboratory diagnosis of oral candidosis may be difficult as it is often difficult to distinguish between pathogenic and commensal forms of* Candida. C. albicans *undergoes yeast to mycelial transformation and this was thought to be representative of a change from commensalism to pathogenicity.* C. albicans *hyphae may be found in mucosa unaffected by oral candidosis and also in infected areas; therefore the presence of hyphae is not always diagnostic of candidosis.*

A number of different forms of oral candidosis can be seen in the oral cavity. These include inflammatory conditions such as chronic erythematous candidosis to the more sinister chronic and plaque-like forms of the infection which may be associated with neoplastic change. In this chapter a classification is described which covers most of the clinical forms of the disease.

The treatment of oral candidosis involves removing or ameliorating the underlying condition followed by the prescription of anti-fungal agents. The anti-fungals used for oral candidosis are the polyenes and the azoles. Used correctly both the polyenes and the azoles can alleviate and, in many cases, resolve oral candidosis.

Bibliography

Calderone, R.A. (1993) Recognition between *Candida albicans* and host cells. *Trends Microbiol.,* **55**, 55–58.

Calderone, R.A. (1994) Molecular pathogenesis of fungal infections. *Trends Microbiol.,* **12**, 461–463.

Gow, N.A.R. and Gadd, G.M. (1995) *The Growing Fungus,* Chapman & Hall, London.

Heykants, J., Can Peer, A., Larvrijsen, K., Meuldermanns, W., Woestnborghs, R. and Cauwenbergh, W. (1990) Pharmacokinetics of oral antifungals and their clinical implications. *Br. J. Clin. Pract.,* **44** (Suppl.71), 50–56.

McCullough, M.J., Ross, B.C. and Reade, P.C. (1996) *Candida albicans:* a review of its history, taxonomy, epidemiology, virulence, attributes, and methods of strain differentiation. *Int. J. Oral Maxillofac. Surg.,* **25**, 136–144.

Odds, F.C. (1988) *Candida and Candidosis,* Balliere, Tindall, London.

Samaranayake, L.P. and McFarlane, T.W. (1990) *Oral Candidosis,* Wright, Oxford.

12

Human immunodeficiency virus and the acquired immune deficiency syndrome

There can be few events in modern microbiology that could match the impact of the human immunodeficiency virus (HIV) on the general population. This virus first started to be mentioned in the early part of the 1980s and has since become the major preoccupation of all governments and the World Health Organization. It has led to more than 6000 papers being published every year on all aspects of the pandemic HIV infection. Best estimates are that around 18 million people are infected with this virus world-wide, but this figure may rise to 20–40 million by the year 2000. Even though in some countries the number of new infections appears not to be increasing, the reservoir of latent carriage of this virus will ensure that it is a major health challenge for years to come.

The human immunodeficiency virus (HIV)

HIV was originally thought to be part of the human T-lymphocyte viruses but has now been classified as part of the human lentovirus (slow virus) and the subfamily Retroviridae. The virus consists of a central protein core (Figure 12.1) containing a protein named p24, a single-stranded RNA core complex and an enzyme reverse transcriptase. Surrounding the core are inner matrix proteins (p17) and a coat of glycoproteins (gp 41 and gp120). The virus is approximately 100–120 nm in size and roughly delta-icosohedral in symmetry.

There are now two main types of HIV, called HIV 1 and HIV 2, which are classified accord-

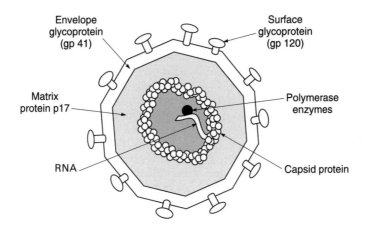

Figure 12.1 Diagrammatic representation of human immunodeficiency virus

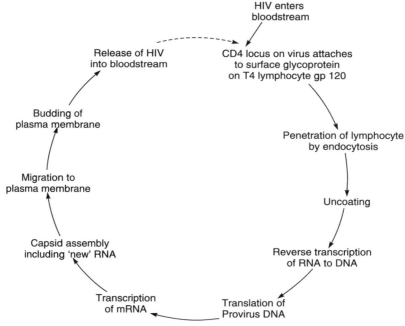

Figure 12.2 The life cycle of HIV in T4 lymphocytes

ing to the differences in glycoprotein envelopes. HIV 1 is distributed widely throughout the world and was the first to be described. HIV 2 was originally confined to Africa but is now also distributed world-wide. HIV has two subtypes: type M (with subtypes A–H) and type O; HIV 2 has five subtypes, A–E. These classifications are used for tracing sources of transmission and for global epidemiology purposes. Both virus types are spread by the same routes of transmission, but in recent experimental and epidemiological studies HIV 2 is acknowledged to be less infective.

The natural history of HIV infection

In order to infect, HIV has to gain access to lymphocytes or macrophages, and this is usually through vaginal or anal intercourse with an infected person. Other routes of transmission of HIV are from an infected mother to her child, *in utero* or at delivery; by breast feeding; exposure to infected blood, blood products or infected tissue and by the use of contaminated needles or syringes. The infectivity of HIV has been measured in experimental animals and it is less infective

than hepatitis B. All the available experimental and epidemiological evidence would support the contention that most exposures to HIV do not result in infection.

In order to understand what happens to patients with AIDS, it is necessary to know how the HIV infect and what effect it has on the immune system. HIV infects predominantly lymphocytes classified as T4 helper cells. Lymphocytes have specific functions in the immune system and are classified accordingly, with a number and a functional description. T4 lymphocytes are called helper cells as their function is to amplify the immune reaction; their activity is regulated by some antagonistic cells called T8 lymphocyte suppressor cells. T8 cells prevent the T4 cells from causing harm to the body by overamplifying the immune reactions. This interplay between T4 and T8 lymphocyte function is important in the development of the acquired immune deficiency syndrome (AIDS) (*see below*). HIV attaches by the glycoprotein gp120 on its surface to a complementary receptor on the lymphocyte called CD4. The interaction between the CD4 receptor on T4 lymphocytes and gp120 has been the subject of intense study as it is recognized that if this attachment could be prevented, then the infectivity HIV could be modulated.

Once attached to T4 lymphocytes, the viral genome and its core, including the enzyme reverse transcriptase, gains entry by endocytosis. The HIV RNA is made into complementary copies of DNA which may, or may not, integrate in the T4 lymphocyte DNA. The generation of DNA from viral RNA is by reverse transcriptase action, and this enzyme also catalyses the reformation of multiple copies of complementary RNA. This 'reverse' process of turning RNA into DNA, and back again, is why HIV is classified as a retrovirus. HIV can then re-enter the bloodstream after assembly of the virus and recoating by a process of budding from the lymphocyte. The life cycle of HIV in T4 lymphocytes is illustrated in Figure 12.2.

This complicated process of HIV reproduction is not without problems. The viral genome of HIV is relatively short, so any mutation can have profound effects on the reproduction of the virus. Small alterations in the viral genome can lead to mutations which can be lethal to HIV. There are advantages, however, to having a small genome as it allows rapid mutation in the presence of anti-HIV agents and the emergence of resistant HIV strains. One recent study has shown the emergence of azothymidine-resistant HIV strains occurs within one month of the start of treatment. This ability to mutate has led to HIV carriers being treated with combinations of agents rather than single antiviral therapies. The ability of the virus to undergo rapid mutations raises the fear that putative vaccines against HIV may have only limited efficacy.

Once the virus has reproduced the second generation of HIV enters the bloodstream and infects more T4 lymphocytes. The timing and stimulus for reproduction of HIV is not known. In some individuals the entry of new virus in the bloodstream from lymphocytes can be very rapid, and in one person took only 10 days. In other individuals it has taken 11 months from inoculation to detect new virus in the circulation. Individuals once infected with HIV are carriers of the virus for life, but about 12 individuals have lost the virus. Most of these people who have lost the virus are being intensely studied, as identification of the reasons for their loss of HIV could offer hope for therapy. Once the newly reproduced virus enters the bloodstream an antibody is detect-

able and individuals used to be described as 'HIV antibody-positive'. The initial inoculation of HIV is usually not of sufficient magnitude to generate an antibody response.

In most patients the infection of T4 lymphocytes is progressive and leads to a decline in their numbers and to a loss of function. This leads usually to acquired immune deficiency syndrome.

Detection of HIV

HIV can be detected in a multiplicity of body fluids:

- Blood
- Saliva
- Semen
- Vaginal fluids
- Perianal secretions
- Tears
- Sweat
- Sputum
- Urine

The virus can be grown in tissue culture, but this is a laborious process and is not usually used for diagnostic purposes. Indirect tests are now commonly used and these include detection of antibody or antigens. Antibody detection is the method of choice for detection of HIV as it is relatively cheap and less labour-intensive. HIV antibody is usually generated in detectable amounts after primary reproduction of the virus in lymphocytes and release into the bloodstream. There is therefore a period where a person may be infected but the antibody cannot be detected; this period is often called the 'window' period. In the window period the individual carrying HIV is infectious. With improvements in the detection of antibody this 'window' period can be reduced to as little as 22 days; formerly this could be up to 11 months. Most HIV infected individuals are identified within 4–6 weeks. Early detection of HIV is important, particularly in the screening of blood products, but also for the mental health of presumptively infected individuals.

In the UK and USA screening is usually done by a simple enzyme linked immunosorbant assay (ELISA) and confirmed using one more specific method. The detection of HIV has been enhanced by the development of specific monoclonal antibodies to the proteins associated with the core of the HIV virus and the nucleocapsid proteins. In particular antibodies to p24 have been developed which can reduce the 'window' period to 4–6 weeks post inoculation.

HIV can be detected in the oral cavity. It is thought that the virus does not remain viable in saliva for long periods, and is not transmitted by salivary contact. There have been a number of studies of families where one member is HIV infected and normal social intercourse has taken place. The virus has not been transmitted in any of these familial studies. HIV can be detected indirectly by the presence of antibodies in gingival crevicular fluid, but the reliability of this method has been questioned.

The testing of an individual for HIV must be done with caution and with full informed consent. Since the detection of HIV has consequences socially, legally and psychologically, the patient must understand and agree to the test. This means careful counselling of the patient by persons trained to understand and deal with any problems resulting from the testing. In most countries the HIV status of an individual is confidential information and there is no statutory obligation to disclose it. A person does not have a legal obligation to tell a healthcare worker of their HIV status. If an individual discloses that they are infected with HIV, then this is privileged information and should be treated with absolute confidentiality, even amongst healthcare workers.

There have been instances where healthcare workers, in particular surgeons, have been found to be infected with HIV. This has led to mass screening and counselling of the patients treated by the surgeons, and a call for all healthcare workers to be screened. The issue of screening of healthcare workers is highly contentious and complicated by legalities. It has been argued that screening in healthcare workers is unnecessary, discriminatory and a waste of resources. The evidence to support such conclusions is that the limited screening studies done on healthcare workers have not shown a higher incidence than the rest of the population. One of the main arguments against screening is that it could coincide with the 'window' period when the person tested would be falsely negative; the tests would therefore not be reliable. The most powerful argument against mandatory screening of healthcare workers is that there have been very few cases when HIV has been transmitted by healthcare workers.

The transmission rate is low unless blood-to-blood contact occurs. Even when significant blood-to-blood contact does occur, the transmission rate has been estimated to be only 0.38%.

Acquired immune deficiency syndrome (AIDS)

Infection with HIV leads to a diminution of the number of T4 lymphocytes and a diminution in immune function. The fall in the population of T4 cells means that the immune reaction is not amplified when an allergen challenge occurs. The situation is made worse by the fact that persons with AIDS still have fully functional T8 suppresser cells which act to further depress what little immune reaction has occurred. The diminution of the immune reaction makes the patient highly susceptible to infection and other disease. This reduction in immune responses may lead progressively to the acquired immune deficiency syndrome (AIDS). If the HIV infected individual has other risk factors then the progression into AIDS can be rapid.

The usual cause of death associated with AIDS is respiratory tract infection, particularly pneumonia and its secondary effects on the cardiovascular system. The cause of pneumonia is usually due to a parasite *Pneumocystis carinii*, which is classified as a protozoan, but recent DNA studies have shown it to be taxonomically closer to fungi. Pneumocystis pneumonia is an example of an opportunistic infection, as it is part of the commensal microflora of normal lungs but in profoundly immunosuppressed AIDS patients it causes disease. Bacteria such as pneumococci and haemophili may also be implicated in pneumonia in AIDS patients.

It is important to realize that AIDS is a syndrome not a disease. A syndrome is a collection of signs or symptoms that may go together. In contrast, a disease has definite signs and symptoms that always go together. Thus, AIDS may lead to multiplicity of signs and symptoms and secondary infections. HIV has also a well described affinity for neural cells and the first signs and symptoms of AIDS may be progressive deterioration of neurological function; this can be misdiagnosed as presenile dementia. The oral signs and symptoms have been divided on the basis of clinical experience into three types and these are shown in Table

Table 12.1 Lesions associated with HIV infection

Group1 Lesions strongly associated with HIV	Group 2 lesions less commonly associated with HIV infection	Group 3 Lesions sometimes associated with HIV
Candidosis Erythematous Pseudomembraneous	Bacterial infections *Mycobacterium tuberculosis* *Mycobacterium avium-intracellulare*	Bacterial infections *Actinomyces israelii* *Eshericha coli* *Klebsiella pneumoniae*
Hairy leukoplakia	Melanotic hyperpigmentation	Cat scratch disease
Periodontal disease Linear gingival erythema Necrotizing ulcerative gingivitis Necrotizing ulcerative periodontitis	Necrotizing stomatitis	Drug reactions
Kaposi's sarcoma	Non-specific ulceration	Fungal infections Cryptococcus Geotrichium Mucor Aspergillus
Non-Hodgkins lymphoma	Salivary gland disease	
	Throbocytopenic purpura	
	Viral infections Herpes type1 Papilloma virus Varicella zoster Herpes zoster	

12.1. The description of non-infective lesions is fully described in contemporary textbooks of oral pathology and only infective lesions will be included in this text.

Oral infective lesions associated with HIV infection

Candida

Candida infections are common in patients with HIV infection. They are an indication of progressive deterioration of immune function, which is reflected in an overgrowth of *Candida* species. The usual initial types of candidiosis are **erythematous** in type (*see* Chapter 11) and found on the hard and soft palate, buccal mucosa and tongue. They may be painless initially, but may progress to form **pseudomembraneous plaques** of **thrush** (*see* Chapter 11). The diagnosis of erythematous candidosis is usually on the basis of clinical presentation and the mycological culture of swabs. It is important to treat oral candidosis in HIV infected individuals as the infection may progress to the pharyngeal area and result in oesophagitis and dysphagia. Oral candidosis may also progress to the trachea causing tracheal infection, which can result in *Candida* lung abscesses.

The early signs and symptoms of oral fungal infections can be treated with topical anti-fungal agents such as nystatin and amphotericin. These latter agents are initially effective as they are fungicidal and resistance to them is very rare. As immune function becomes depressed in HIV infected individuals, systemic anti-fungals are necessary and fluconazole, itraconazole or ketoconazole are used, often in combination with topical agent. Systemic anti-fungals are only fungistatic in their action and can cause serious side-effects (e.g. impairment of liver function). Systemic anti-fungals also have a further disadvantage in HIV infected individuals as they tend to select resistant *Candida* strains. In the past few years, oral azole-resistant *C. albicans* and *C. krusei* strains have been described in terminally ill AIDS patients.

Angular cheilitis

Angular cheilitis is often present in AIDS patients. This lesion is discussed in Chapter 11.

Hairy leukoplakia

Hairy leukoplakia is a hyperakeratotic lesion that classically affects the side of the tongue. It presents as multiple, white keratotic areas which may coalesce and crack; it is usually painless. Hairy leukoplakia is found in other medically compromised individuals and is strongly associated with Epstein–Barr virus. Usually, hairy leukoplakia does not need treatment but aciclovir is sometimes used to limit its spread.

Periodontal infections

Periodontal infections are not uncommon in HIV-infected individuals, particularly where the oral hygiene is poor. The periodontal infections include linear gingival erythema, necrotizing ulcerative gingivitis and necrotizing ulcerative periodontitis. There has been considerable debate as to whether these latter infections are more severe in patients with AIDS, or indeed separate pathological entities; these are discussed in Chapter 7.

Viral infections

Herpes infections due to type 1 and 2 may affect the oral cavity of HIV infected individuals. Both of these viruses produce shallow, small, painful ulcers which may coalesce. In HIV infected individuals herpes infections often persist for long periods of time. In patients with AIDS there is a danger that viraemias may occur with metastatic spread to other life-threatening sites. Early treatment of oral herpetic infections is essential, initially with topical aciclovir, but as the T4 cell count decreases then systemic administration is necessary.

Two other herpes viruses can affect patients with AIDS. Herpes type 4 cytomegalovirus can give large, painful ulceration on any oral surface. This virus is often a sign of disseminating illness elsewhere and is identified by growing it in tissue culture, or by its histological appearance in the lesion. Treatment needs to be prompt and usually involves intravenous ganciclovir or forscarnet (an antiviral with specific activity against cytomegalovirus). Another herpes virus, herpes type 7, has been found in oral leukoplakia-like lesions but its function in this lesion is unknown.

There are two other lesions which are found in AIDS patients in the head and neck region which may have a viral aetiology. **Molluscum contagiosum** gives rise to firm swellings with a white coloration associated with the sebaceous glands of the head and neck. They are usually self-limiting and not treated. Typical 'brick-shaped' pox virus particles can be seen in these lesions; they are a sign of immunosuppression.

The other lesion found in AIDS patients are **papilloma** virus infections. Papilloma virus gives rise to exophytic warts, often at the corners of the mouth.

Management of HIV infected individuals

Patients with HIV infection require a team approach. The primary management of their general condition is usually done by an infectious disease physician. The physician will monitor the differential blood count for any decrease in white cell count. A more precise measure of HIV infection is to count the number of CD4 cells per ml of blood; a diminution is indicative of advancing immunosuppression. Another measure of HIV infection is the CD4/CD8 ratio, which is a measure of T4/T8 cells. This value is usually 0.93–4.50; a low ratio can indicate progress towards AIDS.

The dental management of HIV infected individuals can be done quite safely in general dental practices if the precautions shown in Chapter 14 are observed. The aim of treatment is to remove all sources of oral infection and to encourage good oral hygiene. Extractions can usually be done quite safely without antibiotic cover provided that the white cell count is normal. When an HIV infected individual develops AIDS then their oral management is best done in specialist centres such as oral medicine or oral surgery departments. If interventive oral surgery has to be done then the patient with AIDS needs full assessment and, if necessary, antibiotic cover. Again, this is best done in a hospital.

HIV and dentistry: the case of Dr Acer

One of the events that has caused controversy in AIDS studies is the curious story of Dr Acer, an HIV infected Florida dentist. Dr Acer treated a patient called Kimberley Bergalis shortly before he died of AIDS, carrying out two extractions for her. Ms Bergalis became infected with Dr Acer's HIV strain and her dental treatment was thought to be the source of the problem. Ms Bergalis eventually died of AIDS, but only after her emaciated and ill figure had been seen on television screens world-wide.

Microbiologically, this case raised an enormous number of questions. The first and most important question was whether the virus had been transferred by normal dental treatment and if so by which route? The problems multiplied because subsequently four more of Dr Acer's patients became infected with the same HIV strain that had caused his death.

There was an intensive investigation of Dr Acer's mode of practice, because if HIV was spread by simple dental treatment, then stricter barrier cross-infection measures would be needed.

One of the instruments implicated in the infection were the dental turbines, and it was subsequently shown that HIV could get into simple turbines in sufficient quantities to cause infection. The implication of the handpieces in the infection was the subject of a now infamous, and biased, UK television programme that strongly implicated this as a route of transmission. The exact route of transmission by which Dr Acer infected his patients remains a mystery, but all the evidence supports the fact that normal cross-infection procedures were not to blame. The most plausible and widely held opinion is that Dr Acer mixed some of his own blood with local anaesthetic and injected it in a homicidal act. All the subsequent scientific evidence has shown that HIV is not spread by dental procedures.

Summary

Human immunodeficiency virus infection is now pandemic and unlikely to decrease in the near future. The virus does get into saliva but not in doses sufficient to cause infection. The immmunodeficiency caused by the virus results in secondary infection and ultimately death. The cross-infection control measures commonly practised in dentistry should be sufficient to stop the spread of this infection by dental procedures.

Bibliography

Advisory Committee on Dangerous Pathogens (1995) *Protection Against Blood-borne Infections in the Workplace: HIV and Hepatitis,* HMSO, London.

Busch, M.P., Lee, L.L. and Satten, G.A. (1995) Time course of viral and serological markers preceding HIV-1 seroconversion: implications for blood and tissue screening. *Transfusion,* **35**, 91–97.

Croser, D., Erridge, P. and Robinson, P. (1994) *HIV and Dentistry,* British Dental Association Occasional Paper No. 4, British Dental Association, London.

Expert Advisory Group on AIDS/HIV Infected Healthcare Workers (1996) *Guidance on the Management of Infected Healthcare Workers,* UK Health Department, London.

Health Service Guidelines (1994) *AIDS and HIV Infected Healthcare Workers,* Publication No. (HS)16, Department of Health, London.

Scully, C., Cawson, R.A. and Griffiths, M.J. (1990) *Occupational Hazards to Dental Staff,* British Dental Journal Press, London.

13

Antimicrobial therapy and prophylaxis for oral infections

In 1982 the Editor of *The Lancet* wrote, 'Where antimicrobial agents are concerned, there are two parties to be borne in mind besides the patient – the microbe and the environment.' The journal Editor was drawing attention to the fact that antimicrobial resistance was a major emerging problem, which if not tackled, could cause life-threatening problems. Now, 17 years later, the words in *The Lancet* have proved prophetic. In 1996 the President of the World Health Organization drew attention to the misuse of antimicrobial agents and the emergence of multiply resistant strains as a major problem world-wide. Not only are multiply resistant bacterial strains common in most hospitals, but they are also widely distributed in the community. In addition, the availability of cheap air travel has meant that the vectors of these strains are also distributed world-wide.

Why have multiply resistant strains emerged and become such a problem? The answer to this question is the excessive and inappropriate use of antimicrobial agents. In some countries, antimicrobial agents are freely available for purchase at pharmacies without prescription, and self-medication is the normal practice. This is not, however, the only misuse of antimicrobials. Even in countries where the use of antimicrobials is regulated and they are only available on prescription, their use is often excessive. There is often constant friction between the clinician and the microbiologist, who are at opposite poles of the arguments about antimicrobial usage.

Antimicrobial resistance

In the past 20 years, a great deal of research has led to a fuller understanding of the mechanisms of microbial resistance. Much of the progress in this research has been due to new genetic techniques, which have led to a closer understanding of the methods of DNA encoding for antibiotic resistance. Surprisingly, there has been little research on the basis of antimicrobial resistance in oral micro-organisms, but this is probably a matter of time and resources. Oral microflora has been widely reported to be resistant to some antimicrobials. It is, therefore, highly likely that the methods of resistance in other bacteria apply to oral micro-organisms.

Genetic methods of transfer of antimicrobial resistance

One of the fundamental ways in which resistance is transferred is by **plasmids,** which are pieces of DNA that can be exchanged between bacteria; **resistance plasmids** can be large or small pieces of DNA. Resistance plasmids carry genes that encode for resistance to one or a multiplicity of antimicrobial agents. Resistance plasmids exist as circular pieces of double stranded DNA in the cell, and each bacteria may have more than one type of plasmid. Plasmids are not new; they have been present in bacteria since well before the antibiotic era started. Plasmids can change and acquire new genes; they also mutate and, most importantly, they can be transferred between bacterial cells of the same strain. Plasmids can also be transferred between different bacterial species.

Another method by which plasmids can be transferred is by a form of 'mating' called **conjugation**. The bacterial cell which contains the plasmid produces fimbriae on the surface which attach to the recipient cell. The donor bacterium makes a copy of its plasmid and passes this into the recipient through the fimbriae. This process can occur a multiplicity of times so that whole populations of cells become resistant. The transfer of plasmids can be more complex with small plasmids attaching themselves to larger ones and being transferred into the new recipient cell. Thus, a new population of multiply resistant bacteria can be made if the plasmids encode for antimicrobial resistance.

Another method of transfer of resistance plasmids has been discovered in enterococci. These bacteria secrete **pheromones**, which are substances that attract other enterococci. The pheromones cause two enterococci, called 'mating types', to clump together and exchange plasmids. Streptococci and staphylococci also produce pheromones and exchange plasmids by this method.

Another interesting method of resistance transfer is by **transposons**; these are small pieces of DNA which can attach to plasmids or chromosomes and move from cell to cell. Transposons can move and integrate with host DNA or attach to a plasmid. Transposons are the major method for transfer of resistance between different bacterial species. A good example of this are the pneumococci, which can transfer transposons and resistance to other streptococci.

There is yet another way in which resistance can be transferred and this is by **bacteriophages** (viruses that infect bacteria). These phages attach to specific sites on the bacterial membrane and 'inject' their DNA into the cytoplasm. If the phage does not lyse the bacterium, it can reproduce the DNA and form new phages which can infect other bacterial cells. The phage often leaves copies of its DNA in the bacteria and these can code for resistance. This copy left in the cell can also attach to a transposon and be transferred to another species.

Naked DNA, which could code for antimi-crobial resistance, can be transferred to a recipient bacterium. The bacterium literally takes the DNA into its cytoplasm in a process called **transformation**. The DNA that has been taken into the bacterium usually integrates with that of the recipient.

Mechanisms of antimicrobial resistance

Bacteria have other methods of resisting antimicrobial agents. One method is to stop the entry of the antimicrobial into the bacterial cell. The antimicrobial agents rely on the use of transport systems in the cell wall to gain entry into the bacteria. These transport systems can be modified to stop the transport of the antimicrobial agent into the cell, or slow its entry. This inhibition of entry of an antimicrobial agent can also be linked to increased excretion or transportation of the antimicrobial out of the cell. Thus, although the antibiotic may get into the cell, it will rapidly be excreted before it can do any damage.

Many bacteria inactivate antimicrobial agents by destroying or modifying them with extracellular enzymes. The most well understood example of this process are the penicillinases (or β-lactamases), which cause hydrolysis and cleavage of penicillin molecules. There are about 25 different penicillinases produced by different bacterial species. Similarly there are also enzymes which destroy cephalosporins, and these are called cephalosporinases.

Another method of resisting antimicrobial activity is to modify the agent. Streptomycin, kanamycin and other related aminoglycosides can be chemically modified by bacterial enzymes by the addition of a residue so that they become inactive. Often this additional chemical residue makes the antimicrobial unable to enter the cell, or inactive if it does gain entry.

Bacteria can alter the site of attachment of the antimicrobial within the cell. An example of this is alteration of ribosomes which are the attachment site of erythromycin. The ribosomes have altered protein binding sites for erythromycin, making it unable to attach, and hence it becomes ineffective. This change can be mediated by mutation of the ribosome genes, or the acquisition of plasmids encoding for this modification.

Colonization resistance

It can be seen from the preceding section that bacteria have evolved a number of mechanisms to resist the action of antibiotics. Antibiotics are used if there is an overgrowth of a particular species and an infection ensues. Most of the infections that occur in the oral cavity are **opportunistic** (*see* Chapter 8). In the past decade it has been realized that the best method of preventing opportunistic infection is to stop the overgrowth of any constituent species of the resident microflora. The resident microflora of any particular site displays homeostasis, which prevents the overgrowth by component species, which in turn helps to prevent opportunistic infection (*see* Chapter 4). The resident microflora can usually prevent colonization of that particular site by exogenous pathogens, and this is called **colonization resistance**. Even if the potential pathogen attaches, it will not thrive as it has to compete for nutrients and survive all the adverse factors in the microflora (*see* Chapter 4). It is therefore a good principle to maintain the homeostatic oral flora as this is an essential part of the defence against infection. Unfortunately, one of the most important iatrogenic factors in the destruction of homeostasis, and hence also colonization resistance, are antibiotics, particularly long courses.

The principles of antimicrobial usage for acute oral infections

All acute purulent oral infections need surgical drainage if they are to resolve. In Chapter 8 the use of antibiotics as an adjunct to the surgical treatment of acute purulent infections was discussed. If the antimicrobial is to be successful then the infecting micro-organism must be sensitive to it. The antimicrobial must get into the bloodstream, and hence the affected tissues, in sufficient concentrations to kill or prevent growth of the infecting micro-organism. Antimicrobial agents are either bacteriostatic or bacteriocidal in their action. Bacteriocidal agents kill micro-organisms, whilst bacteriostatic antimicrobials prevent their growth. Ideally bacteriocidal agents should be used but this is not always possible. Microbiologists prefer that the peak concentration of antimicrobial agent in the serum should be at least 4–8 times the minimum inhibitory concentration (MIC) of the infecting micro-organism. This ratio of MIC and peak serum antibiotic has been found by clinical experience and experimental animal studies to be effective. The 4–8 ratio of MIC and peak serum concentration is not always possible to achieve with orally delivered drugs. It can, however, often be attained if the antimicrobial is given intramuscularly, intravenously or by use of a suppository.

The use of bacteriostatic antimicrobials for acute purulent oral infections is not to be routinely recommended as their absorption is often poor and serum and ultimately tissue concentrations are concomitantly low.

The duration of antimicrobials for acute purulent oral infections is still a matter of some controversy. It has been the usual practice to prescribe at least 5 days of antimicrobials, this duration of treatment is being challenged. Recent publications have shown that the duration of antimicrobial therapy can be short. One study looked at a comparison of the use of one or two high doses of amoxycillin and a conventional 5-day course of the same antimicrobial for acute dento-alveolar abscesses. Both regimes were found to be effective if the correct surgical drainage was done. In a recent study of 748 patients with acute dento-alveolar infection, it was found that the 2–3 days of antimicrobial therapy was 98.6% successful. The patients (14) who did not respond had not had successful surgery to drain the pus. There is no need, therefore, for a long course of antimicrobial therapy if the patient shows clinical signs of recovery. These signs of recovery include resolution of swelling and restoration of a normal temperature.

Ideally, the duration of antimicrobial therapy should be judged against the patient's response, and when clinical resolution occurs it should be discontinued. In practice, courses of antibiotics for acute purulent infections are often long and at high doses. Such courses do the patient no good and may be harmful. The longer the course of antimicrobials, the more likely the incidence of side-effects. In addition, long courses of antimicrobials destroy the homeostasis of the oral flora and abolish colonization resistance. All of this compelling evidence for short and effective courses of antimicrobials for acute infections is often ignored by clinicians. Patients are often prescribed long courses of antibiotics and told to finish the full course. One reason that has been advanced for the completion of a course of antimicrobials is that it prevents the emergence of resistant micro-organisms. In fact, finishing a course of antimicrobials may increase the selection of resistant micro-organisms and abolish colonization resistance, quite contrary to the fallaciously perceived aim.

Antimicrobial prophylaxis

Antimicrobial prophylaxis is the prevention of infectious disease by the administration of agents. Approximately one-third of all antibiotic usage is for prophylaxis but much of this is not appropriate. The efficacy of antimicrobial prophylaxis, particularly for the prevention of oral infection, has still to be defined. In general medicine and surgery, the efficacy of antimicrobial prophylaxis is being re-examined, and redefined, and from this work general principles can be clearly made.

There is now general agreement that if infection is to occur it will most likely occur at the time of operation. The pioneering animal work of Burke together with long-term clinical observation has clearly established this fact. Secondary infection, although possible, is in practice extremely rare. It logically follows that if infection occurs at the time of operation the time to have the peak serum concentration of antimicrobials is at operation. The timing of oral antimicrobial administration is best designed from a knowledge of their absorption so that the peak serum concentration is obtained at operation. If the peak serum concentration cannot be attained by an orally administered route, then an intravenous or intramuscular route is to be preferred.

The duration of antimicrobial prophylaxis for the prevention of oral infection is also controversial. It has been the convention to give 5 days of antibiotics. Extensive studies in general surgery have shown that a single dose of an antimicrobial agent before surgery is probably all that is necessary for most procedures. The use of prolonged antimicrobials after surgery is not necessary as it destroys colonization resistance and, ironically, could potentiate secondary infection.

One important principle essential to the effective administration of effective antimicrobial prophylaxis is to define who is at risk and requires prophylaxis.

Three types of patients require prophylaxis. The first is patients with impaired host defence mechanisms; these include patients who are medically compromised and those that are immunocompromised. These patients are discussed in detail in Chapter 13. Surgical procedures in these patients, such as extractions which normally do not require chemoprophylaxis, may need to be covered. These patients must be assessed individually and often in consultation with their physician.

The second group of patients are those undergoing surgery which has a high rate of infectious complications. These patients have a high rate of postoperative infections and are broadly divisible into whether infection is present in the operation site or not. For prophylaxis to be justified then there has to be a real chance of postoperative infection occurring following operation. This infection will be due to endogenous micro-organisms following contamination of the operative field at the time of surgery. When surgery is being done at an infected site with an abscess or cellulitis, then there is the possibility of spreading the infection both locally and systemically; antimicrobials are mandatory in such situations and are really therapy rather than prophylaxis.

The routine removal of third molars, with or without pericoronitis, is often perceived as being associated with a high rate of infection and the routine use of antimicrobial prophylaxis has been advocated. One survey, done a quarter of a century ago, suggested that routine removal of third molars with associated pericoronitis had an incidence of 24% dry sockets, if antibiotics were not given. The incidence of dry sockets could be reduced to 3.6% if phenoxymethylpenicillin was given. Surgical management of third molars has improved and recent surveys have shown that prophylactic antibiotics confer no real advantage in the prevention of postoperative infection. A similar situation pertains in other branches of minor oral surgery such as removal of roots or cysts where bone may be removed. The removal of bone in minor oral surgery is not an indication for antimicrobial prophylaxis. There is no evidence to show that postoperative infection following bone removal, to facilitate extraction of teeth, is prevented by a prophylactic antibiotic.

The third group of patients are those undergoing surgical procedures where the risk of infection is small but the consequences are very serious. The principal patients in this group are those susceptible to infective endocarditis and this condition is discussed below. Other patients in this category are those with orthopaedic joint prostheses. Late, or early, infections in patients with endoprostheses can result in the necessity to remove the prosthesis; unfortunately, such revisions do not have a high success rate. There is, however, very little evidence to link dental treatments which produce bacteraemias with infections of endoprostheses. As a consequence, it is now not regarded as necessary to give patients with endoprostheses antibiotic cover for dental treatments that produce bacteraemias. There is now evidence that poor oral hygiene and incipient oral sepsis could produce constant low grade bacteraemias which could be associated with infections of endoprostheses. The infecting micro-organisms of endoprostheses from oral sources are usually oral streptococci. It is important therefore that patients who have endoprostheses do maintain good oral hygiene.

Infective endocarditis

Infective endocarditis is the infection of the endocardium of the heart by micro-organisms that are present in the bloodstream. The tooth–tissue interface is a unique site in the body for micro-organisms to enter the bloodstream and to potentially infect the heart. The ingress of such micro-organisms is probably frequent but transient, the body's defence mechanisms eliminating them rapidly. Many dental procedures can cause oral micro-organisms to enter the bloodstream and there is often, therefore, an exaggerated link made between patients who develop infective endocarditis and dentistry. The incidence of infective endocarditis following dental procedures in patients predisposed to the condition is extremely low. In the UK about 1000 patients are thought to develop infective endocarditis each year, an incidence that appears not to have changed in the past decade. Of the 1000 patients who develop infective endocarditis each year, probably about 10–15 could be associated with dentistry. For an association with dentistry to be possible, the infecting micro-organism must be commonly found in the oral flora and the dental procedure must have caused ingress into the bloodstream. The 'incubation time' between the dental procedure and the onset of symptoms is usually short, in the case of oral streptococci usually 7–14 days. It can be seen that the link between dental procedures and infective endocarditis is often difficult to prove as much of the evidence is often circumstantial.

Infective endocarditis is usually caused by bacteria, but fungi and other micro-organisms such as Coxiella can infect the heart. Table 13.1 shows the micro-organisms that can infect the heart and it can be seen that oral streptococci are the predominate species isolated from the heart. It used to be thought that, of the oral streptococci, *S.sanguis* caused the majority of cases of infective endocarditis. Since the reclassification and sub-division of the *S.oralis* group, further work is required to precisely identify which of the oral streptococci is the usual cause of infective endocarditis. The major other causative micro-organisms of infective endocarditis are staphylococci derived from the skin. Staphylococcal endocarditis is commonly seen in drug abusers who inject intravenously.

Table 13.1 Micro-organisms isolated from infective endocarditis

Micro-organism	%
Oral streptococci	36
Enterococci	14
Other non-Lancefield group streptococci	12
Staphylococcus aureus	20
Non-coagulase staphylococci	10
Actinobacillus actinomycetemcomitans	3
Coxiella burnetti	1
Candida spp.	1
Other micro-organisms (including viruses)	1

The pathogenesis of infective endocarditis

The pathogenesis of infective endocarditis is still the subject of some debate. Micro-organisms enter the bloodstream and progress to the heart; in patients with a predisposing condition they attach. All of the predisposing conditions cause blood to flow abnormally through the heart. This abnormal blood flow is not uniform and is often described as 'eddy formation'. An eddy formation is when the blood runs back contrary to the main stream and causes a circular whirlpool motion. At the edges of the eddy formation the blood slows and starts to form clots (thrombi), and usually this occurs on the undersides of the heart valves. The sterile clots or vegetations can be colonized as a result of a bacteraemia, and infections of the linings of the heart can result: these infections are infective endocarditis. Such infections are serious as thrombi can break off and occlude the blood supply to a vital organ. Infective endocarditis can cause further bacteraemias and result in infection elsewhere in the body. The infection of the heart may affect its ability to function (heart failure).

It can be seen from Table 13.1 that the principal micro-organisms that cause infective endocarditis are oral streptococci and these have been intensely studied in relation to this disease. Amongst the virulence factors that have been studied is adherence to fibronectin. Oral streptococci can adhere to fibronectin present on the surface of endothelium and multiply to cause infection. Mutants of oral streptococi have been produced that do not adhere well to fibronectin and these have shown a diminished ability to produce infective endocarditis in catheterized animals. The ability to adhere to fibronectin may be an important virulence factor in determining whether an oral streptococcus can cause infective endocarditis.

Another factor that has been postulated to be important is the ability of oral streptococci to produce extracellular polysaccharides (*see* Chapter 5). Mutant oral streptococci were produced and selected for lack of glucosyl-transferase activity. Reinoculation into catheterized animals gave conflicting results. Some mutant strains showed no change, when compared to the wild-type, in their ability to cause infective endocarditis in animals, whilst in others the rate of infection was diminished. The role of oral streptococcal extracellular glucosyltransferases may therefore be important in some strains but not others.

There is considerable recent interest in the ability of oral streptococci to bind platelets which may be present in thrombi on the heart. The mechanism of this adhesion may be by a direct attachment of the streptococcus to the plasma membrane of the platelet. Another form of adhesion may be by a platelet aggregation-associated protein (PAAP) which induces aggregation and activation. When platelets are activated they can release ATP-rich granules; these can be hydrolysed by extracellular ATP-ase and generate energy. This energy is enough to amplify the platelet PAAP reaction and enhance attachment.

When oral streptococci enter the bloodstream they may undergo heat shock and heat-shock protein may be released. Heat-shock protein, as the name implies, is protein that is released only when bacteria undergo sudden changes in temperature or other environmental conditions. Work on the structure of PAAP of oral streptococci has shown that it may be analogous to heat-shock protein found in other bacteria. Recent work on oral streptococci has shown that PAAP is released when bacteria enter the bloodstream during a bacteraemia. PAAP can attach to collagen which may be exposed in damaged endothelium. The expression of PAAP, together with other as yet not completely understood virulence factors such as tissue degrading protease, may be of importance in the development of infective endocarditis. PAAP deficient strains of oral streptococci certainly produce a milder form of infective endocarditis.

Infective endocarditis is a serious life-threatening condition with a 30% mortality rate. It is difficult to diagnose as the initial symptoms, which include tiredness, lassitude, pains in the joints and a mild fever, are non-distinct. It is diagnosed by growth of the micro-organism in blood cultures and by echocardiography, where the clots can be visualized by bouncing sound off them. Infective endocarditis is difficult to treat despite the availability of a variety of antimicrobials. Therapy has to attain high blood concentrations and the aim is to sterilize the vegetations; this requires prolonged intravenous therapy. After the vegetations have been sterilized it may be necessary to replace the damaged heart valves with either mechanical or xenografts. If a person contracts infective endocarditis then there is a 40% probability that it will re-occur. The mortality rate for a recurrent episode of infective endocarditis is greater than 40%.

Prophylactic antibiotics are prescribed to patients with a known predisposition to infective endocarditis. The patients who are 'at risk' are shown in Table 13.2. A consideration of Table 13.1 shows that no single antibiotic would be effective against the whole range of micro-organisms that may be involved in causing infective endocarditis. This makes the choice of an antibiotic difficult and a compromise has to be made. Originally penicillin was the drug of choice, but it has been superseded by orally administered amoxycillin, which is well absorbed and has a good spectrum of activity against bacteria known to be involved in infective endocarditis. Amoxycillin in a single 3 g dose has been shown to attain high serum concentrations for 7–8 hours after administration. Patients who are allergic to penicillin were originally given erythromycin or its derivatives, usually the stearate or the ethyl succinate. Erythromycin is a bacteriostatic antibiotic, and there is some doubt from animal trials about its efficacy in preventing infective endocarditis. Erythromycin and its derivatives have largely been superseded by clindamycin, which is bactericidal and well absorbed.

Table 13.2 Patients at risk from infective endocarditis

Previous infective endocarditis	Rheumatic and other acquired valvular disease
Ventricular septal defects	Patent ductus arteriosus
Coarctation of the aorta	Prosthetic heart valve
Surgically constructed systemic–pulmonary shunts	Persistent heart murmur
Atrial septal defect with a patch	Hypertrophic cardio-myopathy
Marfan's syndrome	

The efficacy of prophylaxis is unproved in humans and it is ethically impossible to do the experiment, as some of the volunteers could die! Most of the data justifying the use of antimicrobial prophylaxis has come from animals, especially rabbits and rats. The animals are catheterized through an artery in the neck. The catheter enters the left ventricle and stops the mitral valve from closing, producing an artificial eddy and clot formation. Two or three days after catheterization a bolus dose of bacteria is put intravenously into the bloodstream and 2 days after this the animal will have infective endocarditis. This experimental approach re-

sembles human infective endocarditis in many respects but it has been criticized as a severe model; it is, however, all that is available to test the efficacy of antibiotic regimes.

There is considerable debate as to which dental procedures actually cause a bacteraemia which may be associated with infective endocarditis. The difficulty in establishing this link makes it difficult to define which dental procedures require antibiotic cover. The problem with defining the procedures is that infective endocarditis is a disease for which no official statistics are kept and therefore advice on antimicrobial prophylaxis comes from reported cases, legal claims and the animal models. The procedures that are associated with infective endocarditis and may require antimicrobial cover are:

- Extraction of teeth
- Scaling of teeth
- Periodontal surgery
- Minor oral surgery
- Incision of abscesses
- Biopsy
- Full mouth periodontal probing
- Surgical endodontics
- Restoration of multiple subgingival lesions
- Radiographic determination of root length for endodontic procedures

Many procedures in dentistry produce bleeding and this is often associated with a risk of infective endocarditis in susceptible patients. Bleeding may, however, produce the opposite effect as it may physically prevent bacteria from entering the bloodstream by flushing them away. The quantity and the frequency of micro-organisms entering the bloodstream may be important. Large numbers of bacteria in the animal models reproducibly produce infective endocarditis and the same may be true for humans. There is another body of opinion that supports the view that repeated low numbers of micro-organisms entering the bloodstream may eventually be responsible for infective endocarditis. Repeated low numbers of micro-organisms enter the bloodstream in cases of untreated periodontal disease, so that it is important that patients at risk from infective endocarditis maintain good oral health.

Summary

The rise in the incidence of antimicrobial-resistant bacteria is a global problem. This rise is principally due to the overuse of antimicrobial agents unnecessarily in medical practice. The methods of resistance amongst bacteria have been extensively studied in non-oral bacteria and mainly involve the transfer of DNA in the form of plasmids.

Antibiotics must be used judiciously if selection of resistant organisms is to be avoided. Recent evidence has shown that short courses of antibiotics are best used for acute infections. Prophylactic antibiotics account for a high proportion of all usage. The use of these agents is best reserved for clinical situations where they have been shown to be effective. Prophylactic antibiotics are best prescribed before the procedure to be undertaken so that the maximum serum levels are present at operation.

Prophylactic antibiotics are prescribed for the prevention of infective endocarditis for some dental procedures. The evidence that infective endocarditis can be prevented relies mainly on animal models. The pathogenesis of infective endocarditis is still not fully understood but is associated with virulence factors such as activation of platelet associated proteins and fibronectin adhesion.

Bibliography

Baddour, L.M. (1994) Virulence factors among Gram-positive bacteria in infective endocarditis. *Infect. Immun.,* **62**, 2143–2148.

British Society for Antimicrobial Chemotherapy (1992) Case against antibiotic prophylaxis for dental treatment of patients with joint prostheses. *Lancet,* **339**, 301.

Editorial (1982) Good antimicrobial prescribing. *Lancet* (Special Suppl.).

Herzberg, M.C., Meyer, M.W., Kilic, A. and Tao, L. (1997) Host–pathogen interactions in bacterial endocarditis: streptococcal virulence in the host. *Adv. Dent. Res.,* **11**, 69–74.

Lacey, R.W., Lord, V.L., Howson, G.L., Luxton, D.E. and Trotter, I.S. (1983) Double blind study to compare the selection of antibiotic resistance by amoxycillin or cephradine in the commensal flora. *Lancet,* **ii**, 529–532.

Levy, S.B. (1992) *The Antibiotic Paradox,* Plenum, London, pp. 67–103.

Lewis, M.A.O., MacFarlane, T.W. and McGowan, D.A. (1986) Short-course high dose amoxycillin in the treatment of acute dentoalveolar abscesses. *Br. Dent. J.,* **161**, 299–302.

Longman, L.P. and Martin, M.V. (1991) The use of prophylactic antibiotics in the prevention of post-operative infection: a reappraisal. *Br. Dent. J.,* **170**, 257–262.

Martin, M.V., Longman, L.P. and Butterworth, M.L. (1997) Infective endocarditis and the dental practitioner: a review of 53 cases involving litigation. *Br. Dent. J.,* **182**, 465–468.

Martin, M.V., Longman, L.P., Hill, J.B. and Hardy, P. (1997) Acute dentoalveolar infections: an investigation of the duration of antibiotic therapy. *Br. Dent. J.,* **183**, 135-137.

Pallasch, T.J. and Slots, J. (1991) Antibiotic prophylaxis for medical-risk patients. *J. Periodontol.,* **61**, 227–231.

Thomas, D.W. and Hill, C.M. (1997) An audit of antibiotic prescribing in third molar surgery. *Br. J. Oral Maxillofac. Surg.,* **5**, 126–128.

14

Cross-infection control

The mouth is a potential source of micro-organisms that could be transferred and cause infection in other persons. The term **cross-infection** refers to the transfer of micro-organisms from a person or object, to another person that results in an infection. It is to be distinguished from **cross-contamination**, which is the transfer of micro-organisms from one person or object to another person that may, or may not, result in an infection. Cross-contamination can also apply to the transfer of potentially infectious micro-organisms from one object to another. It is important in any discussion of cross-infection control to distinguish between the two terms. Many of the procedures that are used in cross-infection control are primarily designed to prevent initial cross-contamination that could ultimately lead to infection. There are many potential routes of transfer in those involved in the care and treatment of the mouth. The highest potential for cross-infection is between dentists, surgery assistants and patients because blood, saliva and contaminated instruments are present. Technicians and ancillary staff could become infected by dental appliances such as dentures, or impressions used to make models of the mouth. In practice, this route is unlikely as the prosthetic materials are usually washed, or disinfected after removal from the mouth.

Proven and well-documented cases of cross-infection originating from the oral cavity are quite sparse in the scientific literature. There are perceived to be a large number of oral micro-organisms that could be involved in cross-infection but there is little evidence that they have actually caused infections. The micro-organisms that have been considered to be involved in cross-infection from the oral cavity are shown in Table 14.1. Ironically, the whole impetus for the procedures that are used in prevention of cross-infection in dentistry came from the AIDS epidemic; ironic because salivary transmission of HIV is exceedingly unlikely and has not been proved in a large number of cohort studies. Even blood transmission of HIV is unlikely, unless a large amount of blood is transferred. Hepatitis B, however, can be a source of cross-infection in dentistry and has caused deaths both to patients and dental personnel. Hepatitis B virus in infected individuals is actively secreted into the mouth by the salivary glands, it remains viable and can reach high concentrations in the saliva. The risk of transmission of hepatitis C is not fully evaluated but dental personnel have a high frequency of antibodies to this virus, suggesting that exposure has occurred. The two new hepatitis viruses F and G are yet to be fully evaluated and remain as potential sources of cross-infection.

Herpes 1 infections are a well-documented source of cross-infection in dentistry. A large proportion of the population carries and sheds herpes 1 into their mouths. Cross-infection from herpes 1 has been described from saliva contamination and contact and from contaminated dental record cards. Prior to the days when gloves were worn, herpetic whitlows on the fingers were not uncommon (Figure 14.1). Herpes 1 is much more infectious than HIV, or the hepatitis viruses. Oral herpes 2 infections are now frequently reported but the primary mode of transmission is thought to be by sexual activity.

The evidence for bacterial cross-infection is scanty. There is convincing evidence that there is maternal transfer of oral streptococci to the infant; this results in colonization (*see* Chapter 4). Ultimately, this colonization could lead to

Table 14.1 The micro-organisms involved in proved cases of cross-infection, their source and route of transmission

Micro-organism	Source	Probable route of transmission	Result
Herpes type 1	Dental hygienist	Hands	Oral herpes
Herpes type 1	Patient	Saliva	Herpetic whitlow
Hepatitis B	Dentist	Non-sterile instruments	Hepatitis B
Hepatitis B	Dentist	Non sterile needles	Hepatitis B
HIV	Dentist	Multiple sharps injury	HIV transmission, AIDS
HIV	Dentist	Contaminated instruments	HIV transmission, AIDS
Hand, foot and mouth disease	Dentists and patients	Bodily contact, secretions	Typical lesions of hand, foot and mouth disease
Mycobacterium tuberculosis	Patients	Contact	Transmission of TB
Staphylococcus aureus (MRSA)	Dentist	Hands	Dental abscesses
Pseudomonas aeruginosa	Dental unit water supplies	Water coolant	Dental abscesses
Other bacteria	Dental procedures	Aerosols, instruments	Occasional reports of infection

opportunistic infection and to dental caries (*see* Chapter 6). Proved cases of cross-infection from other oral bacteria known to cause opportunistic infection have been suggested, but little definitive proof has been presented to support these contentions.

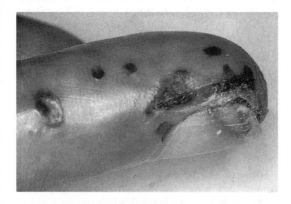

Figure 14.1 An herpetic whitlow on the finger of a dentist caused by herpes type 1 infection. This was quite a common lesion amongst dental personnel prior to the routine use of gloves

The transfer and infection by other known bacterial pathogens has been described. Methicillin resistant *Staphylococcus aureus* (MRSA) has been isolated from the mouths of patients discharged from surgical wards. Two cases of oral infections have been reported by MRSA which originated from a dentist who did not wear gloves; the strains causing the infections had identical antibiotic sensitivities to those from the dentist's hands. *Mycobacterium tuberculosis* is the most worrying of the bacteria that could be a potential source of cross-infection. TB is known to be spread by contact, and by saliva, and other secretions. One dentist who was infected with TB infected 13 of his patients. Many of the strains of TB which are now causing infections have multiple resistance to a number of antibiotics.

The fungi have also been implicated in cross-infection. The differentiation of strains of the imperfect yeast *Candida albicans* has been refined through the use of restriction fragment length polymorphism (RFLP). The use of RFLP techniques has shown that *C. albicans* strains can cause infections in neonatal wards. *C. albicans* can also cause infection immediately *post partum* in infants; the oral cavity of the mother has been implicated in these yeast infections. There is little evidence at present that other yeasts, or fungi, are involved in cross-infection from the oral cavity.

The concept of 'universal precautions'

Ideally, it would be helpful to know what pathogens a person was carrying prior to any form of medical, or dental treatment. In practice this is impossible, as the patient may be an aysmptomatic carrier of the disease, or just 'economical' with the truth. In some countries there is a legal obligation for the patient to notify the dentist of transmissible disease, but this does not always happen. One simple method of overcoming this lack of knowledge of infectious status is to adopt one set of cross-infection measures for all patients: this concept is called **universal precautions**. The concept of universal precautions is not accepted by all countries world-wide. In some countries (e.g. Holland), each dental procedure is assessed for its cross-infection risk, and suitable precautions adopted. Such an approach can be successful but, it is often difficult to accurately assess risk, and two or more dental procedures are often done at one visit. Most countries have therefore adopted one set of cross-infection control precautions for every patient. All personnel involved in the practice of dentistry must understand the risks involved, and should be fully conversant with the procedures employed in cross-infection control.

One exception to the concept of universal precautions is the treatment of potential carriers of transmissible spongiform encephalopathy (TSE). The transmissible agents thought to be responsible for this disease are proteins called prions. In order to destroy prions, steam sterilization (*see below*) for 18 minutes is recommended. The alternative is to destroy all instruments used on a patient suspected of carrying TSE. In practice there are very few patients in this category, and apart from the sterilization procedures the normal universal cross-infection control precautions are applied. TSE is usually identified *post mortem*, but progressive loss of muscular and cognitive function may lead to a presumptive diagnosis. Patients who may be carrying TSE include those who have received pituitary extracts for growth problems, blood relatives of those with TSE, and those who have received transplanted *dura mater*. At present there is no evidence that TSE could be transmitted by simple dental procedures.

Personal protection

There are five elements of cross-infection control that involve personal protection:

Immunization
It is important that all dental personnel are immunized against infectious disease. The immunizations that are required are shown in Table 14.2. These required immunizations apply to all personnel involved in the practice of dentistry, including dental nurses, hygienists, therapists and technicians. It is important to ensure that records of vaccinations are up to date, and that the protective concentration of antibodies for hepatitis B has been achieved.

Table 14.2 Recommended immunizations for dental staff

	Route	Length of protection
Diphtheria	IM	Probably life-long
Hepatitis B	IM	Five years
Pertussis	IM	Probably life-long
Poliomyelitis	Oral	Probably life-long
Rubella	IM	Probably life-long
Tetanus	IM	Probably life-long
Tuberculosis	IM	Probably life-long

Hand protection
Hands are a potential vector and recipient of cross-infection. The protection of the hands from cross-infection is accomplished by three elements: the use of emollient moisturizing cream, systematic handwashing and gloves. The skin of the hands is adversely affected by handwashing and the wearing of gloves; it becomes dry, loses its pliability, may crack and become sore. This loss of pliability can be partially avoided by systematic handwashing, and the use of suitable gloves, but another essential is the use of a moisturizing handcream after every session.

Gloves provide a physical barrier to the contamination of the hands by saliva and blood. It is therefore important to choose gloves that have been tested for the presence of holes and to change them frequently to give the hands a chance to recover from the occlusive effects of being covered. Most gloves are manufactured from latex that may contain protein contaminants. These protein contaminants, if not removed by washing during manufacture, can cause immunological sensitization. This sensitization can vary from the presence of circulating antibodies to anaphylaxis, and can affect clinicians and patients. Estimates of the presence of latex protein antibodies have shown that in the USA they are present in 40% of dental personnel that have been tested. The possibility of sensitization can be minimized by the use of a glove with a low protein content, or those manufactured from a non-latex product. It is also important to avoid gloves that have been dusted with starch powder. Starch can dissipate immunologically active agents into the surgery atmosphere; it can also contaminate wounds during invasive procedures and can cause adhesions to form. Starch can also contaminate the surfaces of restorations such as veneers, and crowns during cementation.

Handwashing must be done systematically prior to any dental procedure to remove contaminants (transient micro-organisms), and some the resident flora (persistent micro-organisms. A liquid soap should be used and followed by thorough rinsing procedure. Leaving soap residues under gloves can cause osmotically adverse effects and contribute to loss of pliability, cracking of the skin, and create potential portals of entry for micro-organisms. The hands should be carefully dried with soft disposable paper towel avoiding abrasion. Handwashing, especially when repeated a multiplicity of times every day, does adversely affect the hands. If the hands are not soiled after treating a patient, then an alcohol hand rub can be used instead of soap. Hand rubs usually contain alcohol and a disinfectant and evaporate quickly from the hands. Hand rubs avoid the removal of hand sebum and abrasion caused by drying, and leave a residue of disinfectant on the hands. Trials of hand rubs have shown that they are as effective in their disinfection action on hands as washing with water.

Eye and face protection

The practice of dentistry involves the generation of aerosols and splatter from saliva. The faces and eyes of operators must be protected by the use of protective, or prescription, spectacles during operative procedures. Spectacles protect the eyes from particles that have been ejected at speed from the mouth, and which have the potential to cause physical damage (*see* Figure 14.2). Spectacles also protect against splatter from aqueous material that could potentially infect. Masks provide similar physical protection to the face, but once wet then micro-organisms can pass through them; for this reason masks should be discarded after single use.

Aerosols are potentially a cause of cross-infection in dentistry, but at present there is no

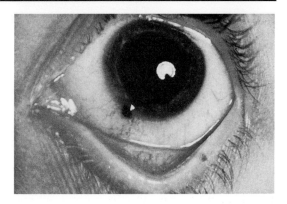

Figure 14.2 A traumatic injury to a dentist's eye. These type of injuries often become infected

definitive evidence to show what infections have been caused by them.

Surgery clothing

There is a wide variety of surgery clothing available. The important two criteria in the selection of surgery clothing are that it must have sleeves that cover the arms, and it must be capable of being washed at temperatures greater than 60 °C. The covering of the arms protects them from splatter. Washing surgery clothing above 60 °C destroys blood-borne viruses such as HIV.

Inoculation injuries

Inoculation (sharps or needlestick) injuries are the most likely causes of cross-infection in dentistry, particularly with the blood-borne viruses. They must be avoided by careful surgery technique, safe disposal of sharps in rigid incineration boxes and wearing thick protective gloves during the clearing up and cleaning of soiled instruments.

A schema for dealing with inoculation injuries is shown in Figure 14.3. If an inoculation injury occurs, then the first action must be to wash it under running water encouraging it to bleed; such action minimizes the risk of inoculation. The wound should then be covered with a waterproof dressing. The hepatitis status of the recipient of the inoculation injury should then be checked and, if necessary, a booster vaccine should be given. A sample of the recipient's serum, for future reference, should be stored in a freezer. This sample can be retrospectively used to check the person's status at the time of injury, should they subsequently be shown to have a blood-borne virus. The

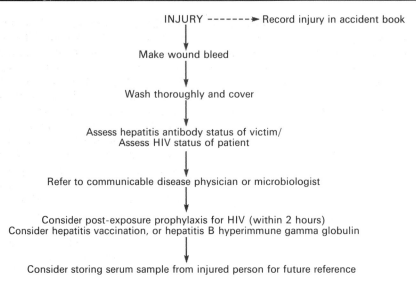

INJURY - - - - - - - ➤ Record injury in accident book

↓

Make wound bleed

↓

Wash thoroughly and cover

↓

Assess hepatitis antibody status of victim/
Assess HIV status of patient

↓

Refer to communicable disease physician or microbiologist

↓

Consider post-exposure prophylaxis for HIV (within 2 hours)
Consider hepatitis vaccination, or hepatitis B hyperimmune gamma globulin

↓

Consider storing serum sample from injured person for future reference

Figure 14.3. Schema for dealing with inoculation injuries

details of the accident should always be recorded. The instrument causing the injury can also be retained, and tested for infectious agents. Some authorities recommend the testing of the patient for blood-borne viruses such as HIV and hepatitis B, but this is not usually practical. If the injured person has received a substantial quantity of blood from a known carrier of HIV, then post-exposure prophylaxis can be administered. To be effective post-exposure prophylaxis must be given within 2 hours. Post-exposure prophylaxis consists of at least three anti-retroviral agents. Inoculation injuries are relatively common in dentistry: one survey showed that every dentist had at least one every year. All inoculation injuries should always be taken seriously.

The surgery design

The design of the surgery for good cross-infection control has been the subject of a number of publications. The surgery should be divided into two zones: one for the operator, the other for the assistant: each should contain a handwash basin. The assistant's zone should have a separate basin for washing instruments. The surgery areas that will be contaminated during operative procedures should be identified as they will require disinfection after every patient. The equipment chosen should be easy to clean, and resistant to commonly used disinfectants.

Surface disinfection

Disinfection is defined as the removal or killing of some pathogens, but usually not spores. Disinfection can be achieved by cleaning, or the use of chemical solutions. The disinfectant agents that are used in dentistry are shown in Table 14.3. A great deal of thought often goes into the choice of chemical disinfectant agent. In practice, the choice of disinfectant is probably not as important as how it is used. The aim of surface disinfection is to reduce opportunistic microbial agents present below a dose that could be infectious, and to kill true pathogens. This is done by a combination of dilution and physical cleaning. The disinfectant is applied and thoroughly wiped off using a vigorous cleaning technique to remove occult blood. The disinfectant is reapplied, and then wiped off. This second application dilutes the micro-organisms present, and leaves residual disinfectant to kill any remaining true, or opportunistic pathogens. A disinfectant should be chosen that has a relatively broad activity and is 'user-friendly'.

Other surgery disinfection

The surgery drains should be disinfected after every session with a non-foaming disinfectant, with a good spectrum of activity. The disinfectant should have rapid cidal properties in order to kill micro-organisms in the presence of blood and other organic detritus that may be present. In drains microbial biofilms may form which are resistant to disinfectants (*see* Chapter 5). Disinfectants used for drains often also contain a detergent to disrupt biofilms, and allow the chemicals to act on the microbes in them.

Table 14.3 The disinfectants that have been used in dentistry

Type	Use
Iodophors	Surfaces, hand disinfection
Aldehydes	Surfaces but only mild aldehydes that do not affect skin
Alcohols	Have been used on surfaces but have poor cleaning properties
Alcohols plus additives	Useful for surfaces
Quaternary ammonium compounds	Have been used on surfaces but have limited efficacy
Peroxygenated compounds	Useful for surfaces and immersion of impressions

The disinfection of impressions, and other laboratory fabricated material, is more difficult and requires immersion. A number of agents for this purpose have been advocated, including hypochlorite, but they are not ideal. The agent chosen must not have a deleterious effect on the dimensional stability of hydrocolloids, and must act in a reasonable time (in practice this is about 15 minutes). The immersion should always be preceded by thorough washing of the item under running water.

Dental unit water supplies

Particular problems occur in dental surgeries with the contamination of dental unit water supplies. This contamination can originate in the water supply. Another common cause of contamination is by backsiphonage through the dental turbine, or the air water syringe, when they are deactivated. This backsiphonage allows bacteria to enter the fine tubing supplying water to the unit. The water in the unit it contains is kept at approximately 37 °C, ideal for the growth of most pathogens. The colonization of the units is in the form of tenacious biofilms (*see* Chapter 5), which can release

planktonic contamination which may be sprayed onto the patient. The types of micro-organisms found contaminating dental unit water supplies principally include species of *Pseudomonas, Klebsiella* and *Moraxella,* but other bacteria and yeasts may be present. *Legionella* species have also been isolated from dental units but there is no proven evidence that they cause infection. The removal of biofilms from dental unit water supplies is difficult, as strong disinfectants are required which can cause damage to the unit tubing. In practice, the contamination of dental unit water supplies does not appear to be significant except in medically compromised patients, where sterile water is required. To reduce contamination of unit water supplies the water is flushed through the unit before each session and this reduces the planktonic contamination. A simple cure for this type of contamination of dental unit water supplies has still to be found.

Sterilization of instruments

Some dental instruments cannot be safely reused (e.g. needles) and should be discarded. Most expert bodies in the world recommend that all other dental instruments used in invasive procedures should be sterilized. Sterilization is the killing of all micro-organisms, or reproducible forms of life including spores. In dental practice sterilization is achieved by steam in an autoclave, or a combination of heated chemicals (chemiclave). Boiling water baths have been used to sterilize instruments, but tests have shown that under the conditions of dental practice they do not reliably work. Hot air ovens can be used to sterilize but their cycle is long (at least 30 minutes), and they damage some dental instruments.

The autoclave is a pressure vessel that uses the latent heat of steam under pressure to sterilize. The autoclave can be filled with steam by simply pumping it in (non-vacuum), or by evacuating the air then introducing steam (vacuum autoclave). Non-vacuum autoclaves are used for unwrapped instruments; vacuum autoclaves can be used for both wrapped and unwrapped instruments. The recommended temperature and time combinations for autoclaves are shown in Table 14.4. Some autoclaves incorporate a drying cycle for the instruments.

Table 14.4 The sterilization times, pressures and temperature combinations used in dental steam autoclaves

Temperature ($^{\circ}$C)	Time (min)	Pressure (lb/in^2)
134	3	30
115	30	15
121	15	15

The chemiclave uses a combination of chemicals and heat to kill micro-organisms. Its chief advantage is that it does not cause corrosion of instruments, or deleterious changes in delicate instruments. The disadvantages of this instrument are that some of the chemicals used in it are known carcinogens, and therefore the scavenger and evacuation mechanisms for the chemiclave have to be efficient.

Prior to sterilization the instruments must be cleaned, either manually or by use of an ultrasonic device or washing machine. Thorough cleaning is necessary as the presence of detritus can protect the micro-organisms against the process of sterilization. After sterilization the instruments should be stored aseptically in dry, lidded containers to prevent contamination.

The sterilization of dental instruments remains a contentious issue. In some countries, for certain dental procedures, disinfection of instruments by mechanical washing is all that is recommended. The scientific validity of such procedures remains to be proved. The sterilization of dental handpieces is also problematical as their efficiency can be affected by this process. There is evidence that handpieces do become internally contaminated during dental procedures and therefore they do need to be sterilized.

Disposal of clinical waste

All clinical waste from procedures that have involved saliva or blood should be considered as potentially infectious. Soft waste (cotton wool rolls, napkins, tissues etc.) should be incinerated, or buried in deep-fill land sites. Sharps should be stored in rigid containers, which are only three-quarters filled, and incinerated.

Summary

Cross-infection control is important in dentistry as it prevents the spread of known and ubiquitous pathogens during dental procedures. The procedures needed for cross-infection control are now defined and include personal protection by immunization, wearing of protective glasses, masks and gloves and the use of steam sterilization. Disinfection also helps reduce microbial load on surfaces and in the biofilms that form in drains. Dental unit water supplies often become contaminated and the only methods of eliminating the biofilms is by the use of strong disinfectants.

Bibliography

Bagg, J. (1996) Tuberculosis: a re-emerging problem for health care workers. *Br. Dent. J.,* **180**, 376–381.

Bagg, J. (1996) Communicable infectious disease. *Dent. Clin. North Am.,* **40**, 385–393.

Fayle, S.A. and Pollard, M.A. (1996) Decontamination of dental unit water systems: a review of current recommendations. *Br. Dent. J.,* **181**, 369–372.

British Dental Association (1999) *Infection Control in Dentistry,* Advice Sheet A12, British Dental Association, London.

Lodi, G., Porter, S.R., Teo, C.G. and Scully, C. (1997) Prevalence of HCV infection in health care workers of a UK dental hospital. *Br. Dent. J.,* **183**, 329–332.

Martin, M.V. (1991) *Infection Control in the Dental Environment: Effective Procedures,* Martin Dunitz, London.

Matthew, I.R. and Frame, J.W. (1997) Sharps injuries involving a sheathed needle. *Br. Dent. J.,* **183**, 70–71.

Scully, C. and Porter, S. (1991) The level of transmission of human immunodeficiency virus between patients and staff. *Br. Dent. J.,* **170**, 97–100.

Index